# Exploring the Benefit of Creative Arts Therapies for Children, Adolescents, and Adults

Nava R. Silton
*Marymount Manhattan College, USA*

A volume in the Advances in Psychology, Mental Health, and Behavioral Studies (APMHBS) Book Series

IGI Global
PUBLISHER of TIMELY KNOWLEDGE

Published in the United States of America by
IGI Global
Information Science Reference (an imprint of IGI Global)
701 E. Chocolate Avenue
Hershey PA, USA 17033
Tel: 717-533-8845
Fax: 717-533-8661
E-mail: cust@igi-global.com
Web site: http://www.igi-global.com



Library of Congress Cataloging-in-Publication Data

Names: Silton, Nava R., 1981- editor.
Title: Exploring the benefit of creative arts therapies for children, adolescents, and adults / edited by Nava R. Silton.
Description: Hershey, PA : Information Science Reference, 2023. | Includes bibliographical references. | Summary: "Exploring the Benefit of Creative Arts Therapies for Children, Adolescents, and Adults discusses the benefits of creative arts therapies for children, adolescents, and adults. The book also looks individually and collectively at the boon of art therapy, dance therapy, music, and drama therapy for improving outcomes for typically developing individuals and for vulnerable populations. Covering key topics such as dance, anxiety, and trauma, this premier reference source is ideal for therapists, social workers, psychologists, mental health counselors, researchers, scholars, academicians, practitioners, instructors, and students"-- Provided by publisher.
Identifiers: LCCN 2023004880 (print) | LCCN 2023004881 (ebook) | ISBN 9781668478561 (hardcover) | ISBN 9781668478608 (paperback) | ISBN 9781668478578 (ebook)
Subjects: LCSH: Art therapy. | Dance therapy. | Art therapy for children. | Dance therapy for children.
Classification: LCC RC489.A7 E98 2023 (print) | LCC RC489.A7 (ebook) | DDC 615.8/5156--dc23/eng/20230406
LC record available at https://lccn.loc.gov/2023004880
LC ebook record available at https://lccn.loc.gov/2023004881
This book is published in the IGI Global book series Advances in Psychology, Mental Health, and Behavioral Studies (APMHBS) (ISSN: 2475-6660; eISSN: 2475-6679)

British Cataloguing in Publication Data
A Cataloguing in Publication record for this book is available from the British Library.
All work contributed to this book is new, previously-unpublished material.
The views expressed in this book are those of the authors, but not necessarily of the publisher.
For electronic access to this publication, please contact: eresources@igi-global.com.

# Advances in Psychology, Mental Health, and Behavioral Studies (APMHBS) Book Series

ISSN:2475-6660
EISSN:2475-6679



**MISSION**

The complexity of the human mind has puzzled researchers and physicians for centuries. While widely studied, the brain still remains largely misunderstood.

The **Advances in Psychology, Mental Health, and Behavioral Studies (APMHBS)** book series presents comprehensive research publications focusing on topics relating to the human psyche, cognition, psychiatric care, mental and developmental disorders, as well as human behavior and interaction. Featuring diverse and innovative research, publications within APMHBS are ideally designed for use by mental health professionals, academicians, researchers, and upper-level students.

**COVERAGE**

- Socialization
- Emotional Health
- Human Interaction
- Treatment & Care
- Cognition
- Mental Health & Disorders
- Substance Abuse
- Eating Disorders
- Psychiatry
- Anxiety



The Advances in Psychology, Mental Health, and Behavioral Studies (APMHBS) Book Series (ISSN 2475-6660) is published by IGI Global, 701 E. Chocolate Avenue, Hershey, PA 17033-1240, USA, www.igi-global.com. This series is composed of titles available for purchase individually; each title is edited to be contextually exclusive from any other title within the series. For pricing and ordering information please visit http://www.igi-global.com/book-series/advances-psychology-mental-health-behavioral/110200. Postmaster: Send all address changes to above address. 

## Titles in this Series

*For a list of additional titles in this series, please visit:*
*http://www.igi-global.com/book-series/advances-psychology-mental-health-behavioral/110200*

***Perspectives and Considerations on Navigating the Mental Healthcre System***
Susan Van Alstyne (Centenary University, USA)
Medical Information Science Reference • © 2023 • 276pp • H/C (ISBN: 9781668450499) • US $305.00

***Combining Exercise and Psychotherapy to Treat Mental Health***
Lara Carneiro (United Arab Emirates University, AI) and Felipe Schuch (Universidade Federal de Santa Maria, Brazil)
Medical Information Science Reference • © 2023 • 300pp • H/C (ISBN: 9781668460405) • US $325.00

***Community Mental Health and Well-Being in the New Normal***
Remya Lathabhavan (Indian Institute of Management, Bodh Gaya, India) and Prabir Chandra Padhy (VIT Business School, Vellore Institute of Technology, Vellore, India)
Information Science Reference • © 2023 • 281pp • H/C (ISBN: 9781668472217) • US $240.00

***Perspectives on Stress and Wellness Management in Times of Crisis***
Rohit Bansal (Vaish College of Engineering, India)
Information Science Reference • © 2023 • 381pp • H/C (ISBN: 9781668485651) • US $245.00

***Facilitating Social Justice, Service Delivery, and Advocacy Through Multicultural Counseling Competencies***
Keith B. Wilson (University of Kentucky, USA) and Si-Yi Chao (University of Kentucky, USA)
Information Science Reference • © 2023 • 315pp • H/C (ISBN: 9781668461556) • US $215.00

*For an entire list of titles in this series, please visit:*
*http://www.igi-global.com/book-series/advances-psychology-mental-health-behavioral/110200*

IGI Global
PUBLISHER of TIMELY KNOWLEDGE

701 East Chocolate Avenue, Hershey, PA 17033, USA
Tel: 717-533-8845 x100 • Fax: 717-533-8661
E-Mail: cust@igi-global.com • www.igi-global.com

*This text is dedicated to my incredible mother, Faye Silton, who has been such a guide and light in my life. Moreover, she introduced me to my love for all things creative!*

# Editorial Advisory Board

# Table of Contents

# Detailed Table of Contents



Art therapy is an effective method of treating behavioral and psychological issues in individuals with dementia and Alzheimer's disease, and has been tested amongst patients as early as the 1980s. Although similar benefits have been seen in populations of people who are not at risk for this disease, studies have shown art therapy to be effective at lowering levels of depression, improving social skills, supplementing verbal communication, enhancing quality of life, and maintaining fine motor skills in participants with dementia and Alzheimer's disease. Additionally, some research has suggested that art therapy may play a role in improving cognition, delaying neuronal decay, and inspiring autobiographical memories, though further research is needed to support these arguments. This chapter will dissect the many studies that suggest various cognitive and psychological benefits, analyze current interventions, examine art's role in a therapeutic setting, and advocate for future studies.

Prison rehabilitation and its impact on different populations, such as women, is not a new concept. Yet, efforts to create healing and non-judgment spaces are continuing to grow and undergoing evaluation. One of these alternative treatments is art therapy. The present review makes use of literature to explore the connection and effective between art therapy, prison rehabilitation, and women. Using the example of how the results of art therapy in treatment spaces can differentiate according to gender, this research shows that mental health among women is more prominent in comparison to men. The results revealed that woman -in general- through different approaches, had effective results emerging from art therapy in prison rehabilitation. In addition, it in most cases, the literature revealed that during prison rehabilitation, women react better to art therapy than men. This chapter argues that the implementation of art therapy as a form of treatment during prison rehabilitation is an effective method for incarcerated women.



The lasting positive impact of Art Therapy on clients is expansive and widely understood, however there has been little research done to quantify this data. The research found that the data that is available shows a significant, positive impact on clients who attend art therapy as a means of treatment for personality, mood, and psychotic disorders as well as those with disorders characterized by varying levels of cognitive deficit. This review analyzes the effects of taking part in an art therapy program on the aforementioned groups and addresses the issue of accessibility to care, weighing the ethics of experiential, self-directed art therapy.

This chapter focuses on how trauma and post-traumatic stress disorder impact children, adolescents, and adults. It explores the history of trauma treatment as well as the benefits of creative arts therapy as a trauma treatment intervention. Creative arts therapy is crucial in the psychological realm, as it uses the building blocks of evidence-based practices to transform the narrative around healing the brain and body. Within the chapter, trauma and PTSD are explained, along with the history of trauma therapy, the history of creative art therapy around the world, and the rise of creative arts therapy in the United States.



Dance and movement therapy has become a quickly growing field in the creative arts therapies, combining psychotherapy and embodiment. Sessions are often available in schools, hospitals, rehabilitation centers, and clinics worldwide. Although dance therapy can be beneficial to individuals of all ages, genders, races, and cultures, the benefit for children is substantial. This chapter will discuss the use of dance and movement therapy with children in the United States and compare it to related practices in other countries. Additionally, approaches and techniques will be analyzed through the lens of best and most practical uses for children. Developmental disorders in children will also be examined to assess the benefits of dance therapy on cognitive, socioemotional, and physical skills. Lastly, this chapter will inspire ideas for future directions to advance the field of dance and movement therapy.

Eating disorders impact a large number of individuals worldwide. Due to a rise in media standards on weight and appearance, prevalence rates of eating disorders are at an incline. Diagnoses include anorexia nervosa, bulimia nervosa, binge eating disorder, and emotional eating. Research in dance movement therapy as treatment for eating disorders suggest that dance movements' creative and physical attributes can positively affect individuals' recoveries from eating disorders as increased body-image satisfaction, self-awareness, and body awareness occurs. Dance movement therapy offers a range of intervention styles that can be tailored through individual therapy or be used to build community in group therapy. Additionally, different intervention designs tackle a myriad of components that plague eating disordered individuals such as attachment style, emotional distress response, and the mind-body connection. Dance movement therapy's treatment has a prominent focus on the therapist/patient relationship, development of physical practice and confidence, and personal reflection.



Music therapy has significant positive effects on stress and stress management. Many individuals suffer from daily and chronic stress. Stress is a risk factor for several ailments and serious diseases. This includes both mental, emotional, and physical stress. Music-based interventions play a significant role in decreasing stress levels. Music is effective in decreasing a variety of different stressors on both the mental and physical levels. Music can support individuals in dealing with uncomfortable stress in a noninvasive and accessible way. This chapter will describe what stress is and why it is so common. Also, it will include the background of music therapy and numerous ways music therapy can help reduce stress. We are only beginning to learn how healing music can be to our nation's current stress epidemic.

A child being put into the foster care system comes with various trials. This begins with the foster child's original household dynamic either consisting of neglect or ill-treatment. Other cases being a parent who may not have the capacity to raise the child. To contextualize the creative arts and how they may benefit foster children, this review uses research collected from previous literature to examine prevalence rates, a child's needs, at-risk youth, how the brain reacts to the creation of art, music therapy, and its effects on foster youth, including after-school programs and support that is provided to children that implement the use of creative arts. Significant findings were compiled about the arts activating parts of the brain, consistently stimulating the same three neurotransmitters (oxytocin, serotonin, and dopamine). Furthermore, the implementation of the arts in foster children's lives can reverse social and developmental delays they may have encountered as a result of trauma.

# Foreword

As I got to know Dr. Silton better, I quickly became aware of her genuine interest in the well-being of others. Dr. Silton is constantly motivated by her undying desire to make things better for others, through research, and education—always leading by example. As an author and educator, Dr. Silton seeks out, and challenges, psychotherapeutic approaches to health. Having worked myself as a dance/movement therapist and by so doing witnessing positive change in individuals and groups, I was ecstatic to find out that Dr. Silton was writing this important book.

As the field of mental health continues to evolve and expand, so does our understanding of the value of integrating creative arts therapies into more traditional forms of therapy. At their core, creative arts therapies utilize the expressive arts to facilitate healing, growth, and transformation for individuals facing a range of challenges. Creative arts therapies have shown to be effective in a variety of settings, from schools and hospitals to private practice and community mental health centers. In recent years, there has been an increasing recognition of the potential for creative arts therapies to complement and enhance traditional forms of therapy.

Integrating creative arts therapies into treatment plans can lead to improved outcomes for clients, including increased self-awareness, reduced symptoms of anxiety and depression, improved coping skills, and enhanced interpersonal relationships, among others. Creative arts therapies can also be effective as standalone interventions, particularly for individuals who may be resistant to more traditional forms of therapy or who have difficulty expressing themselves verbally.

For undergraduate and graduate students interested in pursuing a career in creative arts therapies, this book serves as an invaluable resource for understanding the theoretical underpinnings and practical applications of these powerful interventions. For researchers and clinicians/practitioners already working in the field, this book offers an important overview of the current state of knowledge and practice in creative arts therapies, including emerging trends and promising new directions for research.

This book demonstrates the power of creative arts therapies to facilitate healing and transformation, both in conjunction with traditional forms of therapy and as standalone interventions. I am confident that this book will inspire a new generation of practitioners and researchers to explore the potential of creative arts therapies and to continue pushing the boundaries of what is possible in the field of mental health.

*Jan J. Dijkwel*
*Marymount Manhattan College, USA*

***Jan Dijkwel*** *graduated with a Master of Arts in Dance/Movement Therapy from Drexel University Philadelphia, PA in 1999. His research centered on dance movement therapy practices with those who suffer from Traumatic Brain Injury (TBI).*

# Preface

It turns out that parents need not worry that their college-bound children will dream of a career in the arts rather than in the classic esteemed professions from time immemorial—of medicine, the law, finance, and so many other generally profitable careers.

Moreover, it appears that public and private "lower" schools could substantially benefit from a STEAM (Science, Technology, English, Arts, and Math) curriculum rather than STEM (all of the above minus the arts) since, as will soon become evident, the creative arts can often be used to augment traditional therapies and to lend a voice and an anchor to those who struggle to verbally express themselves and to those who are most vulnerable in our society. The Creative Arts have a great deal to contribute to the well-being of the child, the adolescent, and the elderly, and in our present culture, it can help counter the numbing effects of excessive use of private technology and, most recently, post-COVID-19-induced anxiety.

Readers of this volume will be amazed at the comprehensive research the various authors have collected to describe the broad range of creative arts applications, which, often coupled with talk therapy, can help clients address their mental health challenges, achieve a sense of self-worth and temper their anxiety and stress. They will learn how efficacious the creative arts therapies can be and will glean direct techniques for employing the creative arts with their diverse clientele.

In Chapter 1, Zachary Biron at Marymount Manhattan College is passionate about the field of Art Therapy, especially as it pertains to research in delaying the neuronal deterioration of dementia and Alzheimer's Disease. Though Art Therapy has been in use since the 1980s for treating behavioral and psychological issues, Biron analyzes studies that demonstrate its efficacy in lowering levels of depression, supplementing verbal communication and improving cognition, social and fine motor skills among patients with dementia and Alzheimer's Disease. Biron's chapter will undoubtedly resonate with countless readers who hold out hope for a creative, new solution for dealing with these scourges that threaten the "golden years" and plague even much younger patients.

While Zach Biron critically highlights the ways Art Therapy can help heal older patients who face progressive deficits, in Chapter 2, Dr. Rachel Brandoff, a Board-Certified Art Therapist and Associate Professor and Coordinator of the Art Therapy Concentration in the Community and Trauma Counseling program at Thomas Jefferson University, studies the drastic needs of women, young and old, seeking asylum across the southern border of the USA. Though they lack English language skills, education, legal employment and contend with food insecurity, they often display unusual creativity and perseverance. No surprise, then, that these women are empowered by Art Therapies and, through them, discover gifts that will help them move forward.

Monica Sanchez, a Latina woman herself, and Director of Mental Health Services at LSA Family Health Service, enhances Brandoff's study by specifically detailing therapies (individual, dyad, group psychotherapy and art therapy) for immigrant women who are survivors of significant and complex trauma. Her patients are generally of childbearing age. Students involved in the healing creative arts effort are likely to meet Monica Sanchez at various conferences at regional and national universities.

Dr. Rachel Brandoff appears again in Chapter 3 of our collection. In this chapter, together with Ms. Jacqui Johnson of the Sankofa Healing Studio, they focus on the corrections system in the US (largely concerned with punishment). If the main goals could include rehabilitation, deterrence and restoration, Art Therapy could enhance mental health treatment and provide relief from anxiety, depression and feelings of isolation. For Brandoff and Johnson, this is not a pipe dream. They offer a description of a fascinating pilot study based on an eight-week theme-based art therapy program in a women's county jail in Philadelphia. Authentic artwork from clients, further augment both of Brandoff's impressive chapters.

Brandoff and Johnson are not alone in working tirelessly to improve the treatment of prisoners. In Chapter 4, Giselle B. Caraballo Matos, a graduate of Marymount Manhattan College, researches the intersections between psychology and the legal system, the access of low- income communities to mental health facilities and the possibilities of including the creative arts in standard therapies. One of the surprising findings: women reacted far better than men to these enhanced therapies.

It is possible that some of the participants in Caraballo Matos' prison study suffered from cognitive deficits and/or psychotic symptoms, but in Chapter 5, Emmalynne Knuth of Marymount Manhattan College, a student of Art Therapy and Studio Art, presents a review of the topic because she believes "Art Therapy has the ability to reach a wide range of clients and patients regardless of verbal language, cultural background or socioeconomic status." Knuth, who was featured in a solo exhibition titled, "Lifting the Bell Jar: An Exploration of Art Therapy," also considers the accessibility of care issue and "the ethics and benefits of experiential, self-directed art therapy."

Shira Davis of Lander College for Women, Touro University, hopes to pursue a graduate degree in Neuropsychology. In Chapter 6, she offers her own review of the evolution of Art Therapy from its beginning to the present. Davis presents the "substantial benefits of Art Therapy for the elderly population" but also dives deeper into subgroups such as the incarcerated and those suffering from depression and dementia. Her analysis of Art Therapy techniques and outcomes will be especially welcome.

But this collection moves on from the graphic and "plastic" arts to other diverse forms of art. Clearly, the Improv performances many of us have enjoyed, require a huge dollop of creativity.

In Chapter 7, Dr. Marisa T. Cohen, a relationship researcher, marriage and family therapist and the author of "From First Kiss to Forever," learned Improv and immediately enjoyed the practice of mindful awareness and the joy of play. Later she led virtual improv for self-care groups. Here she considers how to apply the features of Improv to business, education, medical settings and use in therapeutic practice. The reader may very well have seen or heard Dr. Cohen lecture at the 92nd Street Y, the Strand Bookstore or the New York Hall of Science and caught podcasts and radio shows "to discuss the psychology of love and ways to improve our relationships."

For many of us these relationships can be traumatic, but our next researchers, Deanna Alyssa Villetto, LMSW of Columbia University and her sister, Kayla Villetto of SUNY New Paltz, focus on trauma and Post Traumatic Stress Disorder in children, adolescents and adults and specialize in using creative arts therapies in Chapter 8. They believe that the creative arts are "crucial to transform the narrative around healing the brain and body." They will explain what PTSD is and offer a history of trauma therapy and how creative arts therapy can aid in the healing of those who suffer from PTSD.

In Chapter 9, children are definitely the beneficiaries in Jenna Dawn Rivera's Dance and Movement Therapy discussion, though it can be beneficial "for all ages, genders, races and cultures." Already as a high school student, Jenna assisted children with Autism, ADHD, Down syndrome and Cerebral Palsy in Special Education dance classes. At Marymount Manhattan College, after she majored in psychology and minored in dance, she combined her two passions and "discovered the world of dance therapy." She wanted more people to understand the impact dance could have on the developing brain of children. This chapter features an ambitious and fascinating grouping of topics: Dance and movement therapy for children in the US compared to such therapies in other countries, the best and most practical techniques to use with children, how various developmental disorders can benefit from dance in terms of cognitive, socioemotional and physical skills and possible future directions to advance the field of dance and movement therapy.

Yet in Chapter 10, another dance major and fine researcher from Marymount Manhattan College, Heather Kroesche, began this research to help her understand how experts have used dance therapy to help treat eating disorders and disordered eating. Anorexia Nervosa, bulimia nervosa, binge eating disorder and emotional eating are all conditions that have grown in prevalence and severity. Kroesche asserts that "dance movements' creative and physical attributes…[can offer] increased body image satisfaction, self-awareness and body awareness." In fact, they can be "tailored through individual therapy or be used to build community in group therapy." There's much more to savor here pertaining to the development of physical practice, confidence and self-reflection.

In Chapter 11, readers might be least surprised about "The Positive Effects of Music Therapy on Stress." We almost intuitively reach for the nearest medium of choice to listen passively or even sing along. Or we reach for our musical instrument of choice to soothe ourselves in challenging moments. Hunter Rose Lloyd spent over 12 years dancing full time. For Lloyd, it was through dancing that she accessed the healing power of music and movement. She plans on searching for a balance between the deep passions of dance and music to help people. She believes that "music is effective in decreasing a variety of different stressors on both mental and physical levels."

Among significant causes of stress in children are conditions in the foster homes or orphanages that house them. Any book or film featuring an orphan immediately elicits sympathy, since orphans and foster children often encounter multiple traumas that we want so much to help them address. In Chapter 12, Kayleen Cabrera at Marymount Manhattan College, well aware of the tender vulnerabilities of foster children, considered how the arts could be restorative for this population. She sought healing from any trauma they might have endured. Therefore, Ms. Cabrera reviews earlier research to examine…a child's needs…how the brain reacts to the creation of art, music therapy and its effects…how the arts can activate parts of the brain. Amazingly enough, she posits that "the arts in foster children's lives can [even] reverse social and developmental delays!" Dr. Nava Silton, a Developmental Psychologist, Psychology Professor at Marymount Manhattan College and Editor of the textbook, further augments the important developmental discussions in this chapter. She believes that diverse Creative Arts Therapies can be particularly useful for vulnerable populations, in conjunction with traditional therapies or on their own.

Clearly, the creative arts therapies that derive from a clever marriage of the creative arts and efficacious therapeutic approaches offer a canvas, a stage, a movement, a pen, a musical instrument, or other forms of media to help the vulnerable individuals described in this collection express themselves and heal. As for young people aspiring to a meaningful career, they can report to their parents that creative art therapies have already shown great promise and will continue to develop with the continued passionate attention to the practice that is evident in this collection. In the process, they, themselves, will likely bloom and grow.

*Nava R. Silton*
*Marymount Manhattan College, USA*

# Acknowledgment

This text would not have been possible without a wonderful meeting of brilliant minds. First and foremost, I want to gratefully acknowledge all of the esteemed authors who shared their latest engrossing findings in the exciting, diverse and evolving areas of The Creative Arts Therapies.

I look forward to our future correspondence and collaboration.

Secondly, I'd like to graciously thank the peer reviewers who meticulously evaluated the relevance of content, syntax and empirical rigor of each chapter. Thank you.

Additionally, thank you Jocelynn Hessler and Jan Travers for their guidance during the editing process.

Moreover, I would like to thank my incredible husband, Dr. Ariel Brandwein and my charming and hilarious little men, Judah Lior, Jonah Gabriel, and Jacob Zeke Brandwein and my little ladies, Jordana Leah and Juliet Bella, for their good nature, humor, inspiration and patience throughout this endeavor. I want to acknowledge my father, Rabbi Paul Silton and my wonderful siblings, Elana, Michal, Akiva, Tamar, Aviva, and my twin sister Shira for their constant encouragement and support. Finally, I owe the deepest debt of gratitude to a consummate renaissance woman and to one of my absolute greatest heroines, my mother, Faye Silton. Her brilliance, creativity, eloquence, wisdom, patience, kindness, and love know no bounds. I will cherish this text all the more since her brilliant mind and loving hands painstakingly reviewed its contents.

I want to extend a final note of gratitude to all of the educators, academics, and professionals who not only research the important areas of The Creative Arts Therapies (Art Therapy, Dance Therapy, Drama Therapy, Music Therapy, etc.), but who are active clinicians who work hard to enhance the lives of others through these evidence-based practices.

Section 1

# Benefits of Art Therapy

# Chapter 1
# Art in Memory:
## The Positive Effects of Art Therapy on Dementia and Alzheimer's Disease

**Zachary Biron**
*Marymount Manhattan College, USA*

## ABSTRACT

*Art therapy is an effective method of treating behavioral and psychological issues in individuals with dementia and Alzheimer's disease, and has been tested amongst patients as early as the 1980s. Although similar benefits have been seen in populations of people who are not at risk for this disease, studies have shown art therapy to be effective at lowering levels of depression, improving social skills, supplementing verbal communication, enhancing quality of life, and maintaining fine motor skills in participants with dementia and Alzheimer's disease. Additionally, some research has suggested that art therapy may play a role in improving cognition, delaying neuronal decay, and inspiring autobiographical memories, though further research is needed to support these arguments. This chapter will dissect the many studies that suggest various cognitive and psychological benefits, analyze current interventions, examine art's role in a therapeutic setting, and advocate for future studies.*

## INTRODUCTION

*Art therapy* is a term used to encapsulate the practice of utilizing artistic mediums as a form of treatment in a therapeutic setting. Clinicians certified by the state who have acquired their LCAT (Licensed Creative Arts Therapist) use structured approaches backed by the American Art Therapy Association (AATA) and the Art

DOI: 10.4018/978-1-6684-7856-1.ch001

Therapy Credentials Board Inc. (ATCB) to create art in a clinical setting that engages "the mind, body, and spirit in ways that are distinct from verbal articulation alone" (AATA). The field continues to grow as studies examine the correlation between artistic creation and improved behaviors, providing an increasingly solid basis of research and data to support its effectiveness. The present chapter will focus on the applications and known benefits of art therapy on the symptoms of dementia and Alzheimer's disease, highlighting both neurological and psychological improvements the therapy promotes. Furthermore, the current treatments and early interventions used to combat symptoms of dementia and cognitive decay will be discussed and cross-referenced to analyze effectiveness in conjunction with art therapy and promote further research.

## Art as Therapy

The term was first coined in 1942 by World War I artist Adrian Hill, who noted the benefits of creating art while convalescing during his hospitalization for tuberculosis. The practice began to spread in hospitals worldwide following the influential works and findings of Edward Adamson, Margaret Naumburg, and Edith Kramer, respectively. Art therapy has historically been used alongside medicinal and behavioral therapies to treat "development, medical, educational, social, or psychological impairment(s)" (ATCB) and was first used with dementia patients in the 1980s-1990s by practitioner Judith Wald. Wald noted that the artwork created by patients with dementia appeared broken and repetitious, featuring fragmented lines, confused perspectives, and a lack of detail (Wald, 1986, pp. 74-80). Over time, further studies confirmed effectiveness through signs of improved moods, enhanced memory, and decreased symptoms amongst dementia patients utilizing pencil drawing, collage making, and cutting shapes as a form of art therapy (Kahn-Denis, 1997, pp. 194-199). These breakthrough studies launched further research into the application of art therapy as a form of treatment and symptom relief for dementia and Alzheimer's disease throughout the 1990s and 2000s.

Within the past two decades, Art Therapy has become a staple of therapeutic communities worldwide, with at least thirty separate associations and organizations representing the practice across twenty-six countries, including South Africa, Hong Kong, Korea, Israel, The United States, Germany, France, Ireland, Canada, Brazil, and more. The use of the therapy alongside clinical treatments has also increased, gaining notability for use with pediatric (Aguilar, 2017; Clapp, Taylor, Folco, Mackinnon, 2018) and geriatric patients (Shore, 2013; Ciasca, Ferreira, Santana, Forlenza, Santos, Brum, Nunes, 2018). However, setbacks for the field are still present. Much of the public remains ill-informed on the legitimacy of the practice as a genuine form of psychotherapy rather than an exercise for stress relief. This misconception has been aided by the rapid growth of "fake" art therapists over the years who host workshops, sell products, and offer services with no legitimate certifications or "knowledge of both art and therapy (which) are necessary to the art therapist" (Rubin, 1982, pp. 57-58). Though it was Edith Kramer's belief that "all art is therapeutic in the broadest sense of the word" (Kramer, 2001, p. 17), the misrepresentation of the field as a commercial entity diminishes the value and effectiveness of the therapy and misses the "opportunity to offer accurate information and educate the public" (AATA). The continued presence of this issue emphasizes the critical distinction between art as therapy, or a cathartic method of stress relief, and art therapy as a form of psychotherapy, backed by studies collecting empirical data and research (Slayton, D'Archer, Kaplan, 2010). Furthermore, it highlights the continued importance of defining and specifying what art therapy is and is not. For the sake of the present chapter, all references to art therapy are intended to align with the definitions and standards set by professional and educational associations such as AATA and ATCB.

## Structured and Unstructured Approaches

Using structured assessments in art therapy allows for the efficacy of different directives to be cross-referenced and more robust research to be conducted (Deaver, 2002). In structured directive approaches, the therapist determines the theme and tools used in each project. These may include projective techniques such as drawing a bridge (Hays & Lyons, 1981) or a rosebush (Allan & Crandall, 1986) to tap into significant symbolic issues while uncovering powerful feelings that may be difficult to understand in a group setting. A structured approach is often best when working with people just beginning art therapy or with populations who might have difficulty sticking to a self-decided theme, such as individuals with dementia and Alzheimer's disease. This form of diagnostic assessment often involves a series of projects to strengthen assessment and encourage deeper reflection, as seen in the Ulman Personality Assessment Procedure (UPAP) and the Levick Emotional & Cognitive Art Therapy Evaluation & Assessment (LECATA).

Though structured approaches are crucial to the therapeutic process and projective techniques remain in use by art therapists worldwide, non directive art therapy may provide more significant social benefits to group sessions and induce more meaningful resonances as the group "find(s) its own direction and ultimately treat(s) itself" (McNeilly, 1983, p. 211). This form of art therapy allows the participants to choose the theme and tools used as they create their own unguided works of art. Unstructured art therapy provides a stronger sense of personal control and social support when conducted in a group setting, which are vital traits in predicting health outcomes in geriatric populations (Rodin, 1986; Cohen, 2009). Furthermore, some group sessions of unstructured art therapy demonstrate greater benefits in treating elderly patients when compared to alternative forms of treatment, such as verbal therapy (Uttley, Stevenson, Scope, Rawdin, Sutton, 2015). In general, art therapy has been shown to be efficient in improving emotional, social, and psychological issues through a combination of structured and unstructured approaches (Kaimal & Ray, 2016) and proved to be particularly beneficial in elderly populations (Rusted, Sheppard, Waller, 2006), prison inmates (Gussak, 2004), and cancer patients (Monti, Peterson, Kunkel, Hauck, Pequignot, Rhodes, Brainard, 2006).

## Dementia and Alzheimer's Disease

*Dementia* is an umbrella term that categorizes many different memory loss conditions that predominantly affect elderly populations. By far, the most common is Alzheimer's disease, which accounts for 60-80% of all cases of dementia and afflicted more than six million Americans in 2022, according to the Alzheimer's Association. *Alzheimer's disease* is a progressive neurodegenerative disease that causes atrophy of tissue and targets multiple regions of the brain, including the entorhinal cortex, hippocampus, and cerebral cortex. More severe developments can include vascular dementia, which narrows blood vessels and creates blood clots, restricting blood flow and oxygen to the brain. As brain regions are deprived of nutrients and synapses continue to decay, the brain experiences dramatic shrinkage of three to four percent yearly (Fjell, McEvoy, Holland, Dale, Walhovd, 2013; Wang, Hsieh, Wang, 2013). Alzheimer's disease has a high mortality rate, with most patients living four to eight years on average after diagnosis. However, some can live up to twenty years under a caregiver's or clinician's careful watch (Alzheimer's Association, 2023). Deaths from the disease have seen a drastic increase of over 142% from 2000-2018 (Alzheimer's Association, 2020) and are projected to afflict 16 million Americans by 2050 (Mayeux & Stern, 2012).

Across three stages of progression (mild, moderate, and severe), individuals suffering from dementia and Alzheimer's disease experience a rapid decrease in cognitive functioning, including moderate to severe memory loss, difficulty maintaining attention and focus, mood swings and withdrawal, difficulty communicating and socializing, and loss of physical abilities including walking, sitting, and swallowing. This decline in physical and verbal capabilities creates difficulties for nursing staff and caregivers to provide cognitive stimulation and comfort to their worsening symptoms (Wang et al., 2013; Dillehay, 1990). As such, it can be challenging to plan tasks and activities on par with old hobbies to fill the individual's day, often leaving them feeling stripped of identity and pushed to retreat into apathy, "seeing the world with empty eyes" (Zgola, 1987, p. 10).

## Relevant Statistics

Though the prevalence of Alzheimer's disease and dementia in adults aged 70 or older has decreased from 13% in 2011 to 10% in 2019 (Freedman, Cornman, Kasper, 2021), researchers predict cases will rise again as the baby boomer population ages. Currently, the most at-risk populations are adults over 85, with 22% of adults between the ages of 85-89 having a diagnosis of dementia and 33% over the age of 90. 16.4% of Hispanic adults, 16.1% non-hispanic black adults, and 8.5% of non-hispanic white adults indicate that the disease affects people of ethnic and racial minorities more frequently. Further data suggest that women are more likely to suffer from the disease than men, with 11% of this population being women and only 8% being men. (Freedman et al., 2021; Liu, Zhang, Choi, Langa, 2020). Approximately 50% of residents in long-term care facilities, around 750,000 people, have a diagnosis of dementia (Jett, 2018) and often receive substandard care (Mitchell, Mor, Gozalo, 2016; Sachs, Shega, Cox-Hayley, 2004; Joyce, McGuire, Bartels, Mitchell, Gabowski, 2018).

In the United States, nursing facilities that are certified under the Center for Medicare & Medicaid Services (CMS) require the offering of "one or more types of skilled restorative services, e.g., physical or speech therapy" with an emphasis on restorative services (Center for Medicare & Medicaid Services, 2016, p. 18). Though therapy services are required for geriatric patients, a concerning statistic found limited usage of these resources in service facilities. A study conducted in 1994 surveyed all nursing homes in the state of North Carolina, of which 69% reported to offer physical therapy, occupational therapy, speech therapy, or a combination of all three to long-stay residents. However, the number of residents enrolled in such therapies varied from 0-64%. 67% of these administrators stated that the lack of patients with "fair or better rehabilitation potential" limited their provision of such services (Kochersberger, Hielema, Westlund, 1994).

## Neurodegeneration

Crucial to the development of effective interventions and therapies is an understanding of the neuropathology of dementia. Though a growing body of literature continues to be published and plenty of small discoveries have been made, there is not currently an accepted understanding of dementia's underlying causes. All dementias can be categorized as proteinopathies, where abnormal proteins accumulate within the neurons. As toxic changes begin in the brain, an imbalance grows between neurons, astrocytes, and microglia, which work together to transmit action potentials. At the onset of dementia, proteins Beta-amyloid and Tau become toxic to the brain and begin to cause cellular changes. Abnormal Tau accumulations occur in the neuron, forming neurofibrillary tangles (Ball, 1977). At the same time, Beta-amyloid clumps into senile plaques, slowly building up between neurons and damaging synapses. As the level of Beta-amyloid increases, Tau rapidly spreads throughout the brain and shuts down neural networks. Microglial cells begin to fail at clearing away debris, causing chronic inflammation to set in. Some forms of dementia can also affect vascular systems, limiting blood flow and depriving the brain of the glucose needed to power brain activity. As these cellular changes occur and neurons can no longer communicate, the hippocampus begins to shrink (National Institute on Aging, 2017).

The hippocampus is a complex structure located in the temporal lobe, primarily responsible for learning, memory recollection, and spatial navigation (Dhikav & Anand, 2012). As neurons deteriorate within the hippocampus as a result of the disease, individuals lose their ability to think and recall memories. This process may begin as early as six years before the onset of dementia, according to a study conducted by the American Academy of Neurology (Kaye, Howieson, Dame, Moore, Karnos, Camicioli, Ball, Sexton, 1997). As the brain's central hub for learning, the hippocampus undergoes a great deal of structural plasticity throughout an individual's life and is the only structure known in the adult brain to excel at neurogenesis (Lie, Song, Colamarino, Ming, Gage, 2004). A recent study exploring the functions of neural stem cells as a preventative measure for dementia suggests that "many extrinsic factors like dietary intake and physical activity" earlier in life may strengthen neurogenesis, possibly delaying neurodegeneration (Rao, Ganaraja, Murlimanju, Joy, Krishnamurthy, Agrawal, 2022). Further research suggests that utilizing cognitive interventions to further neuroplasticity in the hippocampus can also play a prominent role in preventing the onset of dementia through increasing cognitive reserve (Brown, Chirino, Cortez, Gearhart, Urizar, 2020; Buschert, Bokde, Hampel, 2010; Bugos, Perlstein, McCrae, Brophy, Bedenbaugh, 2007). In both arguments, further research is needed to support the claims and test the efficacy of each possible intervention.

## Current Interventions for Dementia and Alzheimer's Disease

In most cases, non-pharmacological interventions are pursued before medicinal options when treating dementia. A variety of therapeutic approaches are used to treat arising cognitive issues, such as cognitive therapy, aromatherapy, behavioral therapy, and multi-sensory therapies (Ball, Owen-Booth, Gray, Shenkin, Hewitt, McCleery, 2020; Douglass, Walterfang, Velakoulis, Abel, 2018; Vernooij-Dassen, Vasse, Zuidema, Cohen-Mansfield, Moyle, 2010). Though these options may not effectively treat all symptoms of dementia, studies have shown improvements in both behavioral and psychological symptoms that suggest their efficacy in improving quality of life for both patients and family caregivers (Zarit, Femia, Watson, Rice-Oeschger,

Kakos, 2004; Logsdon, McCurry, Teri, 2008; Raglio, Bellelli, Traficante, Gianotti, Ubezio, Villani, Trabucchi, 2008). In pharmaceutical research, current studies hope to combat dementia by inhibiting the production of key-enzyme protein beta-amyloid and cleaning the brain of senile plaques using various antibodies (Panza, Lozupone, Logroscino, 2018; Fan & Wang, 2019). Though some cholinesterase inhibitors are regularly used to reduce some behavioral and cognitive symptoms in mild and moderate cases of dementia and Alzheimer's disease (National Institute on Aging, 2021), no trials have proven successful at combating neuronal decay. One such study hoping to do so evaluated the effectiveness of a beta-amyloid blocker during the prodromal stage of Alzheimer's disease, but was terminated after results indicated the drug contributed to more cognitive decline than the placebo (Egan, Kost, Voss, Mukai, 2019). Research continues into possible pharmacological interventions across all stages of development in Alzheimer's disease.

As an individual approaches the target age for the onset of dementia, most will experience "nonpathological losses in cognitive functioning", or age-related cognitive decline (ARCD), which may increase their potential for developing Alzheimer's disease (Mahncke, Connor, Appelman, Merzenich, 2006). Targeting this issue before it has the chance to develop has yielded promising results, as indicated by studies that used compensatory strategies to induce significant improvements in memory function among individuals with the neurodegenerative disease (Davis, Massman, Doody, 2001; Loewenstein, Acevedo, Czaja, Duara, 2004). Further studies using behavioral-based training programs instead of compensatory strategies found more success in the longevity of improvement amongst participants, citing continued enhancement to memory recollection skills three months after concluding training. Though these trials were conducted on individuals with no symptoms of dementia, the results suggest "intensive, plasticity-engaging training can result in an enhancement of cognitive function in normal mature adults", possibly delaying the onset of the disease altogether (Mahncke et al., 2006).

Though the advancement of Alzheimer's disease can occur quite rapidly after initial diagnosis, the damage to the brain is not uniform, leaving areas responsible for motor skills, personality, and emotional control largely intact until late stages (Stewart, 2004). This suggests a capacity for art therapy as a continued intervention well after dementia's onset. Further research suggests the mental stimulation and increased cognitive reserve induced by active participation in art therapy may stimulate neurogenesis and form new synapses in decaying areas of the brain (Cohen, 2009; Kolb & Whishaw, 1998). In nearly all stages of intervention, art therapy has shown to be reliable at improving general quality of life on a psychosocial level, citing improvements in social support, self-efficacy, happiness, memory recollection, and fine motor skills in Alzheimer's patients (Kaimal & Ray, 2016; Cohen, 2009;

Vernooji-Dassen, 2010; Rodin, 1989; Harlan, 1993; Basting, 2006; Hannemann, 2006; Doric-Henry, 1997).

## Art Therapy as Symptom Relief

Across the three stages of Alzheimer's disease, cognitive functioning declines as symptoms of memory loss, depression, and agitation increase rapidly (Merriam, Aronson, Gaston, Wey, Katz, 1988). Studies have shown that 70-90% of people with a diagnosis of dementia or Alzheimer's disease manifest increasing feelings of anger, depression, restlessness, sadness, and anxiety as the illness progresses, creating more issues for caregivers and generally reducing quality of life overall (Kovach, Noonan, Schlidt, Wells, 2005). Research into art therapy as an effective form of symptom relief has proven beneficial across all stages, including individuals in the most regressed stages of dementia and Alzheimer's disease. Multiple studies have drawn conclusions that suggest art forms such as music can decrease feelings of agitation in more severely demented individuals who do not have the fine motor skills needed to engage with other art therapy directives, increasing their capability for food-intake and mitigating anxieties (Richedson & Neill, 2004; Ragneskog, Asplund, Kihlgren, Norberg, 2001). Further research suggests that the use of individualized music selections for each participant may also help in inducing memories, such as "a particular time of life (childhood) or significant people" (Baird, Garrido, Tamplin, 2019, pp. 155-156). Stimulating memories in this way not only inspires moments of recollecting autobiographical memories, but links an individual back to pieces of their self-identity (Baird et al., 2019, p. 156).

Just as music can help individuals with dementia and Alzheimer's disease reflect inwards, art-making can encourage meaningful changes to a person's outward perspective. Through guided sessions of art therapy, an art therapist can help participants create pieces that stimulate their creativity and expression of personal thoughts and feelings, which, in turn, improve their mental health and combat feelings of depression (Hannemann, 2006; Basting, 2006). Additionally, art therapy is effective at improving communication between participant and caregiver which facilitates further person-centered therapy and activities, combating symptoms of loneliness and withdrawal (Emblad & Mukaetova-Ladinska, 2021). Moreover, this form of connection may not be possible without art as verbal ability declines and individuals begin to feel imprisoned by their own minds. In the battle for control over their shrinking cognitive abilities, art therapy can provide a way to "break through the barrier of the disease" (Kamar, 1997, p. 123) and communicate with their caregivers and loved ones. A study published in the American Journal of Art Therapy demonstrated exactly this, citing the immense benefits that come from providing art as a way to communicate nonverbally, reducing feelings of isolation, tension, and frustration that may have otherwise pushed an individual further into their own apathy (Kamar, 1997).

## Improving Cognition

Few studies have examined the role art therapy can play in improving the cognition of patients with dementia or Alzheimer's disease, instead highlighting symptomatic reliefs or its benefit to caregivers (Emblad & Mukaetova-Ladinska, 2021). When viewing the changes in cognition of participants actively engaged with art therapy across multiple studies, research has suggested improvements in attention, verbal fluency, visual-spatial abilities, and has potentially implied a delay in cognitive deterioration (Stewart, 2004; Eekelaar, Camic, Springham, 2012). Eekelaar et al. (2012) studied the effects of a three-week course in art appreciation in which patients with dementia and Alzheimer's disease created portraits, landscapes, and narrative pieces while actively discussing their experiences and reflections. The results found a significant improvement in each individual's attention span, an 18.6% increase in verbal fluency, and a 5.76% increase in semantic clustering. Though the effects of the study did not show long-term significance after the course concluded, active participation demonstrated a positive trend in cognitive improvement.

As previously discussed, research suggests that an increase in cognitive reserve correlates with the formation of new synapses and increases structural plasticity in the hippocampus (Cohen, 2009; Kolb & Whishaw, 1998). As plasticity increases, there is a greater potential for delaying neuronal deterioration before the onset of dementia in healthy adult brains (Mahncke et al., 2006). However, Stewart (2004) suggested that even patients with severe dementia could somewhat delay further neuronal deterioration through active engagement with exercises such as painting. The participants of this study also seemingly demonstrated improvement in their visual-spatial capabilities as a byproduct of strengthening their creative minds. Though further research is needed to provide empirical data that corroborates the interveners' claims, their suggestions may align with the results found in the healthy adult brain and suggest a degree of efficacy in using art therapy to directly combat cognitive decline. As more sensitive assessment tools and methods are developed, future research will hopefully provide a more accurate evaluation of the effectiveness of art therapy on cognition.

## Fine Motor Skills

In the development of dementia and Alzheimer's disease, the progressively slowing fine motor dexterity associated with self-care is often one of the most challenging losses an individual can face (Paula, Albuquerque, Lage, Bicalho, Romano-Silva,

Malloy-Diniz, 2016). The need for caregivers significantly increases as individuals lose their ability to complete tasks that require precise movement, such as feeding themselves or maintaining good hygiene. The lifestyle adjustment resulting from their decreased capability for self-reliance often arouses feelings of depression, anger, shame, and loss of identity (Kovach et al., 2005; Zgola, 1987). Though no study has produced data that suggests art therapy can restore functioning to fine motor skills after the disease has progressed, some research has highlighted how it can be beneficial in maintaining ability before it is lost. Through hand-brain coordination, the use of art supplies in a therapeutic environment is "conducive to maintaining and developing a patient's coordination and motor skills and strengthening their fine motor skills" (Wang & Li, 2016, p. 108). Cognitive stimulation as a byproduct of creating art has also been found to positively influence fine motor skills, stimulating both the temporal lobe, which affects object recognition and language expression, and the parietal lobe, which controls fine motor functioning in the hand (Frith & Law, 1995).

## Happiness and Social Skills

To a reasonable degree, feelings of depression, anger, and unhappiness afflict everyone diagnosed with a form of dementia (Kovach et al., 2005). As the disease progresses, these feelings often manifest as outbursts or moments of uncontrollable anger as an individual struggles to remain calm. This frustration can be understood by their declining abilities to recall memories of their own life, leaving them victim to "a cruel disease which turns the world into a foreign, unfamiliar place" Klein (1987) starts. "It may be assumed that someone who has been attacked by this disease feels angry about what has happened to (them), and turns (their) anger against whomever is nearest" (Klein, 1987, p. 63). A growing body of research suggests this emotional activity may come from more than just pent-up frustrations, suggesting dysfunction in the right cerebral hemisphere may cause abnormal emotions in patients with dementia or Alzheimer's disease (Holston, 2004). Though it is incredibly unrealistic to propose finding a solution for all negative feelings that come with the onset of this disease, Holston (2004) argues that participation in art activities can regulate mood by targeting the right cerebral hemisphere. This study also discusses the value in the ability to express feelings nonverbally, citing healing factors that come from activities such as painting or drawing, an idea introduced in the section on symptom relief (Kamar, 1997). Negative emotions are significantly reduced when participants form an interest in art therapy and regain a sense of self-accomplishment as they complete their artwork. In turn, this can fulfill an individual's desire to feel self-sufficient and respected, improving quality of life and dissuading potential outbursts (Holston, 2004; Basting, 2006; Hannemann, 2006).

Unfortunately, quality of life has not always been a consistent point of consideration in many studies (Costa, Mercieca-Bebba, Rutherford, Tait, King, 2021), making it difficult to cross-reference findings and replicate results. However, when researchers specify parameters and provide testable statistics backed by empirical research, conclusions suggesting increases in quality of life become far more reliable. In Seifert et al. (2017), researchers conducted a pilot study with 12 dementia patients to measure the effects of art and art therapy on their well-being. Well-being was defined by the questionnaire created to quantify it, composed of many traits under the categories of "mental state and concentration", "corporeal memory", "self-reliance", "self-esteem", and "physicality". All participants actively engaged in sculptural activities once a week for two hours over the course of thirteen weeks. The data received from questionnaires showed significant change in the p-value of most traits under each category when compared against the results of the control group. Their conclusion demonstrates a clear improvement in each participant's overall well-being, measurable through "external assessment for up to six hours after the activity" (Seifert, Spottke, Fliessbach, 2017, p. 11). The happiness of each participant was directly impacted by their participation in an art therapy program, aligning with the expectations of other studies demonstrating similar results (Emblad & Mukaetova-Ladinska, 2021; Seifert et al., 2017; Kamar, 1997; Kaimal & Ray, 2016; Vugt & Dröes, 2017; Cohen, 2009; Vernooji-Dassen, 2010; Rodin, 1989).

Across the board, studies have argued that socialization plays a considerable role in the determination of a patient's happiness, as increases in their social skills consistently correlated with lower levels of depression and decreased agitation (Seifert et al., 2017; Kolanowski & Litaker, 2006; Cohen, 2009; Vugt & Dröes, 2017). Active engagement with socialization helps act as a barrier between stressful circumstances and psychological well-being in all adults, not just individuals with dementia and Alzheimer's disease. In cases of isolation and social withdrawal, however, patients with the disease can experience more significant functional decline and higher mortality rates (Kolanowski & Litaker, 2006; Kiely, Simon, Jones, Morris, 2000; Glass, Leon, Berkman, 2016). Limitations on social engagement due to already declining cognitive capabilities, physical impairments, and environmental obstacles are also associated with greater psychological stress and behavioral problems (Mor, Branco, Fleishman, Haws, Phillips, Morris, Fries, 1995). Several studies introduced earlier in this chapter have demonstrated art therapy's impact on social skills, including Cohen (2009), Tramer (2008), and Ferguson & Goosman (1991). However, few have offered empirical evidence illustrating the contribution of social therapeutic interventions, with one exception.

In Lee et al. (2017), researchers used naturalistic observation to record the effects of socialization in a study they believed to be the first of its kind (Lee, Boltz, Algase, 2017, p. 210). The study observed 110 participants with dementia and Alzheimer's disease over two nonconsecutive days of increased staff-resident interactions to evaluate efficacy. Accounting for variables such as time of day and levels of cognitive function, the data offered empirical evidence that using nonverbal communication to supplement verbal communication significantly improved the patient's quality of life and milieu. The conclusion of this study demonstrates the importance of accounting for both quality and quantity of socialization when managing residential care facilities, offering their data as an argument for "the importance of staff education and performance evaluations that include the ability to interact in a therapeutic manner with persons with dementia" (Lee et al., 2017, p. 210). When aligning this conclusion alongside the conclusions of Cohen (2009), Vugt & Dröes (2017), Seifert et al. (2017), and Tramer (2008), the increased levels of socialization that come as a result of participating in art therapy are linked to a significant increase in the health and well-being of patients with dementia and Alzheimer's disease.

### Supplementing Verbal Ability

With the exception of Eekelaar et al. (2012), little research has offered suggestions that art therapy can increase verbal fluency in individuals with dementia and Alzheimer's disease. Though it can be inferred that the increased use of descriptive language and enriched socialization from engaging with art therapy would bear better results for the longevity of verbal ability than apathy might, further studies must be conducted before a definitive statement can be made either way. A far more agreed-upon argument is that art therapy can offer a bridge for communication between caregivers and individuals with dementia and Alzheimer's disease. Several previously mentioned studies discuss the benefits of using art in this way, as poor verbal fluency does not always equate to the inability to communicate altogether (Kamar, 1997; Lee et al., 2017). Art therapy has, at least in part, proven beneficial in this way, having been developed "as a result of the need to find alternatives to verbal forms of communication, to allow people who have difficulty with words to express themselves and to enable the unsayable to be said" (Miller, 1984, p. 128). There is no one way to communicate, and as the need for nonverbal forms of communication is exacerbated by cognitive decline, the desire for expressive and communicative forms of art increases.

## CONCLUSION

One of the greatest challenges researchers continue to face when reviewing interventions in the development of dementia and Alzheimer's disease is the progression of protein clustering and neuronal degeneration before a diagnosis is given. Though pinpointing the exact beginning of the disease can be difficult due to limited understanding of its underlying causes, the harmful proteins that produce senile plaques can begin accumulating as early as 15-20 years before symptoms manifest (Fan & Wang, 2019). As such, the prodromal symptoms experienced in the "early" stages of dementia and Alzheimer's disease are, in actuality, further in the decomposition phase, or advanced stages, than implied. This highlights the importance of clarifying the difference "between the concepts of the early phase of biology and the early phase of clinical manifestations" (Fan & Wang, 2019, p. 196), as an understanding of how the disease progresses is vital to the development of early interventions that produce therapeutic benefits.

Fortunately, art therapy has been shown to provide positive effects to all communities of seniors, including populations who are not at risk for dementia (Buchalter, 2011; Levine-Madori, 2013, pp. 317-327; Ho, 2012). This could suggest that all individuals between the ages of 70-85 could generally benefit from participation in art therapy services, citing both quality of life improvements and a possibility of delaying an onset of dementia long before symptoms manifest. The findings of Mahncke et al. (2006) and Stewart (2004) may support this possibility, though the strength of their conclusions and short/nonexistent follow-up requires further research to be conducted. As studies continue to explore ways art therapy can be used to contribute to a delay of this kind, researchers must keep the 15-20 year timeline in mind when modeling experiments in hopes of producing data that yields more robust conclusions.

Current research into the efficacy of using art therapy as a cognitive intervention in the development of dementia and Alzheimer's disease leaves much to be desired, and future studies must be conducted using agreed-upon durations, frequencies, and measurements of interventions to offer more conclusive findings. Though the suggestions of improvements to cognition are divisive amongst studies, none dispute the benefits of art therapy on participants' behavioral and psychological symptoms. An overwhelming amount of research suggests that individuals living with dementia and Alzheimer's disease who actively participated in an art therapy program continuously experienced enhanced quality of life, lower levels of depression, and improved social skills, as well as some suggestion for a greater connection to their self-identity, maintenance of fine motor skills, and possible retrieval of autobiographical memories.

Furthermore, the possibility of using art as a form of communication in patients who have experienced a decline in verbal ability due to neuronal decay can be highly valuable for caretakers when assessing that individual's needs. This is in line with the reputation of art therapy in general, which is praised for its ability to "invite alternative modes of receptive and expressive communication, which can circumvent the limitations of language" (AATA) in the lives of all individuals and communities. So long as the potential for creativity is found within people across varying levels of the disease, the value of using artistic interventions to improve their overall well-being remains high (Palmiero, Giacomo, Passafiume, 2012). Thus, the numerous benefits cited above suggest that the symptoms and mental health concerns of individuals with dementia and Alzheimer's disease can be treated more holistically through engagement with art therapy services. Future research will enhance our understanding of these benefits to provide a more informative framework for interventions going forward.

## REFERENCES

Aguilar, B. (2017). The Efficacy of Art Therapy in Pediatric Oncology Patients: An Integrative Literature Review. *Journal of Pediatric Nursing, 36*, 173–178. https://doi.org/ doi:10.1016/j.pedn.2017.06.015

Allan & Crandall. (1986). The Rosebush: a visualization strategy. *Elementary School Guidance & Counseling, 21*(1), 44–51. https://www.jstor.org/stable/42871035

Alzheimer's Association. (2020). 2020 Alzheimer's Disease Facts and Figures. *Alzheimer's & Dementia, 16*(3), 391–460. doi:10.1002/alz.12068

American Art Therapy Association. (2017). *About Art Therapy*. American Art Therapy Association. https://arttherapy.org/about-art-therapy/

Art Therapy Credentials Board, Inc. (2017). *What is Art Therapy?* Art Therapy Credentials Board, Inc. https://www.atcb.org/what-is-art-therapy/

Baird, A., Garrido, S., & Tamplin, J. (2019). Music and Dementia: From Cognition to Therapy. In *Google Books*. Oxford University Press. doi:10.1093/oso/9780190075934.001.0001

Ball, E. L., Owen-Booth, B., Gray, A., Shenkin, S. D., Hewitt, J., & McCleery, J. (2020). Aromatherapy for dementia. *Cochrane Database of Systematic Reviews, 8. The Cochrane Library, 2020*(8). doi:10.1002/14651858.CD003150.pub3 PMID:32813272

Ball, M. (1977). Neuronal loss, neurofibrillary tangles and granulovacuolar degeneration in the hippocampus with ageing and dementia. *Acta Neuropathologica, 37*(2), 111–118. doi:10.1007/BF00692056

Basting. (2006). Arts in Dementia Care: "This is not the end... it's the end of this chapter." *Generations, 30*(1), 16–20. https://www.ingentaconnect.com/content/asag/gen/2006/0000003 0/00000001/art00004

Brown, C. J., Chirino, A. F. C., Cortez, C. M., Gearhart, C., & Urizar, G. G. (2020). Conceptual Art for the Aging Brain: Piloting an Art-Based Cognitive Health Intervention. *Activities, Adaptation & Aging, 45*(1), 39–69. Taylor & Francis Online. doi:10.1080/01924788.2020.1719584

Buchalter (2011). Art Therapy and Creative Coping Techniques for Older Adults. In *Google Books*. Jessica Kingsley Publishers.

Bugos, J. A., Perlstein, W. M., McCrae, C. S., Brophy, T. S., & Bedenbaugh, P. H. (2007). Individualized Piano Instruction enhances executive functioning and working memory in older adults. *Aging & Mental Health, 11*(4), 464–471. Taylor & Francis Online. https://doi.org/ doi:10.1080/13607860601086504

Buschert, V., Bokde, A. L. W., & Hampel, H. (2010). Cognitive intervention in Alzheimer disease. *Nature Reviews. Neurology*, *6*(9), 508–517. doi:10.1038/nrneurol.2010.113 PMID:20717104

Center for Medicare & Medicaid Services. (2018). Survey and Enforcement Process for Skilled Nursing Facilities and Nursing Facilities. In *State Operations Manual*. Center for Medicare & Medicaid Services. https://www.cms.gov/Regulations-and-Guidance/Guidance/Manual s/Downloads/som107c07pdf.pdf

Ciasca, E. C., Ferreira, R. C., Santana, C. L. A., Forlenza, O. V., dos Santos, G. D., Brum, P. S., & Nunes, P. V. (2018). Art therapy as an adjuvant treatment for depression in elderly women: A randomized controlled trial. *Revista Brasileira de Psiquiatria (Sao Paulo, Brazil)*, *40*(3), 256–263. doi:10.1590/1516-4446-2017-2250 PMID:29412335

Clapp, L. A., Taylor, E. P., Di Folco, S., & Mackinnon, V. L. (2018). Effectiveness of art therapy with pediatric populations affected by medical health conditions: A systematic review. *Arts & Health, 11*(3), 183–201. doi:10.1080/17533015.2018.1 443952 PMID:31038441

Cohen, G. (2009). New theories and research findings on the positive influence of music and art on health with ageing. *Arts & Health, 1*(1), 48–62. doi:10.1080/17533010802528033

Costa, D. S. J., Mercieca-Bebber, R., Rutherford, C., Tait, M.-A., & King, M. T. (2021). How is quality of life defined and assessed in published research? *Quality of Life Research: An International Journal of Quality of Life Aspects of Treatment, Care and Rehabilitation, 30*(8), 2109–2121. doi:10.100711136-021-02826-0 PMID:33792834

Davis, R. N., Massman, P. J., & Doody, R. S. (2001). (2001). Cognitive Intervention in Alzheimer Disease: A Randomized Placebo-Controlled Study. *Alzheimer Disease and Associated Disorders, 15*(1), 1–9. https://tinyurl.com/yfwa7h9t. doi:10.1097/00002093-200101000-00001 PMID:11236819

de Vugt, M., & Dröes, R.-M. (2017). Social health in dementia. Towards a positive dementia discourse. *Aging & Mental Health, 21*(1), 1–3. doi:10.1080/13607863.2016.1262822 PMID:28098498

Deaver, S. (2002). What Constitutes Art Therapy Research? *Art Therapy, 19*(1), 23–27. doi:10.1080/07421656.2002.10129721

Dhikav, V., & Anand, K. S.Dhikav & Anand. (2012). Hippocampus in health and disease: An overview. *Annals of Indian Academy of Neurology, 15*(4), 239. doi:10.4103/0972-2327.104323 PMID:23349586

Dillehay, R. (1990). Caregivers for Alzheimer's Patients: What We Are Learning from Research. *The International Journal of Aging and Human Development, 30*(4), 263–285. https://doi.org/ doi:10.2190/2P3J-A9AH-HHF4-00RG

Doric-Henry, L. (1997). Pottery as Art Therapy with Elderly Nursing Home Residents. *Art Therapy: Journal of the American Art Therapy Association, 14*(3), 163–171. doi:10.1080/07421656.1987.10759277

Douglass, A., Walterfang, M., Velakoulis, D., & Abel, L. (2018). Behavioral Variant Frontotemporal Dementia Performance on a Range of Saccadic Tasks. *Journal of Alzheimer's Disease, 65*(1), 231–242. doi:10.3233/JAD-170797 PMID:30040708

Eekelaar, C., Camic, P. M., & Springham, N. (2012). Art galleries, episodic memory and verbal fluency in dementia: An exploratory study. *Psychology of Aesthetics, Creativity, and the Arts, 6*(3), 262–272. APA PsycArticles. https://psycnet.apa.org/doi/10.1037/a0027499

Egan, M. F., Kost, J., Voss, T., Mukai, Y., Aisen, P. S., Cummings, J. L., Tariot, P. N., Vellas, B., van Dyck, C. H., Boada, M., Zhang, Y., Li, W., Furtek, C., Mahoney, E., Harper Mozley, L., Mo, Y., Sur, C., & Michelson, D. (2019). Randomized Trial of Verubecestat for Prodromal Alzheimer's Disease. *The New England Journal of Medicine, 380*(15), 1408–1420. doi:10.1056/NEJMoa1812840 PMID:30970186

Emblad, S. Y. M., & Mukaetova-Ladinska, E. B.Emblad & Mukaetova-Ladinska. (2021). Creative Art Therapy as a Non-Pharmacological Intervention for Dementia: A Systematic Review. *Journal of Alzheimer's Disease Reports*, *5*(1), 353–364. doi:10.3233/ADR-201002 PMID:34189407

Fan, D.-Y., & Wang, Y.-J. (2019). Early Intervention in Alzheimer's Disease: How Early is Early Enough? *Neuroscience Bulletin*, *36*(2), 195–197. doi:10.100712264-019-00429-x PMID:31494835

Ferguson & Goosman. (1991). A foot in the door: Art therapy in the nursing home. *American Journal of Art Therapy*, *30*(1), 2–3. https://pubmed.ncbi.nlm.nih.gov/10114781/ PMID:10114781

Fjell, A. M., McEvoy, L., Holland, D., Dale, A. M., & Walhovd, K. B. (2013). Brain Changes in Older Adults at Very Low Risk for Alzheimer's Disease. *The Journal of Neuroscience : The Official Journal of the Society for Neuroscience*, *33*(19), 8237–8242. doi:10.1523/JNEUROSCI.5506-12.2013 PMID:23658162

Freedman, V. A., Cornman, J. C., & Kasper, J. D. (2021). *National Health and Aging Trends Study Trends Chart Book: Key Trends, Measures and Detailed Tables* (48th ed., Vol. 4). National Institute on Aging., https://micda.isr.umich.edu/research/nhats-trends-dashboards

Frith, C., & Law, J.Frith & Law. (1995). Cognitive and Physiological Processes Underlying Drawing Skills. *Leonardo*, *28*(3), 203–205. https://muse.jhu.edu/pub/6/article/607018/summary. doi:10.2307/1576075

Glass, T. A., Leon, C. F. M. D., & Berkman, L. F. (2016). Social Engagement and Depressive Symptoms in Late Life: Longitudinal Findings. *Journal of Aging and Health, 18*(4). Sage Journals. https://doi.org/ doi:10.1177/0898264306291017

Gussak, D. (2004). Art therapy with prison inmates: a pilot study. *Art Therapy with Prison Inmates: A Pilot Study, 31*(4), 245–259. https://pascal-francis.inist.fr/vibad/index.php?action=getRecordDetail&idt=16112574

Hannemann (2006). Creativity with Dementia Patients. *Gerontology, 52*(1), 59–65. https://doi.org/ doi:10.1159/000089827

Harlan, B. (1993). The Therapeutic Value of Art for Persons with Alzheimer's Disease and Related Disorders. In M. Lahey, R. Kunstler, A. Grossman, F. Daly, S. Waldman, & F. Schwartz (Eds.), *Recreation, Leisure and Chronic Illness.* Routledge. https://www.taylorfrancis.com/chapters/edit/10.4324/9780203058046-13/therapeutic-value-art-persons-alzheimer-disease-related-disorders-jane-harlan

Hays & Lyons. (1981). The bridge drawing: A projective technique for assessment in art therapy. *The Arts in Psychotherapy, 8*(3-4), 207–217. APA PsycInfo. https://psycnet.apa.org/record/1982-26187-001

Ho, B. (2012). *The Effect of Art Therapy Chinese Seniors' Quality of Life in a Residential Setting*. Tati. https://www.tati.on.ca/wp-content/uploads/2012/02/Thesis-Proposal-Bonnie-Ho.docx

Holston, M. (2004). Paintings of the psyche: An innovative hospital program and museum in Rio has nurtured highly acclaimed artists while revealing the healing power of art. *Americas, 56*(2), 6–13. ProQuest. https://www.proquest.com/docview/1797187731/fulltextPDF/374255DB71A54315PQ/4?accountid=10226

Jett, L. (2018). Nursing Homes with Dementia Special Care Units Provide Better Quality of Care. *Harvard Medical School.* https://hcp.hms.harvard.edu/news/nursing-homes-dementia-special-care-units-provide-better-quality-care

Joyce, N. R., McGuire, T. G., Bartels, S. J., Mitchell, S. L., & Grabowski, D. C. (2018). The Impact of Dementia Special Care Units on Quality of Care: An Instrumental Variables Analysis. *Health Services Research, 53*(5), 3657–3679. doi:10.1111/1475-6773.12867 PMID:29736944

Kahn-Denis, K. B. (1997). Art Therapy with Geriatric Dementia Clients. *Art Therapy: Journal of the American Art Therapy Association, 14*(3), 194–199. doi:10.1080/07421656.1987.10759281

Kaimal, G., & Ray, K. (2016). Free art-making in an art therapy open studio: Changes in affect and self-efficacy. *Arts & Health, 9*(2), 154–166. doi:10.1080/17533015.2016.1217248

Kamar, O. (1997). Light and death: Art therapy with a patient with - ProQuest. *American Journal of Art Therapy, 35*(4). ProQuest. https://www.proquest.com/docview/199488748?pq-origsite=gscholar&fromopenview=true

Kaye, J. A., Swihart, T., Howieson, D., Dame, A., Moore, M. M., Karnos, T., Camicioli, R., Ball, M., Oken, B., & Sexton, G. (1997). Volume loss of the hippocampus and temporal lobe in healthy elderly persons destined to develop dementia. *Neurology, 48*(5), 1297–1304. doi:10.1212/WNL.48.5.1297 PMID:9153461

Kiely, D. K., Simon, S. E., Jones, R. N., & Morris, J. N. (2000). The Protective Effect of Social Engagement on Mortality in Long-Term Care. *Journal of the American Geriatrics Society, 48*(11), 1367–1372. doi:10.1111/j.1532-5415.2000.tb02624.x PMID:11083310

Klein. (1987). When the brain betrays the body. *Tel Aviv: Sifriat HaPoalim.*

Kochersberger, G., Hielema, F., & Westlund, R. (1994). Rehabilitation in the nursing home: how much, why, and with what results. *Public Health Reports (Washington, D.C: 1974), 109*(3), 372–376. https://www.ncbi.nlm.nih.gov/pmc/articles/PMC1403501/?page=3

Kolanowski, A., & Litaker, M.Kolanowski & Litaker. (2006). Social Interaction, Premorbid Personality, and Agitation in Nursing Home Residents With Dementia. *Archives of Psychiatric Nursing, 20*(1), 12–20. doi:10.1016/j.apnu.2005.08.006 PMID:16442470

Kolb, B., & Whishaw, I. Q. (1998). Brain Plasticity and Behavior. *Annual Review of Psychology, 49*(1), 43–64. doi:10.1146/annurev.psych.49.1.43 PMID:9496621

Kovach, C. R., Noonan, P. E., Schlidt, A. M., & Wells, T. (2005). A Model of Consequences of Need-Driven, Dementia-Compromised Behavior. *Journal of Nursing Scholarship, 37*(2), 134–140. Sigma. https://doi.org/ doi:10.1111/j.1547-5069.2005.00025_1.x

Kramer, O. (2001). Art as Therapy: Collected Papers. In *Google Books*. Jessica Kingsley Publishers.

Lee, K. H., Boltz, M., Lee, H., & Algase, D. L. (2017). Does Social Interaction Matter Psychological Well-Being in Persons With Dementia? *American Journal of Alzheimer's Disease and Other Dementias, 32*(4), 207–212. doi:10.1177/1533317517704301 PMID:28417644

Levine-Madori. (2013). Utilizing a thematic approach to art therapy with seniors: Enhancing cognitive abilities and social interactions. In P. Howie, S. Prasad, & J. Kristel (Eds.), *Using Art Therapy with Diverse Populations: Crossing Cultures and Abilities* (pp. 317–327). Jessica Kingsley Publishers.

Lie, D. C., Song, H., Colamarino, S. A., Ming, G., & Gage, F. H. (2004). Neurogenesis in the Adult Brain: New Strategies for Central Nervous System Diseases. *Annual Review of Pharmacology and Toxicology*, *44*(1), 399–421. doi:10.1146/annurev.pharmtox.44.101802.121631 PMID:14744252

Liu, H., Zhang, Z., Choi, S., & Langa, K. M. (2020). Marital Status and Dementia: Evidence from the Health and Retirement Study. *The Journals of Gerontology. Series B, Psychological Sciences and Social Sciences*, *75*(8), 1783–1795. doi:10.1093/geronb/gbz087 PMID:31251349

Loewenstein, D. A., Acevedo, A., Czaja, S. J., & Duara, R. (2004). Cognitive Rehabilitation of Mildly Impaired Alzheimer Disease Patients on Cholinesterase Inhibitors. *The American Journal of Geriatric Psychiatry*, *12*(4), 395–402. doi:10.1097/00019442-200407000-00007 PMID:15249277

Logsdon, R. G., McCurry, S. M., & Teri, L. (2008). Time-Limited Support Groups for Individuals with Early Stage Dementia and Their Care Partners. *Clinical Gerontologist, 30*(2), 5–19. Taylor & Francis Online. doi:10.1300/J018v30n02_02

Mahncke, H. W., Connor, B. B., Appelman, J., Ahsanuddin, O. N., Hardy, J. L., Wood, R. A., Joyce, N. M., Boniske, T., Atkins, S. M., & Merzenich, M. M. (2006). Memory enhancement in healthy older adults using a brain plasticity-based training program: A randomized, controlled study. *Proceedings of the National Academy of Sciences of the United States of America*, *103*(33), 12523–12528. doi:10.1073/pnas.0605194103 PMID:16888038

Mayeux, R., & Stern, Y. (2012). Epidemiology of Alzheimer Disease. *Cold Spring Harbor Perspectives in Medicine*, *2*(8), a006239–a006239. doi:10.1101/cshperspect.a006239 PMID:22908189

McNeilly, G. (1983). Directive and non-directive approaches in art therapy. *The Arts in Psychotherapy*, *10*(4), 211–219. https://psycnet.apa.org/record/1984-23708-001. doi:10.1016/0197-4556(83)90021-7

Merriam, A. E., Aronson, M. K., Gaston, P., Wey, S.-L., & Katz, I. (1988). The Psychiatric Symptoms of Alzheimer's Disease. *Journal of the American Geriatrics Society*, *36*(1), 7–22. doi:10.1111/j.1532-5415.1988.tb03427.x PMID:3335733

Miller. (1984). Art therapy with the elderly and the terminally ill. In *Art as Therapy* (pp. 128–129).

Mitchell, S. L., Mor, V., Gozalo, P. L., Servadio, J. L., & Teno, J. M. (2016). Tube Feeding in US Nursing Home Residents With Advanced Dementia, 2000-2014. *Journal of the American Medical Association, 316*(7), 769. doi:10.1001/jama.2016.9374 PMID:27533163

Monti, D. A., Peterson, C., Kunkel, E. J. S., Hauck, W. W., Pequignot, E., Rhodes, L., & Brainard, G. C. (2006). A randomized, controlled trial of mindfulness-based art therapy (MBAT) for women with cancer. *Psycho-Oncology, 15*(5), 363–373. doi:10.1002/pon.988 PMID:16288447

Mor, V., Branco, K., Fleishman, J., Hawes, C., Phillips, C., Morris, J., & Fries, B. (1995). The Structure of Social Engagement among Nursing Home Residents. *The Journals of Gerontology. Series B, Psychological Sciences and Social Sciences, 50B*(1), 1–P8. doi:10.1093/geronb/50B.1.P1 PMID:7757818

National Institute on Aging. (2017). *What Happens to the Brain in Alzheimer's Disease?* National Institute on Aging. https://www.nia.nih.gov/health/what-happens-brain-alzheimers-disease

National Institute on Aging. (2018). *How Is Alzheimer's Disease Treated?* National Institute on Aging. https://www.nia.nih.gov/health/how-alzheimers-disease-treated

Palmiero, M., Di Giacomo, D., & Passafiume, D. (2012). Creativity and dementia: A review. *Cognitive Processing, 13*(3), 193–209. doi:10.100710339-012-0439-y PMID:22438178

Panza, F., Lozupone, M., Sardone, R., Battista, P., Piccininni, M., Dibello, V., La Montagna, M., Stallone, R., Venezia, P., Liguori, A., Giannelli, G., Bellomo, A., Greco, A., Daniele, A., Seripa, D., Quaranta, N., & Logroscino, G. (2018). Sensorial frailty: Age-related hearing loss and the risk of cognitive impairment and dementia in later life. *Therapeutic Advances in Chronic Disease, 10*, 204062231881100. doi:10.1177/2040622318811000 PMID:31452865

Paula, J. J., Albuquerque, M. R., Lage, G. M., Bicalho, M. A., Romano-Silva, M. A., & Malloy-Diniz, L. F. (2016). Impairment of fine motor dexterity in mild cognitive impairment and Alzheimer's disease dementia: Association with activities of daily living. *Revista Brasileira de Psiquiatria (Sao Paulo, Brazil), 38*(3), 235–238. doi:10.1590/1516-4446-2015-1874 PMID:27508398

Raglio, A., Bellelli, G., Traficante, D., Gianotti, M., Ubezio, M. C., Villani, D., & Trabucchi, M. (2008). Efficacy of Music Therapy in the Treatment of Behavioral and Psychiatric Symptoms of Dementia. *Alzheimer Disease and Associated Disorders, 22*(2), 158–162. doi:10.1097/WAD.0b013e3181630b6f PMID:18525288

Ragneskog, H., Asplund, K., Kihlgren, M., & Norberg, A. (2001). Individualized music played for agitated patients with dementia: Analysis of video-recorded sessions. *International Journal of Nursing Practice, 7*(3), 146–155. Wiley Online Library. https://doi.org/ doi:10.1046/j.1440-172X.2001.00254.x

Rao, Y. L., Ganaraja, B., Murlimanju, B. V., Joy, T., Krishnamurthy, A., & Agrawal, A. (2022). Hippocampus and its involvement in Alzheimer's disease: a review. *3 Biotech, 12*(2). doi:10.1007/s13205-022-03123-4

Richedson, N. & Neill, J. (2004). *Therapeutic recreation music intervention to decrease mealtime agitation and increase food intake in older adults with dementia.* Scientific Publishing.

Rodin, J. (1986). Aging and health: effects of the sense of control. *Science, 233*(4770), 1271–1276. doi:10.1126/science.3749877

Rodin, J. (1989). Sense of Control: Potentials for Intervention. *The ANNALS of the American Academy of Political and Social Science, 503*(1), 29–42. https://doi.org/ doi:10.1177/0002716289503001003

Rubin, J. (1982). Art therapy: What it is and what it is not. *American Journal of Art Therapy, 21*(2), 57–58. APA PsycInfo. https://psycnet.apa.org/record/1984-31877-001

Rusted, J., Sheppard, L., & Waller, D. (2016). A Multi-centre Randomized Control Group Trial on the Use of Art Therapy for Older People with Dementia. *Group Analysis, 39*(4). Sage Journals. doi:10.1177/0533316406071447

Sachs, G. A., Shega, J. W., & Cox-Hayley, D. (2004). Barriers to excellent end-of-life care for patients with dementia. *Journal of General Internal Medicine, 19*(10), 1057–1063. doi:10.1111/j.1525-1497.2004.30329.x PMID:15482560

Seifert, K., Spottke, A., & Fliessbach, K. (2017). Effects of sculpture based art therapy in dementia patients—A pilot study. *Heliyon, 3*(11), e00460. doi:10.1016/j.heliyon.2017.e00460 PMID:29264417

Shore (1997). Promoting Wisdom: The Role of Art Therapy in Geriatric Settings. *Art Therapy, 14*(3), 172–177. https://doi.org/ doi:10.1080/07421656.1987.10759278

Slayton, S. C., D'Archer, J., & Kaplan, F. (2010). Outcome Studies on the Efficacy of Art Therapy: A Review of Findings. *Art Therapy: Journal of the American Art Therapy Association, 27*(3), 108–118. doi:10.1080/07421656.2010.10129660

Stewart (2004). Art Therapy and Neuroscience Blend: Working with Patients Who Have Dementia. *Art Therapy, 21*(3), 148–155. https://doi.org/ doi:10.1080/07421656.2004.10129499

Tramer, B. (2008). *Case Study: Geriatric Group Art Therapy in a Nursing Home.* [Thesis, Ursuline College]. https://etd.ohiolink.edu/apexprod/rws_etd/send_file/send?accession=urs1210555128&disposition=inline

Uttley, L., Scope, A., Stevenson, M., & Rawdin, A. (2015). The clinical and cost effectiveness of group art therapy for people with non-psychotic mental health disorders: A systematic review and cost-effectiveness analysis. *BMC Psychiatry, 15*(1), 151. doi:10.118612888-015-0528-4 PMID:26149275

Vernooij-Dassen, M., Vasse, E., Zuidema, S., Cohen-Mansfield, J., & Moyle, W. (2010). Psychosocial interventions for dementia patients in long-term care. *International Psychogeriatrics, 22*(07), 1121–1128. doi:10.1017/S1041610210001365 PMID:20813074

Wald (1986). Fusion of Symbols, Confusion of Boundaries: Percept Contamination in the Art Work of Alzheimer's Disease Patients. *Art Therapy, 3*(2), 74–80. https://doi.org/ doi:10.1080/07421656.1986.10758827

Wang, J.-J., Hsieh, P.-F., & Wang, C.-J. (2013). Long-term Care Nurses' Communication Difficulties with People Living with Dementia in Taiwan. *Asian Nursing Research, 7*(3), 99–103. doi:10.1016/j.anr.2013.06.001 PMID:25030246

Wang, Q.-Y., & Li, D.-M. (2016). Advances in art therapy for patients with dementia. *Clinical Nursing Research, 3*(3), 105–108. doi:10.1016/j.cnre.2016.06.011

Zarit, S. H., Femia, E. E., Watson, J., Rice-Oeschger, L., & Kakos, B. (2004). Memory Club: A Group Intervention for People With Early-Stage Dementia and Their Care Partners. *The Gerontologist, 44*(2), 262–269. doi:10.1093/geront/44.2.262 PMID:15075423

Zgola. (1987). Doing Things: A Guide to Programming Activities for Persons with Alzheimer's Disease and Related Disorders. In *Google Books*. JHU Press.

## KEY TERMS AND DEFINITIONS

**Action potentials:** The sending of information down the axon to trigger an impulse.

**American Art Therapy Association (AATA):** An organization dedicated to growing and developing the profession of art therapy.

**Apathy:** The loss of interest or concern.

**Art Therapy Credentials Board Inc. (ATCB):** An agency ensuring the ethical practice of art therapy through credentialing.

**Astrocytes:** A glial cell that regulates blood flow and transfers mitochondria to neurons.

**Beta-amyloids:** A protein that is normally responsible for neuronal growth and repair, however when corrupted can lead to dementia.

**Center for Medicare & Medicaid Services (CMS):** A division of the Department of Health and Human Services that oversees the medicare and medicaid services.

**Cerebral cortex:** The outermost layer of the brain responsible for higher level processing.

**Cholinesterase inhibitors:** Chemicals that decrease the breakdown of neurotransmitters.

**Chronic inflammation:** Long-term and long-lasting inflammation.

**Cognition:** The acquisition of knowledge and understanding through thought and experience.

**Cognitive reserve:** The capacity for retaining information and resisting damage to the brain.

**Compensatory strategies:** Techniques used to complete tasks in an alternative manner.

**Convalescing:** Recovering strength and health over the course of an illness.

**Corporeal memory:** The hypothesis that the body is capable of storing memories.

**Directives:** A statement or command made by a therapist that specifies or suggests an action the client should perform.

**Efficacy:** The ability to produce a desired outcome.

**Empirical data/research:** Data and research based on verifiable observation rather than theory.

**Entorhinal cortex:** A component of the hippocampal formation that acts as a gateway for incoming and outgoing information.

**Geriatric:** Relating to the elderly, especially relevant in healthcare.

**Hippocampus:** A highly plastic and malleable brain structure located in the temporal lobe responsible for learning and memory.

**Interventions:** An action intended to interfere with or alter the course of a pathological process.

**LCAT (Licensed Creative Arts Therapist):** The license that creative art therapists pursue.

**Levick Emotional & Cognitive Art Therapy Evaluation & Assessment (LECATA):** An assessment developed to evaluate the therapeutic needs of children on the spectrum.

**Microglia:** Immune cells in the central nervous system that combat brain infections and inflammation.

**Milieu:** An individual's social environment.

**Neurodegenerative disorder:** A type of disease in which immune cells in the central nervous system die or stop working.

**Neurogenesis:** The growth of nervous tissue from neural stem cells in the adult brain.

**Neuronal decay:** The death of neurons.

**Neurons:** A brain cell that transmits nerve impulses.

**Prodromal:** The period between the first appearance of symptoms and full development of a disease or illness.

**Proteinopathies:** The abnormal aggregation of proteins within neurons.

**P-value:** A statistical value that measures probability.

**Right cerebral hemisphere:** The right half of the cerebellum which controls muscles on the left side of the body.

**Structural plasticity:** The ability of neural networks to change through growth and reorganization as a result of learning.

**Synapses:** The gap between two neurons across which impulses are transmitted.

**Tau:** A protein involved in stabilizing the internal structure of neurons.

**Temporal lobe:** A pair of lobes located beneath the temples concerned with the understanding of speech.

**Ulman Personality Assessment Procedure (UPAP):** A historical art therapy assessment based on experimental directives that consists of 4 drawings completed in one session.

**Vascular systems:** Circulatory systems composed of vessels that carry blood and lymph fluid throughout the body.

**Visual-spatial abilities:** The ability to decipher where objects are in space.

# Chapter 2
# Art Therapy With Latin-American Immigrant Women

**Rachel Brandoff**
*Thomas Jefferson University, USA*

**Monica Sanchez**
*Little Sisters of the Assumption Family Health Service, Inc., USA*

## ABSTRACT

*Still a melting pot, the United States continues to draw high rates of immigrants from around the world. Significant attention has been given to those entering via the southern border, many of whom are seeking asylum from various countries where their lives and families are at risk. In one social service agency in East Harlem, New York City, a single art therapist has built a thriving mental health program that serves primarily women and families from Latin American countries. These immigrant women face enormous obstacles, including but not limited to profound trauma histories, limited English language skills, lack of education, poverty, food insecurity, and sometimes a lack of ability to seek legal employment. What they also bring with them is fierce love for their children and families, perseverance, and enormous, if sometimes latent creativity. This chapter documents the process towards self-discovery and empowerment in which these women engage through art therapy.*

## INTRODUCTION

A small social service agency in East Harlem, New York City provides a variety of services to a highly traumatized population that remains almost invisible in this crowded city. This chapter presents stories and data that track the impact of art

DOI: 10.4018/978-1-6684-7856-1.ch002

therapy on immigrant women living in New York City; mental health services were offered with the vision that individuals who come to this country with high trauma should not have to endure more trauma. The authors present examples of impactful work drawn from a unique art therapy group delivered in an East Harlem, New York neighborhood. Also presented are suggestions for future directions in art therapy research with immigrant populations.

## BACKGROUND

The immigrant women who comprise the mental health services clientele in East Harlem have suffered extraordinary obstacles. In fact, just holding space for these women to identify their emotional state and share some of the stories that they carry is an overwhelming task; one that commands the therapist to have exceptional self-regulation, personal supports, good supervision, regular therapy, outlets and boundaries, and the ability to make space for burdens without carrying them. The stories of adversity, abuse that is both personal and systemic, and dehumanizing torture are unending.

These clients came to the United States under extremely adverse conditions, often forced from their homes, with limited resources and money. Many have endured family separation, personal and sexual violations, and vocational and financial exploitation both before and after arriving in their new country. Working with clients with extreme abuse histories is intense clinical work. This is a space that challenges even the most courageous and prepared clinicians. In this little agency in East Harlem there has been one consistent professional upholding the mental health services for over eight years. Clinicians come in eager to help and support an underserved, marginalized, devalued community; and in some cases, it is not so long before they start to see the toll it takes on them.

Providing mental health services to a traumatized, immigrant and indigenous population against the backdrop of growing hate speech in America, xenophobia, and extremist nationalist views means treating clients who are regularly degraded and re-traumatized in their daily life. Mental health treatment in this community means constantly vacillating between a state of acute care for mental health first aid and a more reflective post-traumatic stress recovery in psychotherapy. One of the best strategies for working with this population is the use of art therapy, a discipline that inherently cuts across language barriers and transcends embodied trauma, engaging the strength of creativity in helping to re-humanize the client.

## Finding Community

Little Sisters of the Assumption Family Health Service, Inc. (LSA) is a community-based nonprofit organization, founded in East Harlem, Manhattan in 1958, with a mission to address a holistic model of human services consisting of the physical, emotional, educational, and spiritual dimensions of family health. LSA continues to exercise these founding traditions, enhancing them with evidence-based practices derived from medicine, neuroscience, social science and education. LSA helps families meet their most fundamental needs of food, clothing, healthcare, and a safe home through home visits, on site services, support groups and classes. Vulnerable individuals receive the support, instruction, and clinical services needed to allow them to reach and maintain optimal health.

## Mental Health in the Immigrant Community

The need for a full-time mental health counselor at LSA became apparent in 2015 after losing the monthly consultation services of a contract psychiatrist who came once a month to see clients in need of treatment and medication. The psychiatrist performed initial mental health assessments and provided follow-up treatments along with a volunteer part-time social worker. The need for mental health services for the community served by LSA was increasing and there was evidence of severe trauma in clients with no health insurance. There are very limited resources for the uninsured clients in East Harlem. Additionally, the political climate regarding immigration and treatment of southern border immigrants in the United States around this time has not engendered growth in funding for services. It has shed light on some of the traumatic experiences immigrant families face, such as family separation at the border. Barraza, Sanchez, and Solis (2015) discussed the effects of racial/ethnic discrimination against Hispanic/Latino immigrants and its effects on their mental health that can lead to the development of depression, anxiety, and post-traumatic stress disorder.

Immigrant Latinx populations in the United States typically encounter a high likelihood of mental health problems (Falcon & Tucker, 2000). Recent political emphasis on Latin American migrants into the U.S. has augmented the perceptions of this demographic as problematic, and resulted in more ethnic discrimination, reported in nearly 61% of Latinx adults in 2010, up from a report of 50% in 2004 (Lopez, Morin, & Taylor, 2010), raising consideration of the correlation between racial and/or ethnic discrimination and mental health conditions (e.g., depression, anxiety, posttraumatic stress disorder, and suicidality) (Zeiders, Doane, & Roosa, 2012; Barraza et al., 2015).

In January 2015, LSA hired a full time bi-lingual (English and Spanish) Art Therapist and Mental Health Counselor (one of the authors of this chapter) to provide services to their community. Free bilingual individual therapy and therapeutic group support were offered to clients participating in any program at the agency. Mental health services are housed under the umbrella of the *Parenting and Child Development Program* (PCD). The Director of the PCD program supported the new art therapist in establishing a program and protocols to best serve LSA's clients.

PCD works from a two-generational approach to support parents in keeping young children up to eight years of age developmentally, cognitively, and emotionally on track, while promoting parent empowerment through a wide range of services that include financial literacy workshops, supportive groups, educational advocacy, workshops, and a network of referrals. Families with children up to three years old receive home visits and attend socialization groups. Families with children in grades K-5 receive academic enrichment programming after school during the school year and in the summer.

The need for mental health services in the LSA client community was immense and eventually mental health became its own department. The art therapist and director of mental health services took over a long running group called *Building Bridges of Hope*. This group became an art therapy group which felt useful given the variety of languages and trauma history and incorporated cognitive behavioral therapy (CBT) with art therapy.

## Trauma of Latin American Immigrant Women

The *Building Bridges of Hope* group was newly designed specifically for the specific population comprised of low-income women of childbearing age, most of whom are immigrants, who have suffered toxic stress and trauma from domestic violence often in connection with substance abuse, sexual abuse, miscarriage, grief and loss, intergenerational trauma, postpartum depression, anxiety, traumatic family division and reunification processes, and post-traumatic stress disorder. LSA's population also presents with multiple layers of social problems such as, poverty, overcrowded housing, social isolation, difficulty assimilating, limited resources (e.g., healthcare, education, career opportunities, counseling, etc.) and limited access to opportunities (e.g., professional, educational, financial, lifestyle).

In July 2016, LSA received a grant from the New York City Department of Mental Health under Improving Health Equity and Maternal and Infant Health Outcomes also known as the Maternal and Infant Health (MIH) program. The Mental Health Department at LSA took on the charge of providing services for the Toxic Stress and Trauma component of the grant.

## MENTAL HEALTH INTAKE PROCESS

The LSA Mental Health Services Department receives referrals from other departments within the agency and some external referrals from other organizations that work in partnership with LSA. Clients are contacted to arrange the first session, beginning an intake process that typically lasts for two or three sessions; usually an hour to an hour and a half process. The main goal of the intake process is establishing a client's need, appropriateness for treatment, and reason for referral.

This process is complicated by the fact that many clients have not disclosed past trauma before, nor have they talked about the process that brought them to East Harlem and into the circumstance in which they now live. In addition to the complex feelings associated with past trauma, such as shame, guilt, and social stigma, these clients have real concerns pertaining to issues such as legal status, right to live in the United States, trafficking, and family separation. Additionally, despite being in the United States, many clients are still living in dangerous and difficult situations; issues such as maintaining secrecy and learning who to trust are paramount in their lives as well as in therapy.

In the intake process, depression symptoms are assessed through the CES-D (The Center for Epidemiological Studies-Depression; Lewinsohn et al., 1997; Radloff, 1977), and self-esteem is assessed through the Rosenberg self-esteem scale (RSE; Rosenberg, 1965). This scale measures self-esteem by asking participants to reflect on their current feelings and respond to both positively and negatively worded statements.

From intake, clients are referred into short (12-week) or long term (40-week) individual therapy and assigned to a clinician. Typically, group participants are referred by their individual therapist if appropriate. While cognitive behavioral therapy (CBT) is utilized, with clients who identify specific goals, art therapy has been incredibly effective with this population. Despite offering clinical services in both English and Spanish, a language barrier persists among many clients who speak neither, but rather languages of indigenous cultures. Dialects from clients who come from regions of Mexico include Mixtec or Nahuatl, while clients who come from Guatemala sometimes speak Mam or K'iche'.

These clients frequently do not read or write and may have only learned some Spanish when forced to leave their villages and small towns. "Among all post-migration stressors, an inability to communicate in the language of the adopted country is a major challenge" (Lee, 2013, p.56). In cases of language barriers, art can serve as its own communicative tool, and can be transcendent in therapy for immigrants facing psychological distress (Kim et al., 2023).

## THE CASE OF PETRA

In the summer of 2016, Petra reunited with her 12 years old son after 10 years. When Petra's son was just 2-years old, her husband died, and she made the difficult decision to leave her son behind with family while she came to the United States in search of employment and money to support her family. Her home in Guatemala was filled with poverty, housing insecurity, and violent control from illegal criminal gangs. There were no viable opportunities for education or jobs that were available to Petra. After years of working hard, saving and sending money home, and living frugally, Petra found a new love, and also could afford to bring her son to New York. Now her son was here, she was pregnant, and she felt unhappy, worried, and alone. Petra's situation developed into a diagnosis and subsequent treatment for postpartum depression (PPD). Before that happened though, it was the intake process that first revealed her history with suicidal ideation and attempts. Suicide and self-harm assessments are a routine part of the intake (Sommers-Flanagan & Sommers-Flanagan, 1995), and it was where Petra revealed for the first time ever that she had jumped out of the window of her 4th floor apartment. When her husband had picked her up and taken her to the hospital, he reported to the doctor that she had fallen down the stairs; her mental state was not flagged for treatment in the emergency room. The more accurately a clinician knows about a client's past behaviors and motivations, the more precise a client's treatment can be towards their unique situation.

Petra was referred for mental health services through the nursing department in August 2017; she was six months pregnant, and she was concerned about her feelings toward her child and unborn baby. She shared that she was feeling sad and overwhelmed by past events from her childhood and that it was hard for her to feel connected to her son that just arrived from Mexico after being apart for more than ten years; her son was looking to connect with her, and she was having difficulty tolerating his displays of affection, such as hugs. She was feeling disconnected from both her 12-year-old son, and her unborn child. Petra also revealed that she had experience as a victim of domestic violence; she felt angry and confused. Petra's therapy involved a combination of CBT and Art Therapy; through psychoeducation she learned the differences between a feeling and a behavior and how feelings can affect behaviors.

Petra had an extremely limited formal education, as is typical of clients in this East Harlem immigrant community. Using art therapy allowed her to express, describe, and understand her feelings. Petra appreciated a creative exercise called *Exploring Feelings*, where she was provided with a letter-sized piece of white paper with a circle in the middle and various drawing materials. In this directive, Petra was asked to draw her feelings using colors to represent the feeling. Petra worked quietly with two permanent markers for 30 minutes. Petra titled her first drawing (see figure 1) as "Enojada" or Angry, and described her use of the color red saying "I feel that my heart is on fire and it hurts. The blue represents when I talk to my son when I am not screaming at him anymore. When I am not angry anymore." In her second drawing (see figure 2), Petra titled the work "Miedo" or Afraid, and stated her fear that "if I get deported, who is going to stay with my children?"

*Figure 1. "Enojada" or angry*

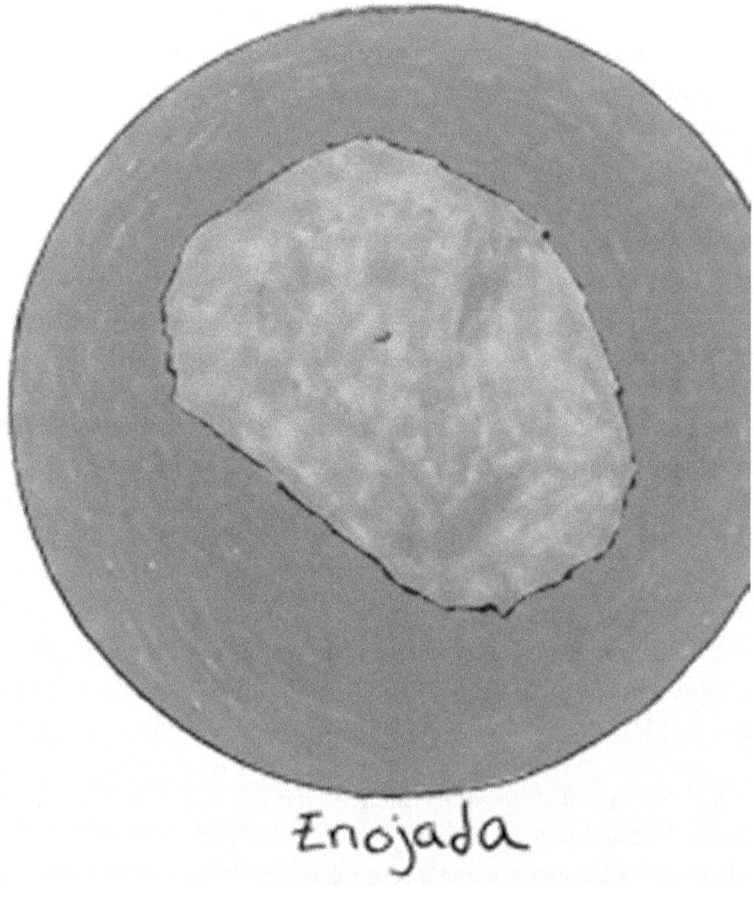

*Figure 2. "Miedo" or afraid*

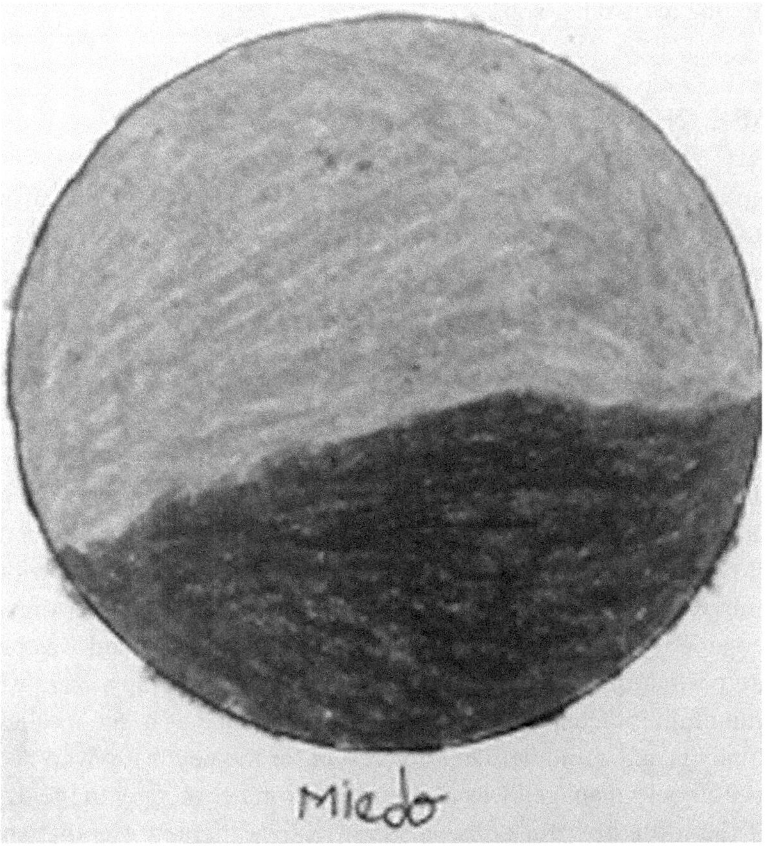


Art therapy directives helped Petra to identify and connect to her feelings of fear about her children, parenthood, and about her childhood sexual abuse experience by which she felt tormented. In addition to her therapy, Petra also enrolled in breastfeeding classes and shared that she felt happy to find other pregnant women and new mothers with similar stories and challenges. She had her baby boy at the end of November and came to therapy with the baby. She continued her treatment as she dealt with the stressors common to new mothers in tandem with her trauma history.

Petra worked hard in therapy, and she allowed herself to recognize the pain that she carried from leaving her baby behind for 10 years; she finally started to process and cope with the emotions of that loss. Upon being reunited with him and pregnant again, Petra's pain was overwhelming for her, and it triggered her memories of trauma. Art therapy helped Petra to identify the losses she carried, and begin the complex processes of self-forgiveness, family reintegration, and learning to express her love. She ultimately embraced the opportunity to heal and have her whole family together. In her last therapy session, Petra shared that she felt therapy had helped her to be loving toward her son.

## THE CASE OF KARA

After completing individual therapy through the Mental Health Department, Kara, a 33- year-old Mexican woman, was referred to the *Building Bridges of Hope* group. Kara immigrated to the USA from Mexico, escaping her abusive husband who claimed her when she was 15 years old. Kara's husband worked as a police officer, and despite having tried to kill her many times, was afforded certain legal protections. To save her own life she was forced to leave her three children, ages 8, 12, and 14, behind with him.

Kara came to the USA and began a new life here, hoping to one day be reunited with her children. When she found out that she was pregnant, Kara was demonstrating suicidal behavior and was hospitalized. Suicidal behavior is not uncommon in immigrant populations with high stress, and especially among those with refugee status (Amiri, 2022). Kara was then referred to LSA from a partner organization. When she came for therapy, she had a three-month-old baby and was presenting with severe postpartum depression (PPD) and PTSD. In therapy, Kara worked on learning mindfulness techniques that she could practice at home to alleviate her PTSD symptoms and could help her be present for the new baby who needed her. Keeping her anxiety managed was a primary task in her therapy in the beginning.

One of the most stressful components of Kara's therapy was that she had to revisit her traumatic memories and document them immediately for the purposes of using them in her legal asylum case. Typically, in trauma-informed therapy, a client would not be rushed in revisiting and facing their traumatic circumstances. In fact, this process may not even happen verbally, and in some cases may take years. Many therapists would consider it a more ideal situation to let the client divulge their trauma history when ready, if at all, and to spend time building safety, relationships, and emotional resources before examining the details of traumatic abuse. But immigrants seeking asylum in the court system do not always get the luxury of this time, or the benefit of waiting until they are emotionally prepared to disclose. This was true in the case of Kara. This was also why her asylum lawyer worked with her therapist, with permission, and encouraged the therapist to help her document her story. In therapy, Kara was able to describe the abuse that she suffered at the hands of the father of her children back in Mexico and prepare for presentation in front of the judge. While Kara relived the horror she endured and used art as a tool to regulate her emotions, examine bits of pain, and bind her anxiety, her therapist diligently wrote down her words. Kara was able to gain asylum through working with a lawyer after processing her trauma history in therapy.

Mental health services for Kara helped her to understand her trauma history and the threats posed to her, identify her life options, develop confidence in her decision-making skills, and reconcile with herself to continue supporting her children from a distance and waiting patiently to be reunited with them. She continued in her process toward obtaining her green card and found a supportive and healthy relationship.

Kara participated with 12 other women in a *Building Bridges of Hope Group* where she had the opportunity to work with clay in one project directive. Clay has been shown in art therapy to have a grounding effect on clients, and to help clients achieve a state of creative flow (Chilton, 2013; Lee, 2013; Lee, 2015). It has also been used in art therapy with immigrant groups to examine issues pertaining to acculturation (Salom, 2015). After being given a large, handful-sized piece of clay, clients were asked to sculpt an animal that they identify with. Kara sculpted a whale (see Image 3) and said, "I started making a dolphin, but it transformed into a whale. Dolphins are like me, calm. The whale symbolizes the transformation that I have had in my life. I transformed into a powerful whale, a good and powerful mother." Kara used the transformative power of artmaking, and in this case clay, to explore her own transformations.

*Figure 3. Kara's Whale*

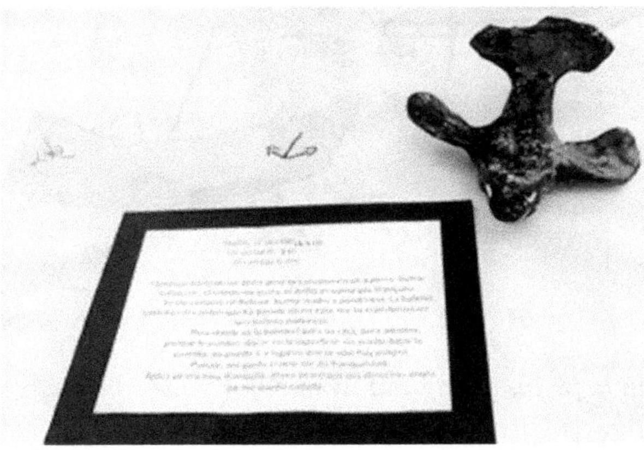

## *BUILDING BRIDGES OF HOPE* ART THERAPY GROUP

The *Building Bridges of Hope* art therapy group ran multiple times in 15-week cycles. Typically, clients were referred to the group by their treating therapist. Clients quickly established a trusting space for sharing the emotions associated with complex trauma histories and sustaining many major life challenges simultaneously. Emphasis in the group was placed on creating a safe space for clients to process their trauma, while avoiding re-traumatization. This was accomplished by specifically providing education about psychotherapy and group therapy, inviting sharing, measuring and limiting disclosures, providing specific referrals to clients when necessary for other services (e.g., nursing, legal, children's therapy, immigration support, court preparation, medical translation, etc.), and establishing group rituals and norms (Guerra et al., 2022; Kira et al., 2012; Reading & Rubin, 2011).

Group participants explored complex topics like trauma and identity through an art therapy process. In one creative phototherapy narrative project, group participants explored facets of their story by answering questions such as *What does it mean to be an immigrant woman for you?* (See figure 4). Interventions including phototherapy have been demonstrated to be effective tools in facilitating disclosure, building connections (Shechtman & Tsegahun, 2004), and exploring fractured identity markers, processing past trauma, and aspects of immigrant assimilation (Canul, 2017; Choi, 2021; Sadeghi, 2018).

*Figure 4. Phototherapy immigrant narrative*

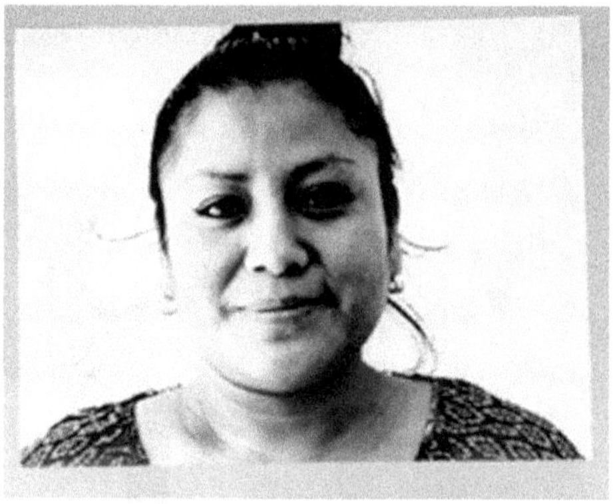

*What does it mean to be an immigrant woman for you?*

*¿Qué significa ser una mujer Inmigrante para ti?*

*"It is a hard question because we leave our family behind, we leave everything behind. I said goodbye to my family and came crying because it was about life and death. I didn't know if I was going to be able to cross over or not and will never be able to see my family again."*

In another project that employed multimedia dollmaking (see figure 5), art therapy group participants reported feeling increased confidence and having found their voice. Dollmaking as a clinical intervention has been known to facilitate reminiscence (Winslow, 2018), identity construction, grief processing (Feen-Calligan, Mcintyre, & Sands-Goldstein, 2009), relationship exploration (Ignacio & Cupchik, 2021), and trauma processing (Homer, 2015; Stace, 2014).

*Figure 5. Mila's doll*

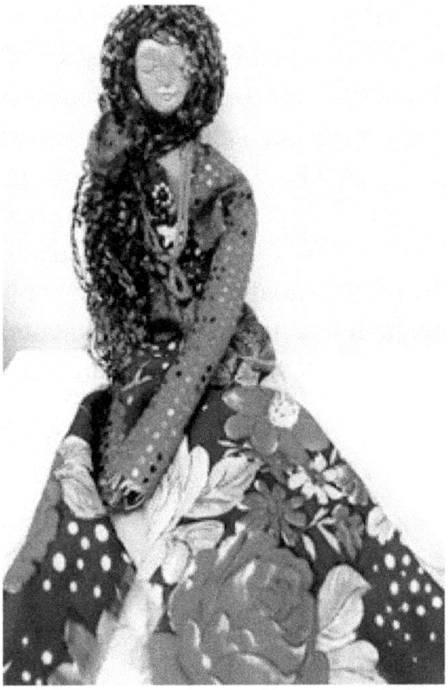

The *Building Bridges of Hope Group* allowed participants to gain support from peers, and to provide support to other members. Through shared experience, artmaking, and processing of their creative experience, group members reported a reduction in feelings of shame and guilt, and in feeling isolated. Clients in the group learned about the impact of toxic and chronic stress and intergenerational trauma, as well as stress management tools and practical coping skills.

Dollmaking has emerged as a favorite and meaningful directive for every cycle of the Building *Bridges of Hope* client group. Clients have been provided with a variety of art materials, including tissue paper, fabric, yarn, and little stones and beads to construct jewelry and accessories. Textile materials may foster creativity through both a culturally relevant art form, and the relationship to the materials as sensory stimuli (Collier, 2011; Reynolds, 2004).

First, clients were instructed to write a message, a mantra, a prayer, or a dedication in the paper that will become the head of their doll. This message is only for them to see and is not shared with the larger group. Then clients are given access to materials and provided with visual instructions to build a form for their doll (see figure 6). Clients then dress and decorate their dolls. Finally, the clients were asked to give their doll a name and to share her story with the group. Dolls can be powerful symbols, access many cultures, and are one of the world's oldest toys. Kara, the client mentioned above, said the following about her doll (see Figure 7): "My doll's name is Hope. I never had a doll when I was a little girl. My mother did not have money to buy me one. Finally, I have one and her name is Esperanza, because I still have faith to have a better life and achieve what I want." Dolls have a unique accessibility for women and female-identifying persons due to the gendered roll traditionally imposed on them. This can enhance their effectiveness as therapeutic tools for women's therapy groups (Alden, 2000; Cohen, 2013; Moya-Raggio, 1984). Dolls help to carry on the rituals and traditions of some cultures, and they lend themselves to a dramatic interaction that can be pivotal in advancing issues of relationship in therapy (Agosin, 2014; Feen-Calligan et al., 2009; Garlock, 2016; Krystyniak, 2020; Rickerl, 1996).

*Figure 6. Doll instructions*

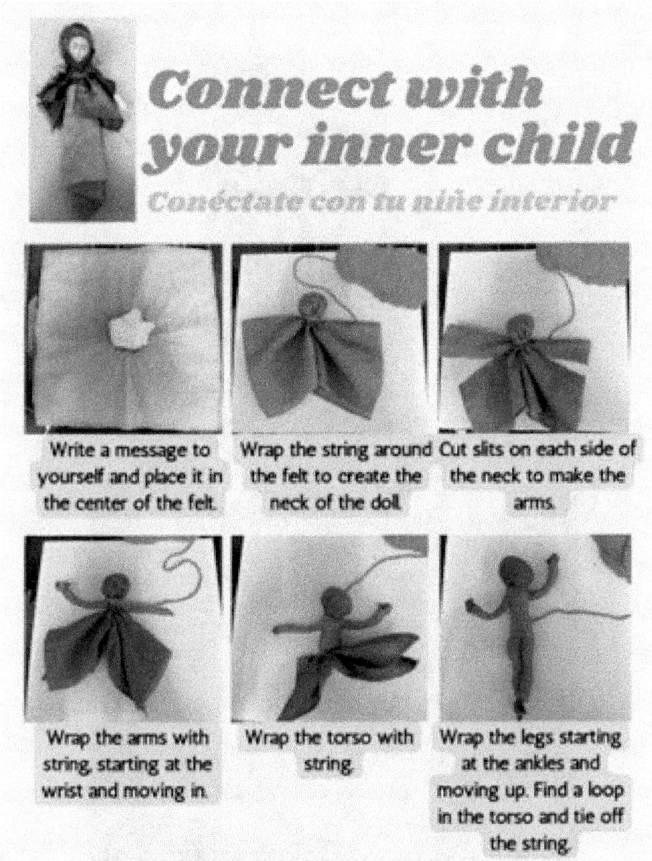
Connect with your inner child
Conéctate con tu niñe interior
Write a message to yourself and place it in the center of the felt.
Wrap the string around the felt to create the neck of the doll.
Cut slits on each side of the neck to make the arms.
Wrap the arms with string, starting at the wrist and moving in.
Wrap the torso with string.
Wrap the legs starting at the ankles and moving up. Find a loop in the torso and tie off the string.

*Figure 7. Kara's doll*

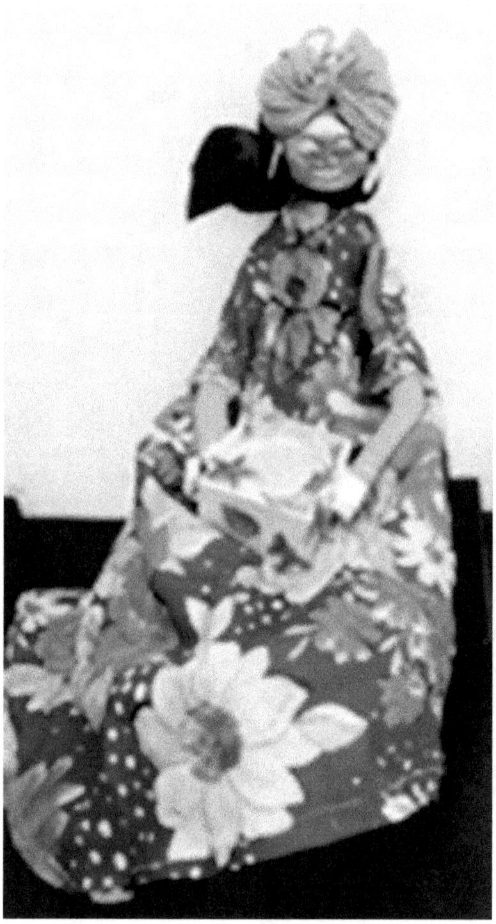

In the *Building Bridges of Hope* art therapy groups, clients were exposed to a range of different art materials and creative techniques. Clients worked with clay and explored self-concept through photography. Clients experienced creating flowers and hearts through felting, which is used to safely release aggression. *Building Bridges of Hope* art therapy group has successfully engaged clients that demonstrate an understanding of their own feelings and thoughts, which allows them to acquire coping skills to better manage their stress. This in turn helps them to decrease symptoms of anxiety and depression. Clients expressed that having a safe space for them to create and express helped them to understand the importance of letting their children explore and express themselves independently in their own environment. This in turn, promoted a healthy attachment style between mothers and children.

After weeks of special projects, building connections, and processing trauma, each *Building Bridges of Hope* art therapy group comes to an end; the ending is marked with a celebration. The art therapy group concludes with an event attended by all group participants, and they can extend it to family and friends. The celebration includes music, an art show of work selected and arranged by the clients, refreshments, and honor certificates which are a testament to the clients' bravery, commitment, and hard work. Agency staff attend to demonstrate steadfast support, and the therapist is present to share poignant words about the creative and therapeutic processes engaged in throughout the group. The celebration is a meaningful and ritual end to a group where so much happened in just 15 weeks.

## DISCUSSION

Art therapy can be a great resource with immigrant populations. Art can serve as a tool to help clients cross cultural barriers including language to forge connections and express themselves. Art making taps into expressive tools that are inherent in all humans, and that are still a regular part of indigenous and old-world cultures. Creative expression serves in many Latinx and indigenous cultures as a tool for communication, storytelling, record keeping, and the documentation of history (Agosin, 1996; Carocci, 2010; Charland, 2011; Garlock, 2016; Mujica, 1997). In preserving traumatic memories through art, individuals can reclaim their past.

The *Building Bridges of Hope* art therapy group uses directives that elicit an exploration from outside to the inside. One of the first directives in groups is working with clay where clients are asked to create an animal or symbol that they identify with, and then to create a mural where they paint the animals or symbol's environment. The program includes some gentle movements designed to help clients to connect with their body and bring head, heart, and body together. Van Der Kolk (2014) states in his seminal text "scientific methods have confirmed that changing the way one breathes can improve problems with anger, depression, anxiety and that yoga can positively affect such wide-ranging medical problems as high blood pressure, elevated stress hormone secretion, asthma and low- back pain" (p. 269). Stevens and Spears (2009) state, "Mind-body interventions use a variety of techniques designed to increase the mind's ability to affect bodily function and symptoms" (p. 4). Trauma can be a disembodying experience and can contribute to feelings of disassociation; grounding and mindfulness practices can help to counter this impact.

Creating a sense of emotional safety within both the therapeutic space, and the community center or agency is essential to successfully making a space for expression and support; a space where the hard work of processing trauma can be achieved. The nature of the *Building Bridges of Hope Group* encouraged parents to explore through art, which helps them develop confidence in letting their children explore and take advantage of agency services and groups. This helped participants to develop independence, healthy risk taking, and helped promote a healthy family attachment style. LSA also offers mother-child dyad art therapy services; The mother-child relationship in the context of creative play with art materials allows the duo to make images which strengthens the parent-child relationship and allows a restructuring to happen (Hall, 1991). Creating environments where young children can work creatively and productively with their parents helps to promote a positive familial interaction; this can strengthen their attachment (Hosea, 2006). This is something that all families can benefit from, but also those in East Harlem, living in poverty in the wake of the COVID-19 pandemic. East Harlem, like many immigrant communities, remains in a state of crisis of mental health, community violence, substance abuse, suicide, poverty, and inadequate social service resources. The *Building Bridges of Hope* art therapy group has perhaps become more essential than ever as a lifeline to its participants.

## FUTURE DIRECTIONS

The art therapy services at LSA demonstrate how art therapy can help immigrant women to reconnect with their own stories- both uplifting history and trauma ridden. Through creative materials and directives that inspire imagination and links to history, clients can describe in very eloquent and clear ways how the treatment supports them to heal and grow. Art Therapy has been essential for these clients to connect with parts of themselves that they forgot that they had.

Future art therapy services might consider incorporating qualitative, quantitative, and arts-based measures that examine the benefits and challenges of group processes for victims of complex trauma. While so many of the clients served by the mental health department at LSA did experience benefits from the art therapy groups, it is also clear that not every client can tolerate group work, and it may at times be contraindicated for an individual or overwhelming for the rest of the group. There is little research that qualifies what these factors are beyond identifying them as judgements that are at the discretion of the group leader or treating therapist. The community might be better served by research that helps us understand what qualities might exempt a person from group work, and particularly group work that can be re-traumatizing.

As more research explores the impact of intergenerational trauma (Swain, 2019), there is ample opportunity to examine both the impact of parents' trauma on their children, and also the impact of a parent's post-traumatic growth on their children. The impact of having a parent in therapeutic treatment may help us better understand the long-term benefits for the youth who are indirectly affected by trauma. In addition, future research could take a more targeted look at the benefits of dyad art therapy, as is offered at LSA, and assess the impact for the mother and child participants. These services may impact the maternal relationships including the attachment style and quality of connection, the ability to reconnect if separated, and the degree and type of parentification that is frequently present in immigrant families.

Some concepts for future research have emerged from the inclusion of certain directives or materials. Frequently in dollmaking, clients will create what they describe as a spirit doll. Clients will explore through the doll an abstract concept and personify an idea that needs acknowledgment in their life, for example femininity or ancestry. In some cases, clients created a doll to represent lost loves, lost children, or their own lost childhood for which they yearned. By employing an allegory in the form of a doll, clients are able to explore ideas much larger than themselves which have been influential in their lives. Allegories are an old concept in art (Fletcher, 2012; Shore, 2014), and allegory doll making in art therapy might benefit from further exploration.

The immigrant community of East Harlem, New York, is filled with survivors of extreme trauma who have braved inhumane atrocities to bring themselves and their families to safety in the United States. They are strong, proud, and in need of services to help facilitate the processing of trauma and the assimilation that will assist them in living in this culture. Art therapy is a way of providing access to therapy that transcends language barriers, cultural differences, and trauma symptoms. Increased services can help support immigrant families and communities.

## ACKNOWLEDGMENT

This research received no specific grant from any funding agency in the public, commercial, or not-for-profit sectors.

This research was supported (non-monetary provision of supplies and art materials) by LSA Family Health Service (https://littlesistersfamily.org/), the New York based non-profit and host site for mental health and art therapy services.

## REFERENCES

Agosin, M. (1996). *Tapestries of hope, threads of love: The arpillera movement in Chile, 1974–1994* (C. Kostopulos-Cooperman, Trans.). University of New Mexico Press.

Agosin, M. (2014). *Stitching resistance: Women, creativity, and fiber arts*. Solis Press.

Alden, A. (2000, June 30). Sewing comfort out of grief. *Midwifery Today, 43*(54).

Amiri, S. (2022). Prevalence of suicide in immigrants/refugees: A systematic review and meta-analysis. *Archives of Suicide Research*, *26*(2), 370–405. doi:10.1080/13811118.2020.1802379 PMID:32780682

Appleton, V. (2002). Avenues of hope: Art therapy and the resolution of trauma. *Art Therapy: Journal of the American Therapy Association*, *5*, 6–13.

Barraza, E., Sanchez, C., & Solis, C. (2015). *An arts-based exploration of immigration and acculturation through the lenses of first, second, and third generation clinical art therapists*. [Theses, Loyola University].

Buchalter, S. (2015). *Raising self-esteem in adults: An eclectic approach with art therapy, CBT. and DBT-based techniques*. Jessica Kingsley Publishers.

Canul, G. D. (2017). Genealogical-PhotoTherapy as a tool for integrating my Mayan and Spanish origins. *MindConsiliums, 17*(3), 1-16. https://mindconsiliums.org/pub/2017/03/2017-03-Canul-G-D-genealogical-phototherapy-integrating-my-mayan-and-spanish-origins.pdf

Carnwell, R. (2017). Essential differences between research and evidence-based practice. *Nurse Researcher*, *8*(2), 65–68.

Carocci, M. (2010). Textiles of healing: Native American AIDS quilts. *Textile (Oxford)*, *8*(1), 68–84. doi:10.2752/175183510X12580391269986

Charland, W. (2011). War rugs: Woven documents of conflict and hope. *Art Education*, *64*(6), 25–32. doi:10.1080/00043125.2011.11519149

Chilton, G. (2013). Art therapy and flow: A Review of the literature and applications. *Art Therapy: Journal of the American Art Therapy Association*, *30*(2), 64–70. doi:10.1080/07421656.2013.787211

Choi, S. S. (2021). *Foreigner to Third Culture Kid: Exploring Intersectional Self-Identity through Phototherapy*. [Thesis, Pratt Institute]. ProQuest Dissertations & Theses Global. (2555973384). https://www.proquest.com/dissertations-theses/foreigner-third-culture-kid-exploring/docview/2555973384/se-2

Cohen, R. A. (2013). Common threads: A recovery programme for survivors of genderbased violence. *Intervention (Amstelveen, Netherlands)*, *11*(2), 157–168. doi:10.1097/01.WTF.0000431118.16849.0c

Collier, A. F. (2011). The well-being of women who create with textiles: Implications for art therapy. *Art Therapy: Journal of the American Art Therapy Association, 28*(3), 104–112. doi:10.1080/07421656.2011.597025

Feen-Calligan, H., Mcintyre, B., & Sands-Goldstein, M. (2009). Art Therapy Applications of Dolls in Grief Recovery, Identity, and Community Service. *Art Therapy: Journal of the American Art Therapy Association, 26*(4), 167–173. doi:10.1080/07421656.2009.10129613

Fletcher, A. (2012). *Allegory: The theory of a symbolic mode*. Princeton University Press. doi:10.1515/9781400842049

Garlock, L. R. (2016). Stories in the cloth: Art therapy and narrative textiles. *Art Therapy: Journal of the American Art Therapy Association, 33*(2), 58–66. doi:10.1080/07421656.2016.1164004

Guerra, C., Toro, E., Taylor, E. P., Lobos, P., & Pinto-Cortez, C. (2022). Design considerations for group interventions for adolescent victims of interpersonal violence in Chile. *Journal of Aggression, Maltreatment & Trauma, 31*(10), 1318–1336. doi:10.1080/10926771.2022.2089864

Homer, E. (2015). Piece work: Fabric collage as a neurodevelopmental approach to trauma treatment. *Art Therapy: Journal of the American Art Therapy Association, 32*(1), 20–26. doi:10.1080/07421656.2015.992824

Hosea, H. (2006). The Brush's Footmarks": Parents and infants paint together in a small community art therapy group. *International Journal of Art Therapy, 11*(2), 69–78. doi:10.1080/17454830600980317

Ignacio, A., & Cupchik, G. (2021). Therapeutic benefits of adult doll play. *Imagination, Cognition and Personality, 41*(1), 5–30.. doi:10.1177/0276236621989227

Kim, S.-Y., Lee, J. S., & Choi, H. (2023). The Effects of art therapy on anxiety and distress for Korean–Ukrainian refugee: Quasi-experimental design study. *Health Care, 11*(4), 466. doi:10.3390/healthcare11040466 PMID:36833000

Kira, I. A., Ahmed, A., Wasim, F., Mahmoud, V., Colrain, J., & Rai, D. (2012). Group therapy for refugees and torture survivors: Treatment model innovations. *International Journal of Group Psychotherapy, 62*(1), 69–88. doi:10.1521/ijgp.2012.62.1.69 PMID:22229369

Krystyniak, J. (2020). *The Use of Dolls and Figures in Therapy: A Literature Review*. [Thesis, Lesley University]. 321. https://digitalcommons.lesley.edu/expressive_theses/321

Lee, S.-Y. (2013). "Flow" in art therapy: Empowering immigrant children with adjustment difficulties. *Art Therapy: Journal of the American Art Therapy Association, 30*(2), 56–63. doi:10.1080/07421656.2013.786978

Lee, S.-Y. (2015). Flow indicators in art therapy: Artistic engagement of immigrant children with acculturation gaps. *Art Therapy: Journal of the American Art Therapy Association, 32*(3), 120–129. doi:10.1080/07421656.2015.1060836

Lewinsohn, P. M., Seeley, J. R., Roberts, R. E., & Allen, N. B. (1997). Center for Epidemiological Studies-Depression Scale (CES-D) as a screening instrument for depression among community-residing older adults. *Psychology and Aging, 12*(2), 277–287. doi:10.1037/0882-7974.12.2.277 PMID:9189988

Linesch, D., Quezada, P., Acevedes, P., Trochez, M., & Zuniga, E. (2012). An art therapy exploration with Latino families. *Art Therapy: Journal of the American Art Therapy Association, 29*(3), 120–126. doi:10.1080/07421656.2012.701603

Moya-Raggio, E. (1984). —Arpilleras||: Chilean culture of resistance. *Feminist Studies, 10*(2), 277–290. doi:10.2307/3177867

Mujica, B. (1997). Tapestries of hope, threads of love: The arpillera movement in Chile 1974-1994/Ashes of revolt. *Americas, 49*(5), 62–63.

Najavits, L. (2002). *Seeking safety: A treatment manual for PTSD and substance abuse*. Guilford Press.

Pifalo, T. (2007). Jogging the cogs: Trauma-focused art therapy and cognitive behavior therapy with sexually abused children. *Art Therapy: Journal of the American Art Therapy Association, 24*(4), 170–175. doi:10.1080/07421656.2007.10129471

Radloff, L. S. (1977). The CES-D scale: A self report depression scale for research in the general population. *Applied Psychological Measurement, 1*(3), 385–401. doi:10.1177/014662167700100306

Reading, R., & Rubin, L. R. (2011). Advocacy and empowerment: Group therapy for LGBT asylum seekers. *Traumatology, 17*(2), 86–98. doi:10.1177/1534765610395622

Reynolds, F. (2004). Conversations about creativity and chronic illness II: Textile artists coping with long-term health problems reflect on the creative process. *Creativity Research Journal, 16*(1), 79–89. doi:10.120715326934crj1601_8

Rickerl, K. (1996). Quilting a new tradition. *Journal of Psychosocial Nursing and Mental Health Services, 34*(4), 40–43. https://search-proquestcom.ezproxy.philau.edu/docview/102413 3953. doi:10.3928/0279-3695-19960401-14

Rosenberg, M. (1965). *Rosenberg Self-Esteem Scale (RSES)* [Database record]. APA PsycTests., doi:10.1037/t01038-000

Rubin, J. (Ed.). (2001). *Approaches to art therapy: Theory & technique* (2nd ed.). Brunner-Routledge.

Sadeghi, S. (2018). *Photovoice, a Long of Belonging Among Iranian Immigrants.* [Thesis, Notre Dame de Namur University]. ProQuest Dissertations & Theses Global. (2377675269). https://www.proquest.com/dissertations-theses/photovoice-long-belonging-among-iranian/docview/2377675269/se-2

Salom, A. (2015). Weaving potential space and acculturation: *Art therapy at the museum. Journal of Applied Arts & Health, 6*(1), 47–62. doi:10.1386/jaah.6.1.47_1

Shechtman, Z., & Tsegahun, I. (2004). Phototherapy to enhance self-disclosure and client–therapist alliance in an intake interview with Ethiopian immigrants to Israel. *Psychotherapy Research, 14*(3), 367–377. doi:10.1093/ptr/kph030

Sholt, M., & Gavron, T. (2006). Therapeutic Qualities of Clay-work in Art Therapy and Psychotherapy: A Review. *Art Therapy: Journal of the American Art Therapy Association, 23*(2), 66–72. doi:10.1080/07421656.2006.10129647

Shore, A. (2014). Art therapy, attachment, and the divided brain. *Art Therapy: Journal of the American Art Therapy Association, 31*(2), 91–94. doi:10.1080/07421656.2014.903827

Sommers-Flanagan, J., & Sommers-Flanagan, R. (1995). Intake interviewing with suicidal patients: A systematic approach. *Professional Psychology, Research and Practice, 26*(1), 41–47. doi:10.1037/0735-7028.26.1.41

Stace, S. M. (2014). Therapeutic doll making in art psychotherapy for complex trauma. *Art Therapy: Journal of the American Art Therapy Association, 31*(1), 12–20. doi:10.1080/07421656.2014.873689

Stevens, R., & Spears, E. (2009). Incorporating photography as a therapeutic tool in counseling. *Journal of Creativity in Mental Health, 4*(1), 3–16. doi:10.1080/15401380802708767

Swain, G. (2019). The Healing Power of Art in Intergenerational Trauma: Race, Sex, Age and Disability. *Canadian Journal of Disability Studies, 8*(1), 15–31. doi:10.15353/cjds.v8i1.469

Van der Kolk, B. (2014). *The Body Keeps the Score: Brain, mind and body in the healing of trauma.* Viking.

Vick, R. M. (1999). Utilizing prestructured art elements in brief group art therapy with adolescents. *Art Therapy: Journal of the American Art Therapy Association*, *16*(2), 68–77. doi:10.1080/07421656.1999.10129670

Winslow, L. E. (2018). *Creating reminiscence through art therapy doll making with older women*. [Thesis, Notre Dame University]. ProQuest Dissertations & Theses Global. (2164378232). https://www.proquest.com/dissertations-theses/creating-reminiscence-through-art-therapy-doll/docview/2164378232/se-2

## KEY TERMS AND DEFINITIONS

**Art Therapy:** The use of creativity and artistic expression facilitated by a trained art therapist in the service of meeting health and wellness goals, including, but not limited to, increasing self-awareness, improving self-esteem, learning communication skills, practicing interpersonal strategies, building trust, coping with symptoms, and recovering from trauma.

**Healing:** The process of improving individual functioning and recovering from one's wounds, whether physical, psychological, or emotional.

**Immigration:** Movement of a people or community from one country or territory to another; can happen for a wide variety of reasons including escape from poverty, oppression, and lack of opportunity.

**Mental Health:** The state of being that describes psychological wellness or illness within a person.

# Chapter 3
# Art Therapy With Incarcerated Women

**Rachel Brandoff**
*Thomas Jefferson University, USA*

**Jacqui Johnson**
*Sankofa Healing Studio, USA*

## ABSTRACT

*The corrections system in the United States is largely focused on punishment. Trauma-informed therapeutic services were particularly absent during the COVID-19 pandemic lockdown. This chapter discusses the importance and benefits of providing incarcerated persons with mental health treatment such as art therapy. The authors highlight one pilot study, which conducted an 8-week theme-based art therapy group in a women's county jail in Philadelphia, Pennsylvania. Participant benefits from the group correlated with three of the main goals of the incarceration system: rehabilitation, deterrence, and restoration. Participants reported multiple benefits including decreased symptoms of anxiety, depression, and feelings of isolation. A decrease in reported jail infractions among participants was also noted. The authors discuss directions for future research with this population.*

## INTRODUCTION

Art therapy is an effective way for incarcerated individuals to express themselves and process their emotions and experiences, and especially in cases where traditional talk therapy may be challenging due to illiteracy, organicity, or difficulties with verbal communication. Art therapy can be a cost-efficient way to combat behavioral problems

DOI: 10.4018/978-1-6684-7856-1.ch003

linked to mental illness and decrease symptoms of depression among incarcerated individuals. Art therapy provides a safe and acceptable way for individuals to express and release potentially destructive feelings such as anger and aggression, leading to an overall positive increase in mood and fewer infractions (Erikson, 2008).

Society benefits from providing incarcerated people with mental health treatment; this might include opportunities for personal growth, insight, reflection, reconciliation, and reparations. Providing incarcerated women with access to medical and mental health care, pre- and post-natal care, drug-treatment and STD treatment is not only humane, but it also is a step towards acknowledging racial justice inequalities, interrupting cycles of oppression and intergenerational trauma, and helping inmates return to society in a better condition than when they left. The intentions behind the design of our corrections system were to be both punitive, and constructive in the shaping of more desirable social behavior. Research supports that collaborative healthcare and consistent social services for incarcerated people results in better interpersonal behavior, increased resiliency, decreased complaints, better coping skills, decreased recidivism, and an increased likelihood of life success after incarceration (Gold & Marcus, 2008; Ha & Robinson, 2011). Addressing inmates' mental health needs decreases suicide attempts, emergency room visits, and overall correctional costs (Morrissey, et al., 2006). Investing in our incarcerated population benefits the social order, most significantly perhaps by interrupting cycles of violence and oppression.

The shame and stigma associated with incarceration can have significant negative impacts on mental health and well-being, including increased rates of depression, anxiety, and post-traumatic stress disorder (PTSD; Harner & Riley, 2013; James & Glaze, 2006; Mignon, 2016). "Mental health is likely to worsen in jail/prison settings due to increased stress, fear, isolation from loved ones, limited access to mental health services, and substandard treatment by health and correctional staff" (Tadros, et al., 2021, para 5). It is important to recognize the humanity of incarcerated individuals and to work towards creating a more just and equitable criminal justice system that prioritizes rehabilitation and restoration over punishment (Herman, 2023). Therapists working with incarcerated individuals should be aware of the impact of shame and stigma, and the increased likelihood of mental illness. Jails are not designed for mental health, and they lack adequate resources to ensure that inmates are getting humane healthcare treatment. Nevertheless, there is much that can be achieved within a jail setting that will bring skilled clinicians, and therapeutic services to the inmate population and better serve the goals of corrections (Rice & Jennings, 2014).

This chapter showcases the impact of art therapy on the well-being of incarcerated individuals; a pilot study showcasing the participation of 32 incarcerated people in a structured, theme-based, 8-week art therapy group in a county women's jail.

The findings of this study highlight some of the most optimal benefits of providing trauma-informed mental health care to incarcerated persons. The authors present future directions in art therapy research with an incarcerated population.

## BACKGROUND

Incarcerated women represent a vulnerable and underserved population in the United States. They have little mental health support, exposure to clinical interventions, and relationships with qualified psychotherapists (Bloom & Covington, 2008; Erikson, 2008). Lack of mental health support and minimal therapeutic treatment for incarcerated women perpetuates social injustice and systemic racism, maintains family separation, keeps families in poverty, and exacerbates the impact of trauma and adverse experiences on individuals and their families (Bronson & Berzofsky, 2011; Nair, et al., 2021; Walker et al., 2016). Over 80% of jail detainees in a Chicago-based study including 1272 women were identified as meeting criteria for one or more lifetime psychiatric disorder. This jailed population demonstrated higher rates than the general population for all disorders except for schizophrenia; and over 33% met criteria for post-traumatic stress disorder (PTSD). This psychiatric prevalence in this study supports the need for greater clinical mental health treatment services in the jails (Teplin, et al., 1996).

The inequalities of the incarcerated female population, compared with male inmates, result in undue medical burden and mental health issues caused in part from inadequate treatment and care (Mignon, 2016; Springer, 2010). Some of the traumatic stress caused by incarceration, as well as other mental health symptoms can be addressed through the incorporation of art therapy into inmate services (Rubin, 2010; Wadeson, 2010). Art therapy is a form of psychotherapy that through combining artmaking with a commitment to social justice principles provides opportunities for empowerment to individuals and communities who have been marginalized or oppressed due to systemic inequalities. This approach to healing works by creating space for self-expression and social change. Research supports the use of art therapy in alleviating physical and mental distress, and in promoting effective reflection and discourse (Gussak & Rosal, 2016). It can be used in a variety of settings, including community organizations, schools, hospitals and healthcare settings, and carceral settings.

## ADVERSE CHILDHOOD EXPERIENCE (ACES)

While individuals who are incarcerated are often labeled as the oppressors, most were victims first. Incarcerated women have extensive histories of adverse childhood experiences (Aday, Dye, & Kaiser, 2014) which when untreated, are associated with significantly increased risk for chronic physical illness (Mignon, 2016), social dysfunction (Connolly, 2020), mental illness (Aday, Dye, & Kaiser, 2014), and increased suicidality (Felitti et al., 1998). This statement highlights the fact that many individuals who are incarcerated have experienced significant trauma and adversity throughout their lives, beginning in childhood. Research has shown that adverse childhood experiences (ACEs), such as physical or emotional abuse, neglect, and household dysfunction, are associated with a range of negative outcomes later in life, including increased risk for chronic illness, mental health issues, and involvement with the criminal justice system (Karlsson & Zielinski, 2020). While a history of trauma is not a defense for illegal activity, it does in part explain the compounded negative social impacts for individuals whose experience has been marginalized and includes tremendous systematic discrimination.

For incarcerated women in particular, the prevalence of ACEs is high (Belknap, 2020). Many women who are incarcerated have experienced domestic violence, sexual abuse, and other forms of trauma that can contribute to their involvement with the criminal justice system (Aday, Dye, & Kaiser, 2014). These experiences can also contribute to the development of mental health issues, such as depression, anxiety, and PTSD. While ACE scores for incarcerated women vary, research has consistently shown that women who are incarcerated have higher rates of ACEs than the general population (Stensrud, Gilbride, Bruinekool, 2019).

These high rates of ACEs among incarcerated women highlight the need for trauma-informed care and support services that can help women address the underlying issues that contribute to their involvement with the criminal justice system (Levenson & Willis, 2019; Stensrud, Gilbride, Bruinekool, 2019). By providing access to mental health services, substance abuse treatment, and other forms of support, it is possible to improve outcomes for incarcerated women and reduce their risk of future involvement with the criminal justice system.

Providing access to whole-person mental health services and trauma-responsive care is essential for catalyzing positive forward movement. Incarcerated females with extensive trauma histories often have an inherent mistrust of verbal disclosure, particularly in the context of therapy or counseling. Gussak (2006) promoted the idea that expression of intense emotion through art may be more socially acceptable for incarcerated clients and limit the risk of negative consequences of externalization. Art therapy can engage inmate populations through creativity despite the presence of emotional resistance (Gussak, 2004). Alternative forms of therapy can be effective for individuals who may have difficulty expressing themselves through spoken language. Art therapy allows individuals to communicate through creative expression rather than relying solely on verbal communication (Stevenson & Orr, 2013; Young & Bernak, 1996).

The development of neuroscience has helped to substantiate what clinicians see every day: trauma has a dramatic and lasting impact. Neuroimaging studies support the understanding that traumatic memories may be harder to speak of and share. Using PET scan technology with patients diagnosed with PTSD, two studies noted heightened activity in brain centers which control emotional arousal, such as the amygdala and medial temporal lobe. Conversely, these studies noted decreased activity in Broca's area, believed to be the part of the brain that helps us to translate understanding of and convey personal experience (Rauch, et al., 1996; Shin et al., 1999). Similarly, studies that have employed the use of functional magnetic resonance imaging (fMRI) scans with patients with PTSD also show a significant decrease in activity, and change in activity, of brain centers responsible for organizing visual data, emotional regulation and responsiveness, maintaining and cataloging memory, and feeling fear (Bremner, et al., 2005; Frewen, et al., 2017; Hughes & Shin, 2011, van der Kolk, 2000).

## TRUST

Individuals who have experienced trauma in their lives, including betrayal by loved ones, typically struggle to trust others, and may have a difficult time working with authority figures. This can pose a multi-layered dilemma. It is not uncommon for individuals who are incarcerated to have a general distrust of correctional officers and other staff members who work in prisons and jails. This distrust may stem from a variety of factors, including early life trauma, past negative experiences with staff members, a perception of staff members as being part of a repressive system, and a lack of transparency in the correctional system (Young & Haynie, 2022). Significantly disproportionate prevalence of sexual assault victimization, known to highly correlate with mistrust, exists in the incarcerated female population; this was over that of incarcerated men and community sampled women (Karlsson & Zielinski, 2020).

Lack of trust in a corrections system is problematic, and trauma-informed correctional care is only starting to be introduced (Miller & Najavits, 2012; Levenson & Willis, 2019). It can contribute to a tense and hostile environment within prisons and jails, which can make it more difficult for staff members to do their jobs effectively. Additionally, a lack of trust between incarcerated individuals and staff members can lead to a lack of cooperation and a breakdown in communication, which can make it more difficult to maintain safety and security within correctional facilities. Lastly, a lack of trust between inmates and staff can impede efforts toward healing and rehabilitation in cases where staff want to foster these goals (Bender, 2023).

Therapists working with incarcerated individuals should acknowledge the presence of distrust and work with clients to strategize dealing with it. One way to do this is to emphasize the importance of building positive relationships with individuals who are trustworthy and who can provide support and assistance; this may involve some consideration of how to deem if individuals are trustworthy. Learning to determine trustworthiness is an important goal both in and out of an incarcerated setting. Therapists can work with clients to develop communication and conflict resolution skills that can help them navigate challenging interactions, and eventually foster trust.

Trust is a foundational aspect of any therapeutic relationship. Therapists must work to establish trust with their clients from the beginning of therapy, and they must continue to maintain that trust throughout the therapeutic process. When clients trust their therapist, they are more likely to engage in therapy, share their experiences and emotions, and make progress towards their goals. Building a safe space in therapy, where clients feel safe to share their thoughts, emotions, and experiences can be challenging in the best of circumstances. Without trust, clients may feel hesitant or guarded, making it difficult for them to open to connection, share their experiences, and make progress in therapy. Creating an environment of trust. Ultimately, building an environment of trust in a jail requires a commitment to treating all individuals with dignity and respect, and a willingness to work collaboratively to create a safe and supportive environment for everyone. By focusing on transparency, communication, consistency, positive reinforcement, and mental health services, it is possible to create a person-centered environment that is conducive to rehabilitation and positive change. Trust allows clients to communicate openly and honestly with their therapist. When clients feel that their therapist is trustworthy, they are more likely to share their innermost thoughts and feelings, which can lead to greater insight and understanding. When clients feel stigmatized or ashamed about past actions or current circumstances, including the incarceration itself, they become hesitant to disclose personal information. This is a barrier to active engagement in therapy.

For many incarcerated women, there is good reason for mistrust. Some may fear retaliation from other inmates or prison staff if they disclose certain information. Cultural factors may also play a role in the mistrust clients feel that inhibits verbal disclosure. For example, some incarcerated individuals may come from backgrounds or families where privacy is highly valued, even essential. Additionally, traumatic experiences sometimes are accompanied by threats of harm if secrecy is broken. Sharing personal information with unknown people may be seen as inappropriate or disloyal.

## ART THERAPY IN JAIL

Art therapy has great benefits in the incarcerated community; in fact, the creative process is so inherently beneficial, that art is often found in the cell areas of the incarcerated (Johnson, 2007). The effects of art therapy can directly be seen and measured in incarcerated clients who have demonstrated an increase in self-esteem (Gussak, 2009), decrease in continued violence or abusive behavior (McGinn et al., 2016), increase in ability to relax (Czamanski-Cohen & Weihs, 2016; Gross & Haynes, 1998), reduction in stress (Curl, 2008), and greater insight and increased self-awareness (AlDabbagh, 2014).

With the help of a trained, compassionate, and trauma-responsive art therapist, incarcerated clients can learn to employ their own creative process as a tool for mindfulness (Peterson, 2014), to explore personal feelings (Hanes, 2008), and to transform their mood (Dalebroux, Goldstein & Winner, 2008; Smolarski, Leone, & Robbins, 2015). Additionally, the use of art making and engagement of creative process can help an incarcerated client to explore their grief and loss (Ferszt, Hayes, DeFedele, & Horn, 2004; Graves-Alcorn, 1994) and process the residual impact of past trauma (Kometiani, 2020). The inclusion of art therapy in the mental health treatment for individuals with trauma has demonstrated great benefits (Brewster, 2014; Hass-Cohen & Findlay, 2009).

While some prisons and jails do offer various programs in mental health care, education, rehabilitation, fitness, and wellness, many do not. The parameters around such programs and jail regulations govern who can participate, and from one facility to the next they can vary greatly. Perhaps some of the greatest disparities in the incarceration system exist between the prisons, typically larger privately managed facilities run by corporations, and the jails, often crowded, under-funded, under-resourced, city-run institutions with limited social service structures.

In the city of Philadelphia, Pennsylvania, the city jail serves as a holding cell for up to two years; some people are held much longer while they await charges, a hearing, or bail money. During that time there are virtually no therapeutic, educational, or wellness services available to the person. There is an important need here that is not being met. If society is going to call this system one of corrections, and not simply punitive segregation, then there should be efforts put towards helping people to adjust to family separation, employing mental health first aid, and assessing for acute care mental health needs. Various sources identify goals of the corrections systems as deterrence, incapacitation, rehabilitation, retribution, (Kifer, Hemmens, & Stohr, 2003) restitution, (University of Minnesota Libraries. n.d.), reentry (Stohr & Walsh, 2020). The problem is that our current system of jailing people long-term without charge, representation, or trial, while not giving them access to proper mental healthcare does not promote anything except incapacitation and further mental decline. Denying people, even those incarcerated for committing crimes (alleged and untried, in the case of most holding jails), access to mental health care amounts to cruelty and inhumane treatment.

## METHODOLOGY AND PARTICIPANTS

In an effort to explore the potential impact and possible benefit of mental health care on the jailed population, one art therapist conducted a mixed methods (Creswell, 2014) pilot study with 32 females, aged 19-59 years. Participants engaged in an 8-week structured art therapy group which included a self-report survey with demographic and detailer questions, an ACEs questionnaire, and two other surveys (The OQ®-GRQ – Group Climate Questionnaire (MacKenzie, 1990), Devereux Adult Resilience Survey (DARS) (Mackrain, 2008). In addition to this data, participants attended the therapy group, made artwork, and then proceeded to show their artwork, share their experience, and derive meaning from their experiences.

The 32 participants were adult women who all had experienced significant trauma during their childhood, and all had experienced physical and/or sexual violence prior to incarceration. For most of the women, their presence in the jail was their first arrest. Most of them were primary caregivers for children under the age of 12, lived within zip codes noted as being high crime areas and having high levels of community violence. Half of them did not have a high school diploma. A significant majority of them were housing insecure and lived below the poverty line. This group of incarcerated women had an average self-report ACE questionnaire score of eight. This is significantly higher than the general population, which demonstrates that 60% of the population has experienced at least one ACE, over 16% experienced 4 or more ACEs, and that females show significantly higher prevalence of ACE scores than males (Merrick et al., 2019; Giano et al., 2020).

The 8-week art therapy group was run on a curriculum of themes. Participants explored topics of personal identity, personal responsibility, self-care, past reflection, interconnectedness, making plans, and setting goals. Each week, the group started with some sort of check-in, and included some lessons and practice around breathwork, meditation, and increasing mindfulness by becoming attuned to one's own body, as has been demonstrated to have benefit in short term art therapy (Tripp, 2007). Participants made art each week and were given small gifts of art materials to carry their creative energy and output through the week until the next group; the jail sanctioned these materials and allowed the inmates to keep the materials when they returned to their cells. Inmates were encouraged to engage in creative journaling between group therapy sessions, which has demonstrated great benefits for individuals with histories of trauma that included relationship abuse, such as domestic violence (Ikonomopoulos, et al., 2017).

Several shared themes emerged during the group, and shared in this chapter are some pieces of artwork made in group that are emblematic of these themes. These themes were categorized in terms of abuse and empowerment. Themes of abuse included (a) the fear of being taken advantage of (again); (b) the internalized belief of being powerless; (c) the pressure to quickly "get over" traumatic experiences; and (d) the desire and efforts toward breaking cycles of abuse. Themes pertaining to empowerment included (a) the comparison of art therapy to traditional mental health services that they had experienced; (b) the inherent freedom experienced when having been given art materials; (c) questions about the self and what they feel and experience inside; and (d) understandings and assertions of what they may have wanted in the past and of what they now want.

## OUTCOMES AND RECOMMENDATIONS

As is often the case in group art therapy, participants leaned into the sense of community that group participation brought them (Riley, 2001). Women in jail with histories of trauma are dually isolated; living in incarceration makes isolation from others your daily reality. Living with and sustaining the impacts of trauma, including things like relationship abuse and sexual violence, creates an emotionally isolating reality. As happened in this group, art therapy often serves to decrease participants' experience of isolation (Tutty et al., 2016). It also supported the findings of Skop, et al. (2022), who learned that group art therapy helped survivors of trauma to build resilience, reclaim empowerment, use metaphor through art, and create connections.

Through a growing understanding that the trauma of their early and developing lives has greatly impacted who they are and current circumstances, the participants in this group set out to be the support system for each other that they had rarely ever had in life. By learning to ask the important questions of *What Happened to You?* (Winfrey & Perry, 2021), instead of the old trauma paradigm- *What's wrong with you?* - participants could begin to move forward toward healing and empowerment (Bloom, 1995; van der Kolk, 1996).

Incarcerated individuals may use rigid defenses such as silence and aggression for survival. Defense mechanisms such as avoidance and denial can serve as protective behaviors. By addressing the underlying issues that contribute to the use of these defense mechanisms, it is possible to support incarcerated individuals in developing healthier coping strategies and behaviors (Gussak, 2004). In the Philadelphia jail, art therapy was effective at decreasing depressed mood amongst participants. Furthermore, it was viewed as a safe and acceptable way to express, release, and cope with potentially destructive feelings since inmates who participated were accused of and received fewer infractions during and after the group.

Some of the lessons derived from this study included an increased understanding of the prevalence of trauma and human trafficking experiences among the incarcerated female population. While many participants in the group had experienced histories of sexual trauma and abuse, several of those individuals did not self-identify as rape victims or see themselves as being the victim of a reportable crime. This may be due to misinformation and misunderstandings about what constitutes rape, who has the right to consent or object to sex acts, or to complications pertaining to identity and adopting the moniker of victim.

The art made by individuals who have encountered and are continuing to encounter major life traumas quickly brought up multiple intense themes (note that some artwork is shown in the next section). A common approach in both group therapy and trauma therapy is to carefully monitor and regulate emotional and traumatic content disclosures to maintain the emotional safety of clients. It might be discouraged to allow a client to share too much, too soon. In this group, participants engaged quickly into a deep dive into trauma content. While the facilitating art therapist had to monitor the possibility and outcomes associated with one group member triggering a trauma response in another with intense imagery or verbally shared memories, this was also balanced against the overwhelming good for individuals of simply having the group. Group members routinely expressed their feelings of being completely starved of attention, relationships, and services. Context is everything. While it may be beneficial, in many group therapy settings, to prevent the early deep dive into trauma content, in a jail setting where residents have a unique combination of too much time on their hands and too little time of therapeutic value and processing with a trained mental health professional, there is value in reconsidering typical recommendations.

## ARTWORK

The following images comprise some of the artwork made in this art therapy group. All images are shared proudly with the consent of the artists, each of whom adopted the identity of artist.

*Figure 1.*
*Artwork Title: Traditional Therapy*
*Materials: Crayon and pencil*
*Art by: Sankofa Art Therapy participant*
*Directive: Experience with Traditional Therapy*
*Notes: This participant discussed her experience with and perception of traditional talk therapy. She spoke of the contrast of those experiences with her unique relationship with art therapy.*

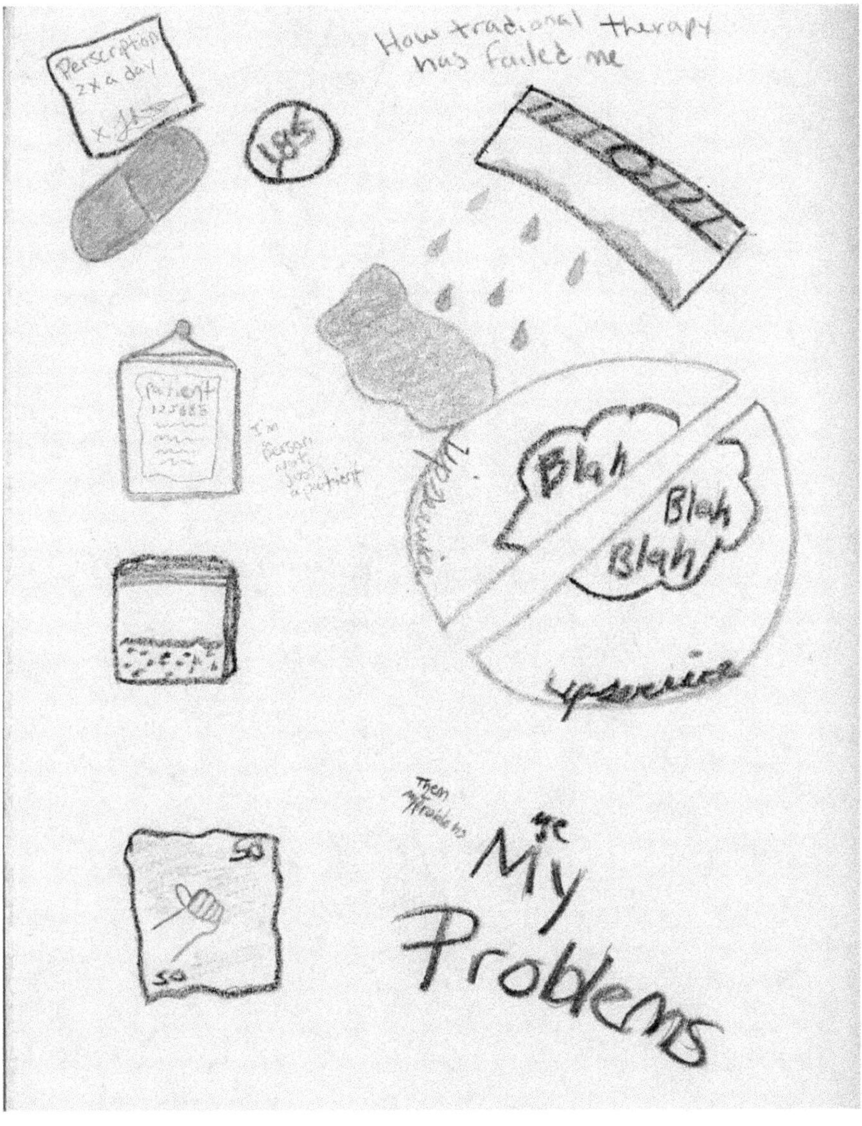

*Figure 2.*
*Artwork Title: Capacity*
*Materials: Crayon and pencil*
*Art by: Sankofa Art Therapy participant*
*Directive: Create a picture of your self-care.*
*Notes: This participant discussed how this image illustrates the struggle she faces of being a caretaker for others with little or no time to care for herself.*

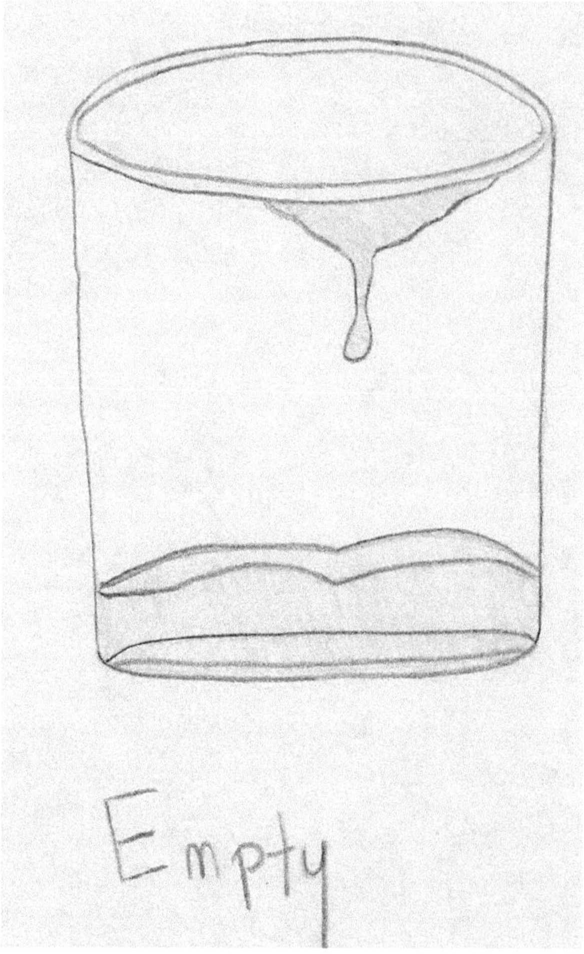

*Figure 3.*
*Artwork Title: Versions of Me*
*Materials: Crayon and pencil*
*Art by: Sankofa Art Therapy participant*
*Directive: How do people see you?*
*Notes: This participant described how she felt as though she was seen as a binary, either good or bad, which was determined by the choices she made.*

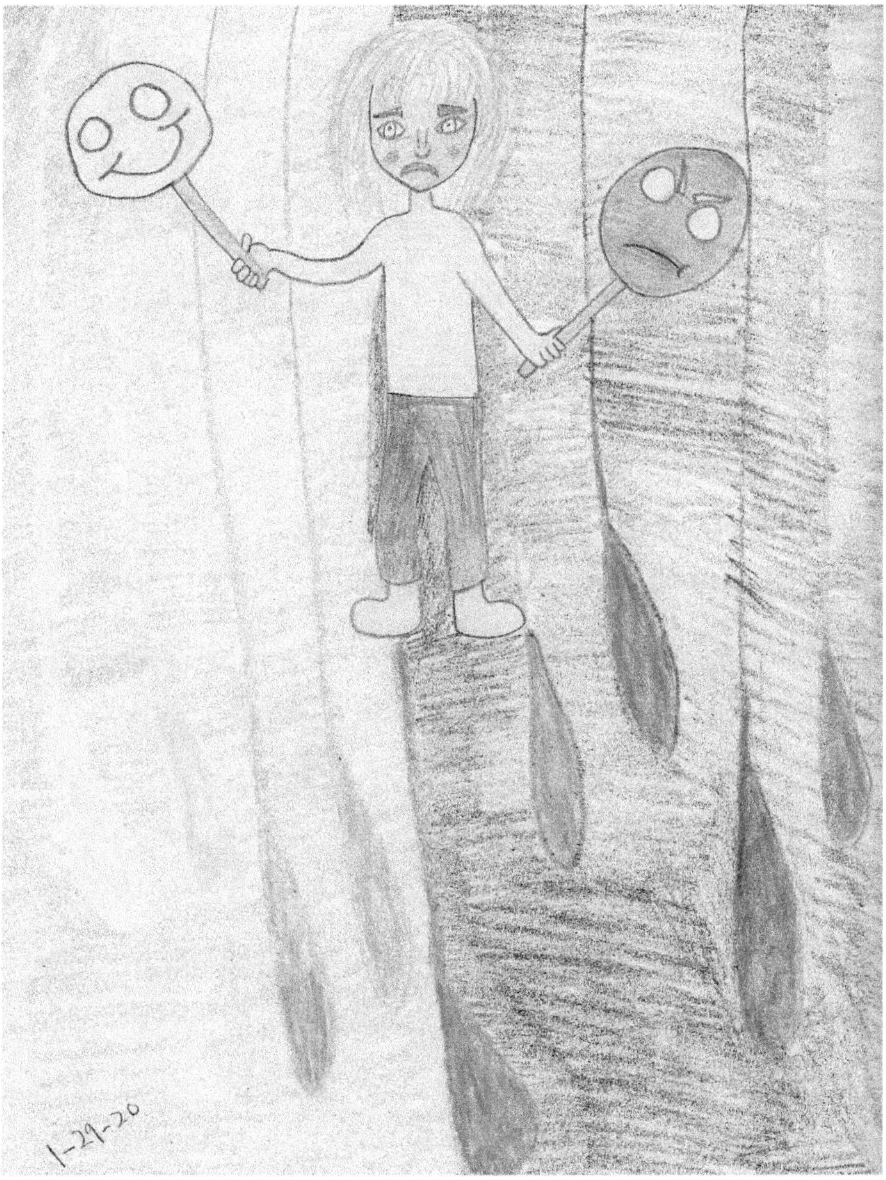

*Figure 4.*
*Artwork Title: Emotional Sound*
*Materials: Crayon and pencil*
*Art by: Sankofa Art Therapy participant*
*Directive: How can you use your voice?*
*Notes: This participant spoke of how she is able to tell her story through art and use colors to express her emotions.*

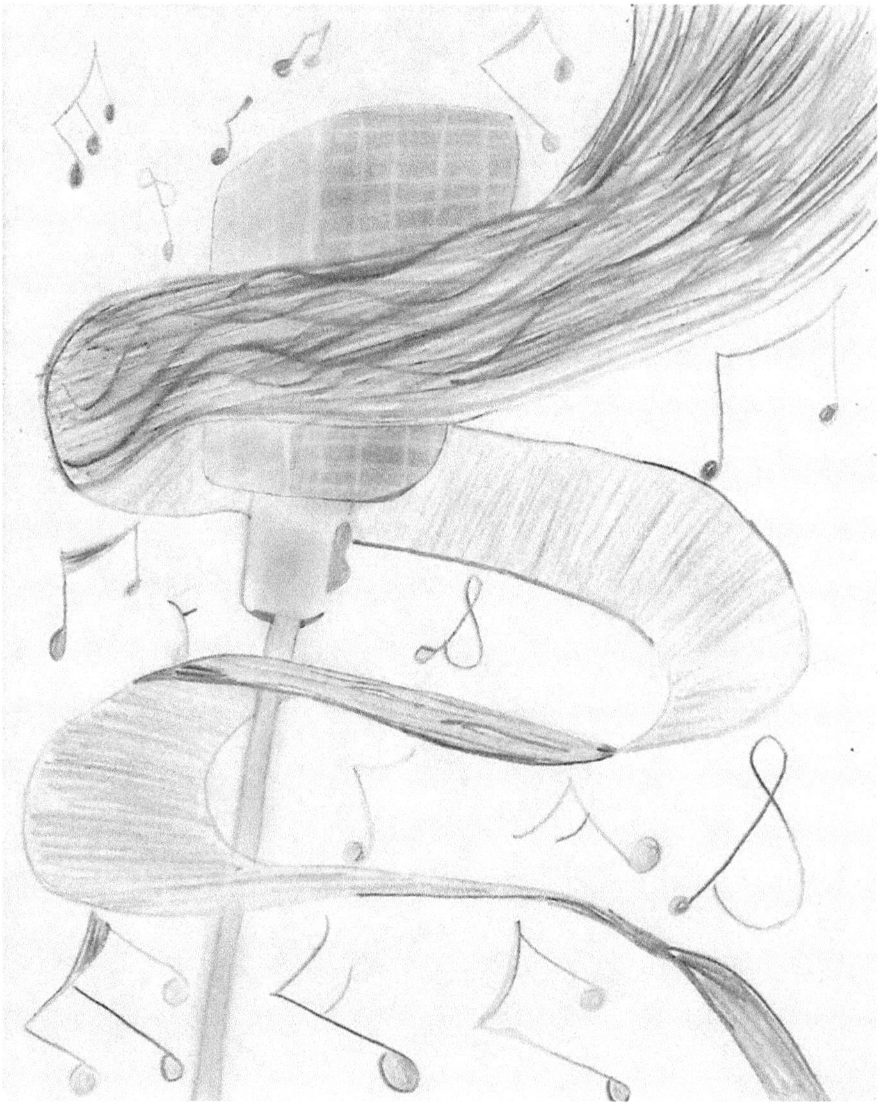

*Figure 5.*
*Artwork Title: Keep Out*
*Materials: Crayon and pencil*
*Art by: Sankofa Art Therapy participant*
*Directive: Create a safe container*
*Notes: This participant created a container that houses her memories and asserted that she is the only one with the key to unlock it.*

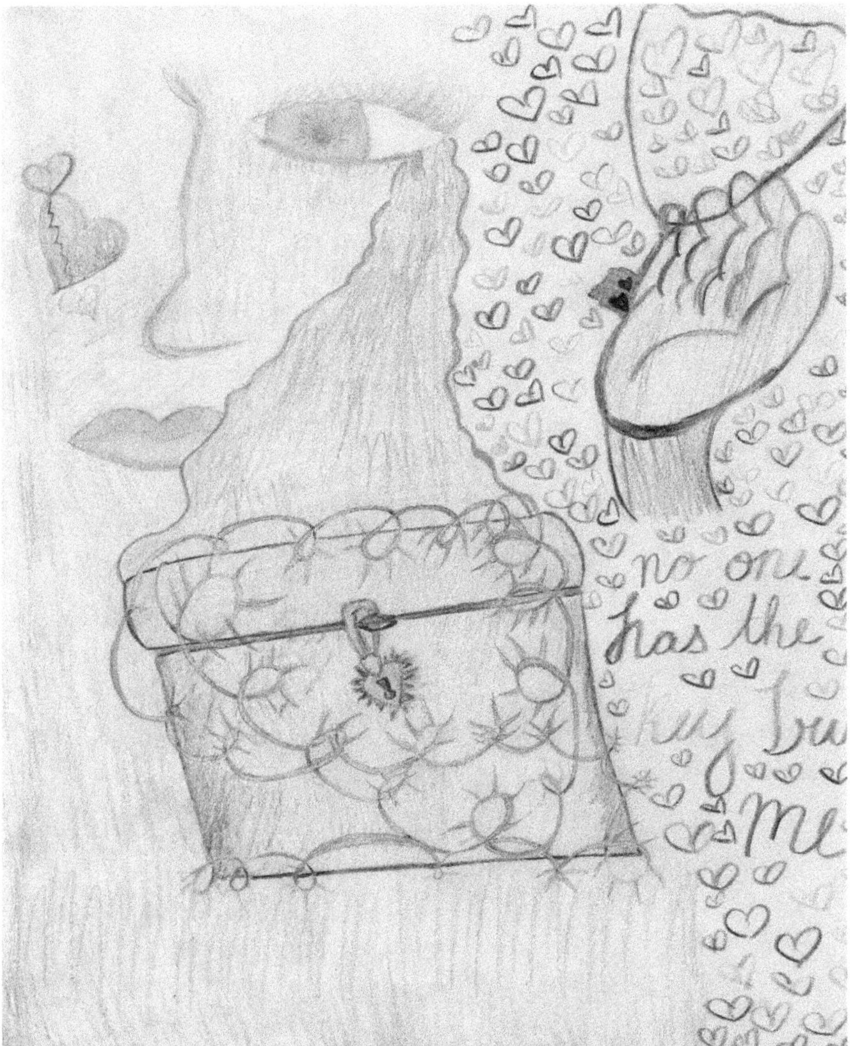

*Figure 6.*
*Artwork Title: Compliant Smile*
*Material: Pencil*
*Art by: Sankofa Art Therapy participant*
*Directive: Experience with Traditional Therapy*
*Notes: This participant created a depiction of her road to recovery and her frustrating experience with mandated talk-therapy programs where she did not feel treated as an individual.*

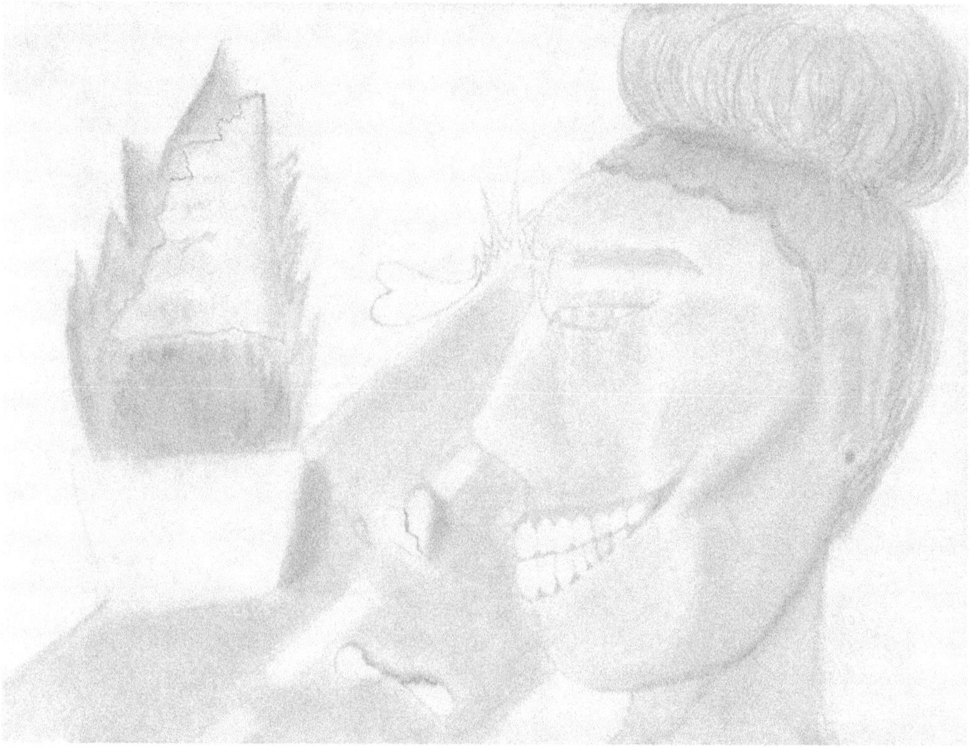

*Figure 7.*
*Artwork Title: Mending Heart*
*Materials: Colored pencils and graphite pencils*
*Art by: Sankofa Art Therapy participant*
*Directive: What does healing look like?*
*Notes: This participant created a wounded heart with a needle and thread available. She discussed this as a demonstration of her resiliency despite her circumstances.*

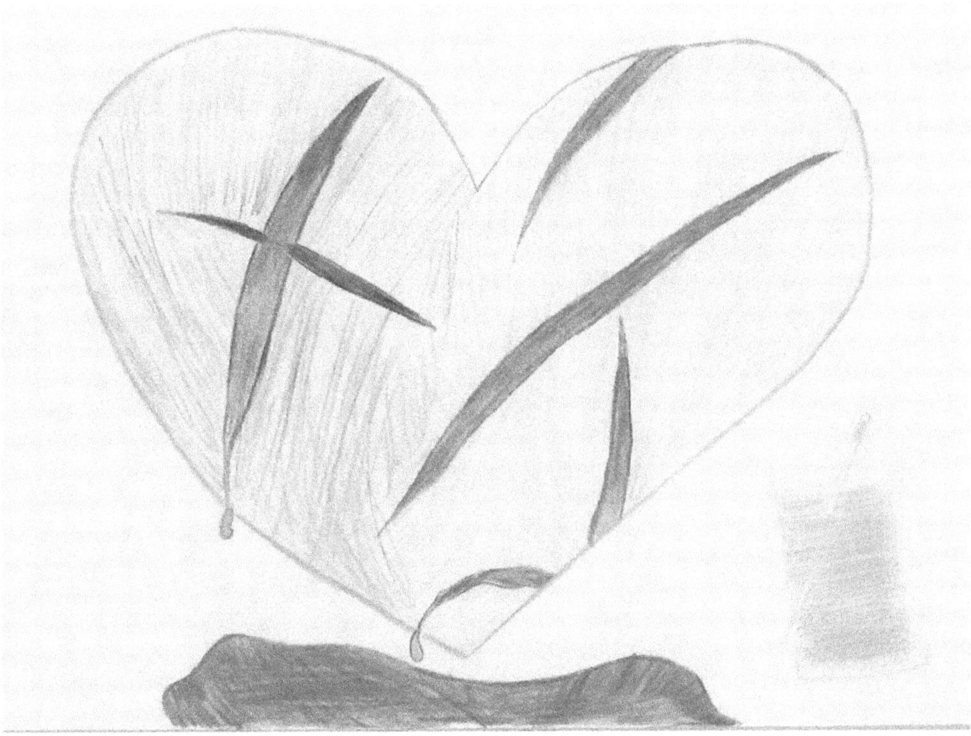

*Figure 8.*
*Artwork Title: Breaking the Cycle*
*Materials: Crayon and pencil*
*Art by: Sankofa Art Therapy participant*
*Directive: Break the Cycle of Power and Abuse*
*Notes: This participant created an illustration that she now has tools that are needed for her to break the cycle of power and abuse in her life.*

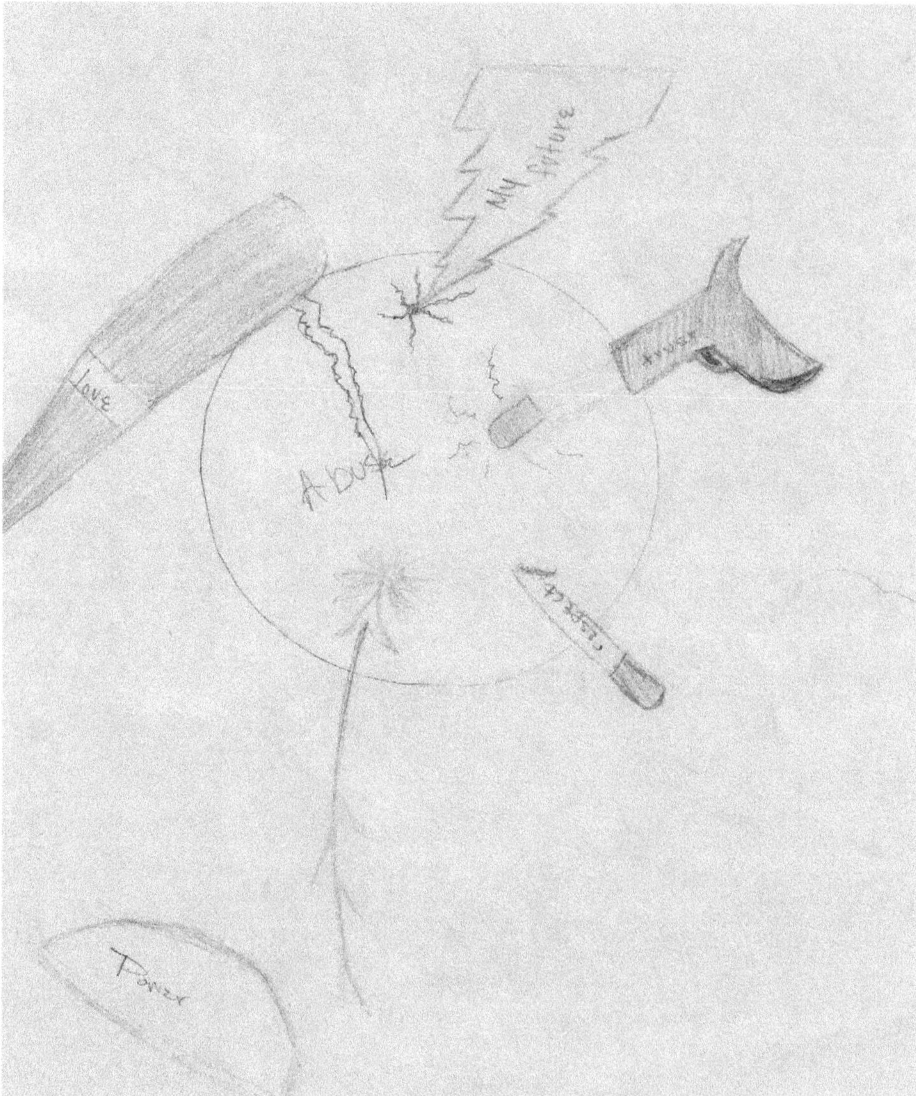

*Figure 9.*
*Artwork Title: Worthy*
*Materials: Crayon*
*Art by: Sankofa Art Therapy participant*
*Directive: Who are you?*
*Notes: This participant gained insight that she can be the hero of her story and that she has the power to make herself happy.*

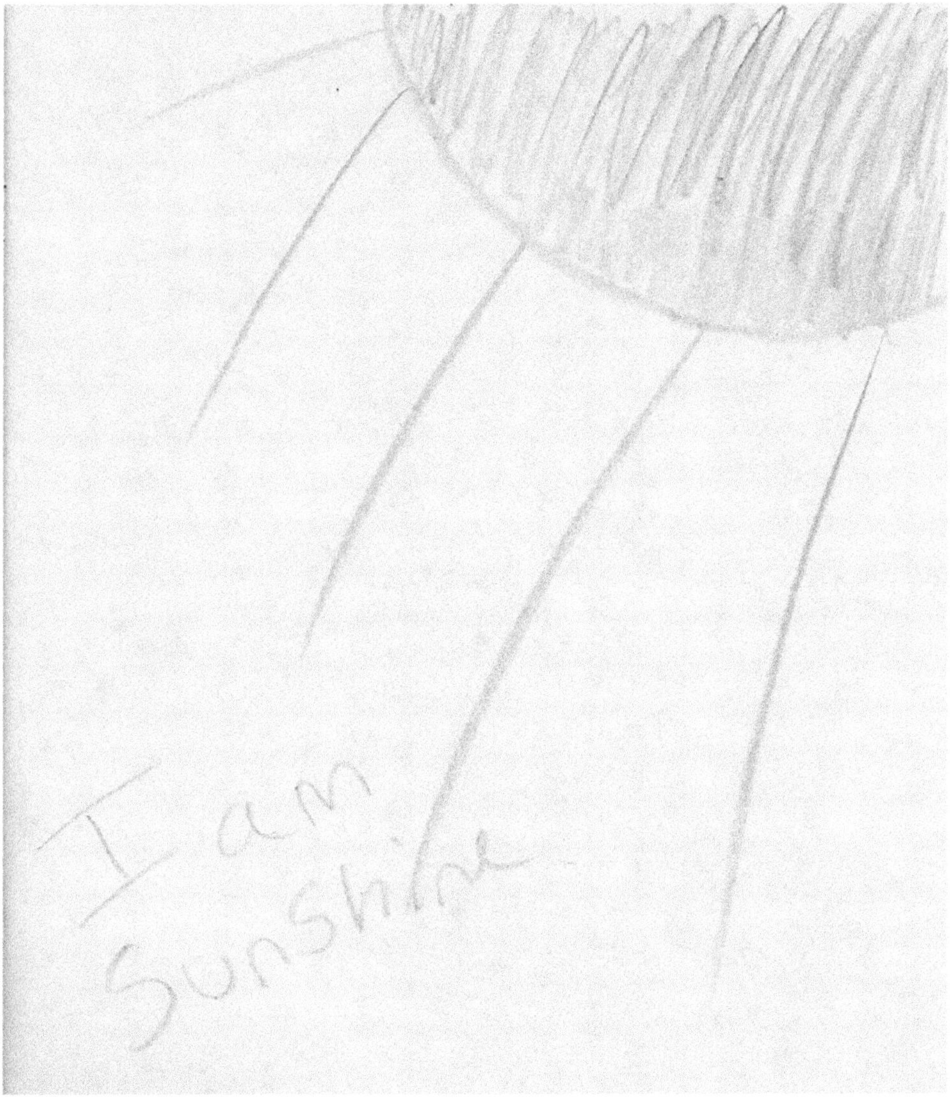

*Figure 10.*
*Artwork Title: Stolen Dreams*
*Materials: Colored pencils, watercolor paint, and pencil*
*Art by: Sankofa Art Therapy participant*
*Directive: Who are you?*
*Notes: This participant reflected that as a young child, she had dreams of being a ballerina. The shadow of sexual abuse and human trafficking stole those dreams.*

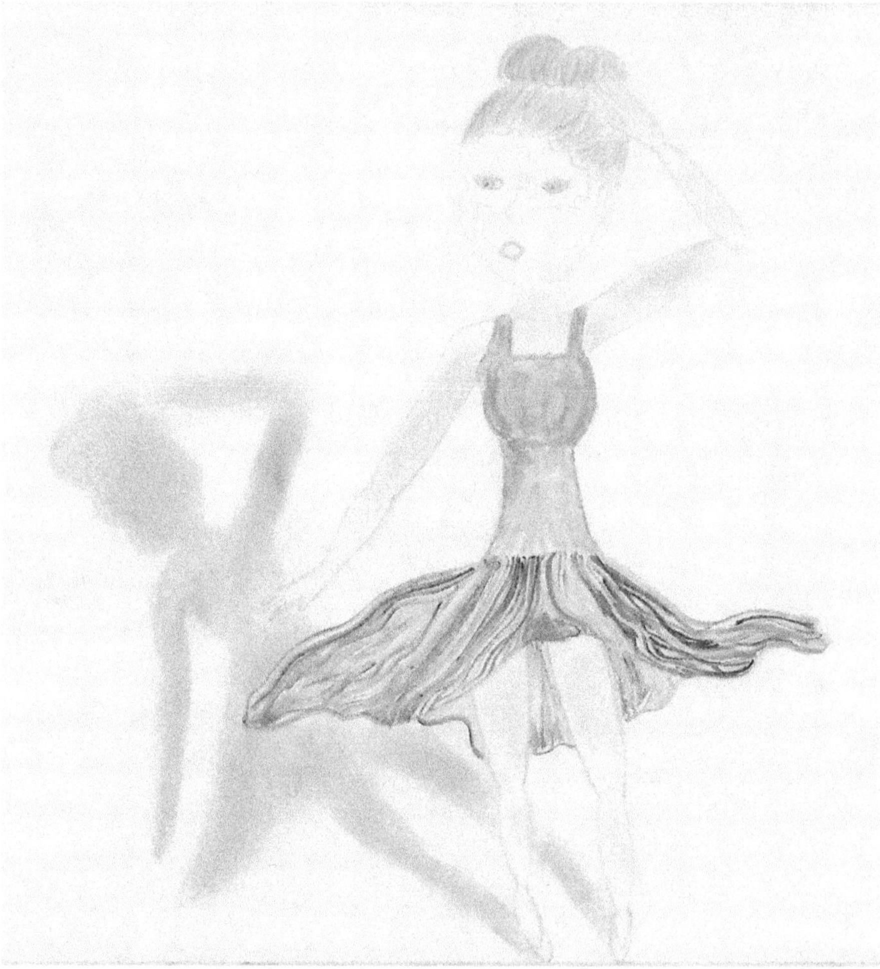

*Figure 11.*
*Artwork Title: Stolen Dreams*
*Materials: Colored pencils, crayons, and pencil*
*Art by: Sankofa Art Therapy participant*
*Directive: Who could you ask for help?*
*Notes: This participant created an illustration of feeling lost in a system that is dark and cold. She is struggling to hold on to the hope and light inside of her so that she won't be completely engulfed by the pain.*

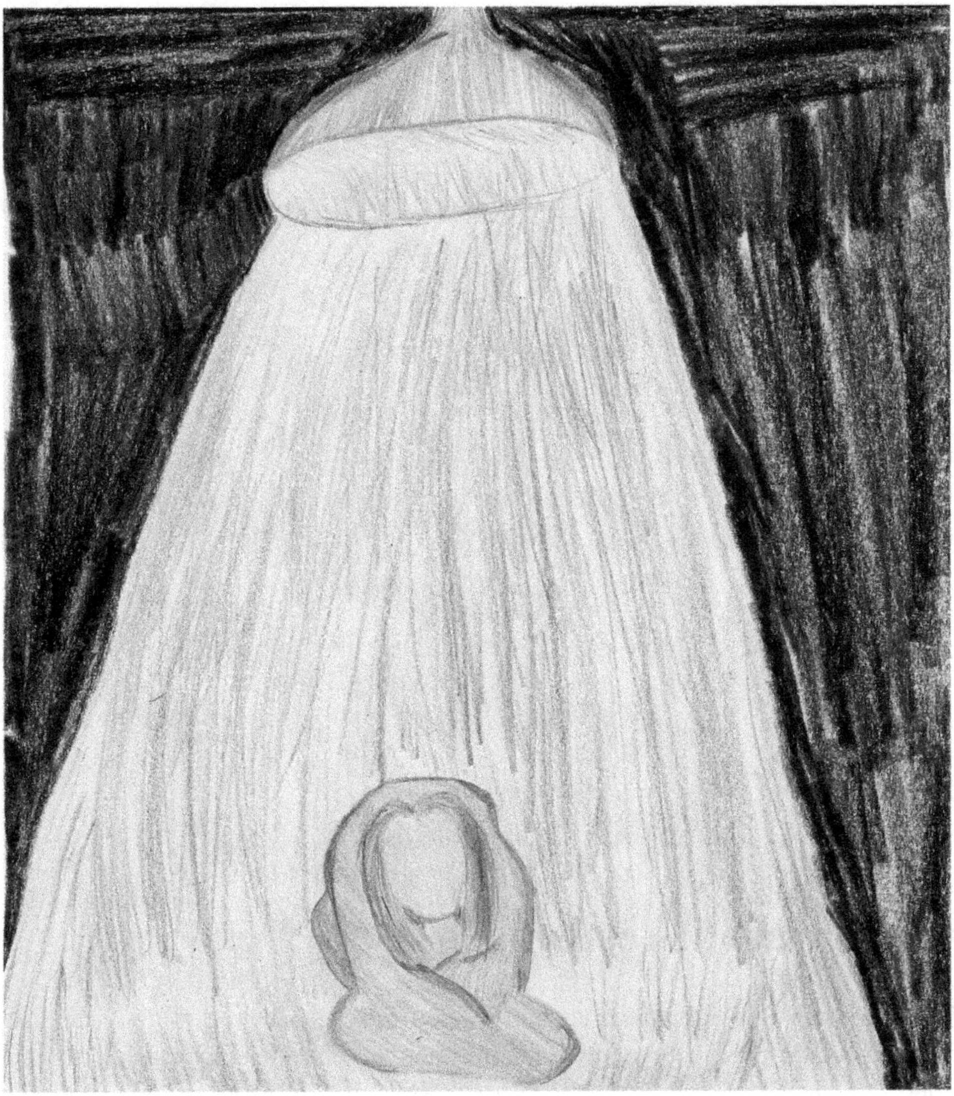

*Figure 12.*
*Artwork Title: More than meets the eye*
*Materials: Colored pencils, watercolor paint, and pencil*
*Art by: Sankofa Art Therapy participant*
*Directive: How do you see yourself?*
*Notes: This participant created a representation of the complexity of her emotions through the use of colors.*

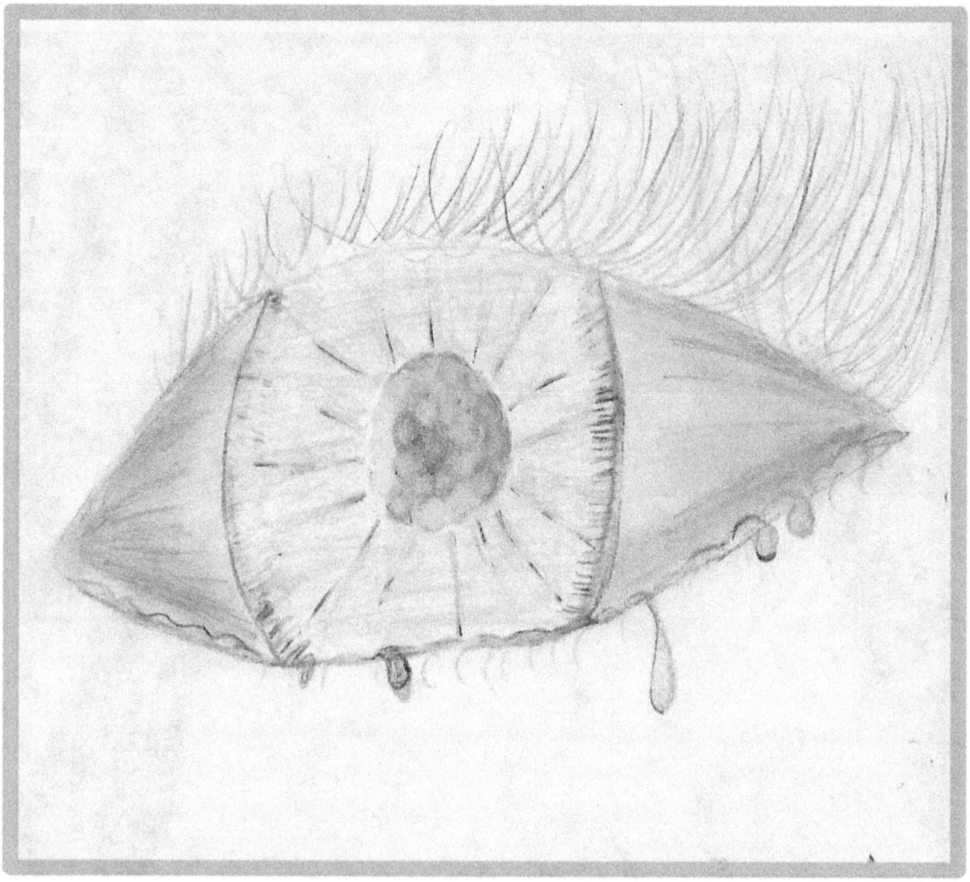

## FUTURE RESEARCH DIRECTIONS

Further research involving incarcerated women and the use of art therapy can lead to more specific practical recommendations about factors like approach, duration, group size, interventions, goal setting, and assessment of outcomes. Incarceration rates in the United States provide ample opportunities to examine and improve upon the practices surrounding imprisonment. People of all ages, genders, racial and cultural backgrounds who are locked up can still benefit from increased quality and quantity of mental health services. These mental health services can aid in the process of rehabilitation and constitute humane treatment. Increased mental health services includes psychoeducation which can help individuals to cope with the stressors of family separation and life behind bars, and prepare individuals for eventual release and re-immersion into the community. Art therapy is a viable tool for effecting change in incarcerated persons, and especially in those who have complex trauma backgrounds. Participation in the art therapy group contributed to a decrease in the number of disciplinary reports written on inmate participants, as presented in this chapter.

There is a great need for future research to further the understanding of how therapeutic interventions can benefit incarcerated individuals, as well as their children and communities. While the art therapy study presented in this chapter was conducted over 8 weeks, there are benefits to pursuing longer-term interventions as well as long-term follow up on individual participants. Longevity studies could help explain how art therapy groups might impact incarcerated women over time. It would also allow for the tracking of intergenerational benefits in the cases of incarcerated women who are parents or caregivers.

Families and particularly children of incarcerated women are deeply impacted in ways that are not fully explored in literature. Future research should consider the impact of art therapy groups for the children and/or families of incarcerated females. This may help develop an understanding of how art therapy could support families who are separated, and aid in the family reunification process.

This research revealed that the use of certain defense mechanisms by some group participants, such as rationalizing, denying, and downplaying abuse, served as a critical survival tool. While these strategies can be adaptive and useful at times, future research might consider if they may promote detrimental health effects over the long-term.

Clients in art therapy often place value on the establishment and maintenance of certain rituals in the context of treatment. This group created their own rituals that helped to provide a safe container for vulnerability and sharing. Future research could examine the value of shared rituals in incarcerated populations, and in creating customs as a strategy for engaging changes in social dynamics.

Art Therapy groups provided for women who were recently released from incarceration may help former inmates to process their experience of incarceration and readjust to the responsibilities of society. Art therapy could be a vital tool in reducing recidivism. The authors also believe that art therapy groups prior to incarceration may be the missing component of a successful diversionary program.

## CONCLUSION

There are many problems with the United States corrections system, including but not limited to the excessive use of incarceration, holding people in jail who have not been charged, the disproportionate rate of incarceration of Black people, and the privatization of the carceral industry. This has resulted in a for profit model that incentivizes the continued incarceration of people over any other model, such as those that emphasize education, rehabilitation, reparations, community service, or continued family connectedness.

Participants in this research on art therapy in an urban jail reported a variety of benefits after participation in art therapy groups. These benefits included decreased feelings of isolation, anxiety, and depression. They also reported feeling empowered to take on leadership roles within their community, and an eagerness to share their previously untold stories. The women participants in this group experienced benefits significant enough that they requested a continuation of art therapy, and a desire to have their children participate in a similar group.

There is a need for more practice and research on therapeutic health care initiatives in the jail setting. This is even more true with incarcerated women. This art therapy group pilot study conducted in a Philadelphia jail provides some insight into the benefits of providing mental health treatment for inmates.

## ACKNOWLEDGMENT

This research received no specific grant from any funding agency in the public, commercial, or not-for-profit sectors.

This research was supported (non-monetary provision of supplies and art materials) by Sankofa Healing Studio, a Philadelphia-based non-profit organization focused on social justice issues and therapeutic intervention.

## REFERENCES

Aday, R. H., Dye, M. H., & Kaiser, A. K. (2014). Examining the traumatic effects of sexual victimization on the health of incarcerated women. *Women & Criminal Justice*, *24*(4), 341–361. doi:10.1080/08974454.2014.909758

AlDabbagh, M. (2014). Positive Art Impact On healing therapy "Review Study". Brewster, L. *The Impact of Prison Arts Programs on Inmate Attitudes and Behavior: A Quantitative Evaluation*.

Belknap, J. (2020). *The invisible woman: Gender, crime, and justice*. SAGE Publications.

Bender, K. A. (2023). Incarcerated Women's Perceptions of the Role Model Prison Officer as Procedurally Just. *International Journal of Offender Therapy and Comparative Criminology*, *0*(0), 0306624X2211442. Advance online publication. doi:10.1177/0306624X221144287 PMID:36601909

Bloom, B., & Covington, S. (2008). Addressing the mental health needs of women offenders. In R. Gido, L. Dalley, & D. McDonald (Eds.), *The unmet mental health needs of women across the criminal justice system*. Prentice-Hall/Pearson.

Bloom, S. L. (1995). Creating sanctuary in the school. *Journal for a Just and Caring Education*, *1*(4), 403–433.

Bremner, J. D., Vermetten, E., Schmahl, C., Vaccarino, V., Vythilingam, M., Afzal, N., Grillon, C., & Charney, D. S. (2005). Positron emission tomographic imaging of neural correlates of a fear acquisition and extinction paradigm in women with childhood sexual-abuse-related post-traumatic stress disorder. *Psychological Medicine*, *35*(6), 791–806. doi:10.1017/S0033291704003290 PMID:15997600

Brewster, L. (2014). The Impact of prison arts programs on inmate attitudes and behavior: A Quantitative evaluation. *Justice Policy Journal, 11*(2). https://repository.usfca.edu/cgi/viewcontent.cgi?article=1008&context=pna

Bronson, J., & Berzofsky, M. (2011). *Indicators of mental health problems reported by prisoners and jail inmates*. U.S. Department of Justice. https://www.bjs.gov/content/pub/pdf/imhprpji1112.pdf

Creswell, J. W. (2014). *Research design: Qualitative, quantitative and mixed methods approaches* (4th ed.). Sage.

Curl, K. (2008). Assessing stress reduction as a function of artistic creation and cognitive focus. *Art Therapy: Journal of the American Art Therapy Association*, *25*(4), 164–169. doi:10.1080/07421656.2008.10129550

Czamanski-Cohen, J., & Weihs, K. L. (2016). The bodymind model: A platform for studying the mechanisms of change induced by art therapy. *The Arts in Psychotherapy*, *51*, 63–71. doi:10.1016/j.aip.2016.08.006 PMID:27777492

Dalebroux, A., Goldstein, T. R., & Winner, E. (2008). Short-term mood repair through art-making: Positive emotion is more effective than venting. *Motivation and Emotion*, *32*(4), 288–295. doi:10.100711031-008-9105-1

Erickson, B. J. (2008). *Art therapy treatment with incarcerated women* [Unpublished doctoral dissertation, University of Central Florida].

Felitti, V. J., Anda, R. F., Nordenberg, D., Williamson, D. F., Spitz, A. M., Edwards, V., Koss, M. P., & Marks, J. S. (1998). Relationship of childhood abuse and household dysfunction to many of the leading causes of death in adults: The Adverse Childhood Experiences (ACE) Study. *American Journal of Preventive Medicine, 14*(4), 245–258. doi:10.1016/S0749-3797(98)00017-8 PMID:9635069

Ferszt, G. G., Hayes, P. M., DeFedele, S., & Horn, L. (2004). Art therapy with incarcerated women who have experienced the death of a loved one. *Art Therapy: Journal of the American Art Therapy Association, 21*(4), 191–199. doi:10.1080/07421656.2004.10129695

Frewen, P., Thornley, E., Rabellino, D., & Lanius, R. (2017). Neuroimaging the traumatized self: fMRI reveals altered response in cortical midline structures and occipital cortex during visual and verbal self- and other-referential processing in women with PTSD. *European Journal of Psychotraumatology, 8*(1), 1314164. doi:10.1080/20008198.2017.1314164 PMID:28649298

Giano, Z., Wheeler, D. L., & Hubach, R. D. (2020). The frequencies and disparities of adverse childhood experiences in the U.S. *BMC Public Health, 20*(1), 1327. doi:10.118612889-020-09411-z PMID:32907569

Gold, K. J., & Marcus, S. M. (2008). Effect of maternal mental illness on pregnancy outcomes. *Expert Review of Obstetrics & Gynecology, 3*(3), 391–401. doi:10.1586/17474108.3.3.391

Graves-Alcorn, S. L. (1994). *Expressions of healing: Embracing the process of grief.* Bookbaby.

Gross, J., & Haynes, H. (1998). Drawing facilitates children's verbal resorts of emotion laden events. *Journal of Experimental Psychology, 4*, 163–179.

Gussak, D. (2004). Art therapy with prison inmates: A pilot study. *The Arts in Psychotherapy, 31*(4), 245–259. doi:10.1016/j.aip.2004.06.001

Gussak, D. (2006). Effects of art therapy with prison inmates: A follow-up study. *The Arts in Psychotherapy, 33*(3), 188–198. doi:10.1016/j.aip.2005.11.003

Gussak, D. (2009). Comparing the effectiveness of art therapy on depression and locus of control of male and female inmates. *The Arts in Psychotherapy, 36*(4), 202–207. doi:10.1016/j.aip.2009.02.004

Gussak, D. E., & Rosal, M. L. (Eds.). (2016). *The Wiley Handbook of Art Therapy*. John Wiley & Sons, Inc.

Ha, B. C., & Robinson, G. (2011). Chronic care model implementation in the California state prison system. *Journal of Correctional Health Care*, *17*(2), 173–182. doi:10.1177/1078345810396859 PMID:21525120

Hanes, M. J. (2008). Signs of suicide: Using road drawings with inmates on suicide observation at a county jail. *Art Therapy: Journal of the American Art Therapy Association*, *25*(2), 78–84. doi:10.1080/07421656.2008.10129418

Harner, H. M., & Riley, S. (2013). The impact of incarceration on Women's mental health: Responses from women in a maximum-security prison. *Qualitative Health Research*, *23*(1), 26–42. doi:10.1177/1049732312461452 PMID:23034774

Hass-Cohen, N., & Findlay, J. C. (2009). Pain, attachment, and meaning making: Report on an art therapy relational neuroscience assessment protocol. *The Arts in Psychotherapy*, *36*(4), 175–184. doi:10.1016/j.aip.2009.02.003

Herman, J. (2023). *Truth and repair: How trauma survivors envision justice*. Basic Books.

Hughes, K. C., & Shin, L. M. (2011). Functional neuroimaging studies of post-traumatic stress disorder. *Expert Review of Neurotherapeutics*, *11*(2), 275–285. doi:10.1586/ern.10.198 PMID:21306214

Ikonomopoulos, J., Cavazos-Vela, J., Vela, P., Sanchez, M., Schmidt, C., & Catchings, C. V. (2017). Evaluating the effects of creative journal arts therapy for survivors of domestic violence. *Journal of Creativity in Mental Health*, *12*(4), 496–512. doi:10.1080/15401383.2017.1328290

James, D., & Glaze, L. (2006). *Mental health problems of prisons and jail inmates*. U.S. Department of Justice. http://bjs.ojp.usdoj.gov/content/pub/pdf/mhppji.pdf

Johnson, L. M. (2007). Jail wall drawings and jail art programs. *International Journal of Criminal Justice Sciences*, *2*(2), 66–84. https://citeseerx.ist.psu.edu/document?repid=rep1&type=pdf&doi=5368e93862bd61fd4898fa6de09cde0bb100273b

Karlsson, M. E., & Zielinski, M. J. (2020). Sexual Victimization and Mental Illness Prevalence Rates Among Incarcerated Women: A Literature Review. *Trauma, Violence & Abuse*, *21*(2), 326–349. doi:10.1177/1524838018767933 PMID:29661117

Kifer, M., Hemmens, C., & Stohr, M. K. (2003). The Goals of corrections: Perspectives from the line. *Criminal Justice Review*, *28*(1), 47–69. doi:10.1177/073401680302800104

Kometiani, M. K., & Farmer, K. W. (2020). Exploring resilience through case studies of art therapy with sex trafficking survivors and their advocates. *The Arts in Psychotherapy*, *67*, 101582. doi:10.1016/j.aip.2019.101582

Levenson, J. S., & Willis, G. M. (2019). Implementing trauma-informed care in correctional treatment and supervision. *Journal of Aggression, Maltreatment & Trauma*, *28*(4), 481–501. doi:10.1080/10926771.2018.1531959

McGinn, T., Taylor, B., McColgan, M., & Lagdon, S. (2016). Survivor Perspectives on IPV Perpetrator Interventions: A Systematic Narrative Review. *Trauma, Violence & Abuse*, *17*(3), 239–255. doi:10.1177/1524838015584358 PMID:25964277

Merrick, M. T., Ford, D. C., Ports, K. A., Guinn, A. S., Chen, J., Klevens, J., Metzler, M., Jones, C. M., Simon, T. R., Daniel, V. M., Ottley, P., & Mercy, J. A. (2019). Vital signs: Estimated proportion of adult health problems attributable to adverse childhood experiences and implications for prevention — 25 States, 2015–2017. *MMWR. Morbidity and Mortality Weekly Report*, *68*(44), 999–1005. doi:10.15585/mmwr.mm6844e1 PMID:31697656

Mignon, S. (2016). Health issues of incarcerated women in the United States. *Ciencia & Saude Coletiva*, *21*(7), 2051–2060. doi:10.1590/1413-81232015217.05302016 PMID:27383339

Miller, N. A., & Najavits, L. M. (2012). Creating trauma-informed correctional care: A balance of goals and environment. *European Journal of Psychotraumatology*, *3*(1), 17246. doi:10.3402/ejpt.v3i0.17246 PMID:22893828

Morrissey, J. P., Steadman, H. J., Dalton, K. M., Cuellar, A., Stiles, P., & Cuddeback, G. S. (2006). Medicaid enrollment and mental health service use following release of jail detainees with severe mental illness. *Psychiatric Services (Washington, D.C.)*, *57*(6), 809–815. doi:10.1176/ps.2006.57.6.809 PMID:16754757

Nair, S., McGreevy, J. E., Hutchinson-Colas, J., Turock, H., Chervenak, F., & Bachmann, G. (2021). Pregnancy in incarcerated women: Need for national legislation to standardize care. *Journal of Perinatal Medicine*, *49*(7), 830–836. doi:10.1515/jpm-2021-0145 PMID:34167182

Peterson, C. (2014). Mindfulness-based art therapy. *Mindfulness and the art therapies. Theory into Practice*, 42–58.

Rauch, S. L., van der Kolk, B. A., & Fisler, R. E. (1996). A symptom provocation study of posttraumatic stress disorder using positron emission tomography and script-driven imagery. *Archives of General Psychiatry*, *53*(5), 380–387. doi:10.1001/archpsyc.1996.01830050014003 PMID:8624181

Rice, K., & Jennings, J. L. (2014). The ROC program. *Journal of Correctional Health Care, 20*(1), 59–69. doi:10.1177/1078345813505067 PMID:24226289

Riley, S. (2001). *Group process made visible: Group art therapy*. Brunner-Routledge.

Rubin, J. A. (2010). *Introduction to art therapy: Sources & resources* (2nd ed.). Routledge.

Shin, L. M., McNally, R. J., Kosslyn, S. M., Thompson, W. L., Rauch, S. L., Alpert, N. M., Metzger, L. J., Lasko, N. B., Orr, S. P., & Pitman, R. K. (1999). Regional cerebral blood flow during script-driven imagery in childhood sexual abuse-related PTSD: A PET investigation. *The American Journal of Psychiatry, 156*(4), 575–584. doi:10.1176/ajp.156.4.575 PMID:10200737

Skop, M., Darewych, O. H., Root, J., & Mason, J. (2022). Exploring intimate partner violence survivors' experiences with group art therapy. *International Journal of Art Therapy, 27*(4), 159–168. doi:10.1080/17454832.2022.2124298

Smolarski, K., Leone, K., & Robbins, S. J. (2015). Reducing negative mood through drawing: Comparing venting, positive expression, and tracing. *Art Therapy: Journal of the American Art Therapy Association, 32*(4), 197–201. doi:10.1080/07421656.2015.1092697

Springer, S. A. (2010). Improving healthcare for incarcerated women. *Journal of Women's Health, 19*(1), 13–15. doi:10.1089/jwh.2009.1786 PMID:20088653

Stensrud, R. H., Gilbride, D. D., & Bruinekool, R. M. (2019). The Childhood to prison pipeline: Early childhood trauma as reported by a prison population. *Rehabilitation Counseling Bulletin, 62*(4), 195–208. doi:10.1177/0034355218774844

Stevenson, M., & Orr, K. (2013). Art therapy: Stimulating non-verbal communication. *Nursing and Residential Care, 15*(6), 443–445. doi:10.12968/nrec.2013.15.6.443

Stohr, M. K., & Walsh, A. (2020). Corrections: From research, to policy, to practice. *Sage (Atlanta, Ga.)*.

Tadros, E., Barbini, M., & Kaur, L. (2021). Collaborative healthcare in incarcerated settings. *International Journal of Offender Therapy and Comparative Criminology, 0*(0), 0306624X2110589. doi:10.1177/0306624X211058952 PMID:34784803

Teplin, L. A., Abram, K. M., & McClelland, G. M. (1996). Prevalence of psychiatric disorders among incarcerated women. I. Pretrial jail detainees. *Archives of General Psychiatry, 53*(6), 505–512. doi:10.1001/archpsyc.1996.01830060047007 PMID:8639033

Tripp, T. (2007). A short-term therapy approach to processing trauma: Art therapy and bilateral stimulation. *Art Therapy: Journal of the American Art Therapy Association, 24*(4), 178–183. doi:10.1080/07421656.2007.10129476

Tutty, L. M., Babins-Wagner, R., & Rothery, M. A. (2016). You're not alone: Mental health outcomes in therapy groups for abused women. *Journal of Family Violence, 31*(4), 489–497. doi:10.100710896-015-9779-6

University of Minnesota Libraries. (n.d.). *The purposes of punishment.* https://open.lib.umn.edu/criminallaw/chapter/1-5-the-purpose s-of-punishment/

van der Kolk, B. (2000). Posttraumatic stress disorder and the nature of trauma. *Dialogues in Clinical Neuroscience, 2*(1), 7–22. doi:10.31887/DCNS.2000.2.1/bvdkolk PMID:22034447

van der Kolk, B. A. (1996). The body keeps the score: Approaches to the psychobiology of post-traumatic stress disorder. In B. A. van der Kolk, A. C. McFarlane, & L. Weisaeth (Eds.), *Traumatic stress: The effects of overwhelming experience on mind, body and society* (pp. 214–241). Guilford Press.

Wadeson, H. (2010). *Art Psychotherapy* (2nd ed.). John Wiley & Sons, Inc.

Walker, L. E. A., Pann, J. M., Shapiro, D. L., & Van Hasselt, V. B. (2016). A Review of best practices for the treatment of persons with mental illness in jail. In: Best Practices for the Mentally Ill in the Criminal Justice System. SpringerBriefs in Psychology (BRIEFSBC). Springer, Cham. doi:10.1007/978-3-319-21656-0_5

Winfrey, O. & Perry, B. D. (2021) *What Happened to You? Conversations on Trauma, Resilience, and Healing*. Flatiron Books: An Oprah Book.

Young, J. T. N., & Haynie, D. L. (2022). Trusting the untrustworthy: The Social organization of trust among incarcerated women. *Justice Quarterly, 39*(3), 553–584. doi:10.1080/07418825.2020.1807588

Young, M. E., & Bemak, F. (1996). The Role of Emotional Arousal and Expression in Mental Health Counseling. *Journal of Mental Health Counseling, 18*(4), 316–332.

## KEY TERMS AND DEFINITIONS

**Adverse Childhood Experiences (ACEs):** A specific type of adverse experience that occurs during childhood and can have significant impacts on a person's development and functioning throughout their lifespan. ACEs can include experiences such as physical, emotional, or sexual abuse, neglect, household dysfunction, and exposure to violence or substance abuse.

**Art Therapy:** The intentional use of artistic expression facilitated by a mental health provider that has advanced specialty training in Art Therapy to process grief, recover from trauma, manage symptoms, enhance self-awareness, improve communication with self or others, or to achieve other defined therapeutic goals.

**Corrections:** The process of or institution established to facilitate changing behavior by stopping and punishing identified negative behaviors and learning and implementing positive behaviors; most used in discussion of individuals who violate the normal social order, including breaking laws and challenging typically accepted social structures.

**Healing:** The individual process of improving one's functioning and recovering from one's wounds, whether physical, psychological, or emotional.

**Mental Health:** The state of being that reflects how psychologically healthy or unwell a person thinks and feels that they are, including the identification and management of symptoms, coping strategies, relationships, and engagement in life.

**Mental Wellness:** An individual's journey to obtain their mental health goals.

**Person-Centered Therapy:** Emphasizes the importance of empathy, unconditional positive regard, and authenticity in the therapeutic relationship. The therapist strives to create a space where the individual feels heard, understood, and valued as a unique and complex individual.

**Rehabilitation:** The process of, or institution established to facilitate the process of change and positive growth within a person, which may exist on many levels, including psychological, behavioral, social, and emotional.

**Social Justice:** The process and goal of examining history, institutions, current societal structures, community services, and attitudes for equity, equality, integrity, fairness, and respect for dignity, and making changes that will move towards these ethical principles.

# Chapter 4
# Rehabilitation Through the Arts:
## How Art Therapy Impacts Incarcerated Woman

**Giselle Caraballo-Matos**
*Marymount Manhattan College, USA*

## ABSTRACT

*Prison rehabilitation and its impact on different populations, such as women, is not a new concept. Yet, efforts to create healing and non-judgment spaces are continuing to grow and undergoing evaluation. One of these alternative treatments is art therapy. The present review makes use of literature to explore the connection and effective between art therapy, prison rehabilitation, and women. Using the example of how the results of art therapy in treatment spaces can differentiate according to gender, this research shows that mental health among women is more prominent in comparison to men. The results revealed that woman -in general- through different approaches, had effective results emerging from art therapy in prison rehabilitation. In addition, it in most cases, the literature revealed that during prison rehabilitation, women react better to art therapy than men. This chapter argues that the implementation of art therapy as a form of treatment during prison rehabilitation is an effective method for incarcerated women.*

DOI: 10.4018/978-1-6684-7856-1.ch004

## INTRODUCTION

Prison rehabilitation is a resource to help create a healing space for inmates with trauma and/or mental illness. This program's focus is to re-shape and re-educate inmates, in hopes of reducing recidivism by providing them with resources to cultivate a healthier lifestyle and to improve relations with the self and others. These resources often include traditional psychotherapy. However, these resources are often lacking in prison. Fortunately, alternative treatments or therapies, such as art therapy, are available for these at-risk populations. Many individuals, who are incarcerated, can benefit from art therapy in prison rehabilitation, since the positive outcome of art therapy outweighs the neutral outcome. The present literature review focuses on the impact of art therapy techniques in prison rehabilitation for incarcerated women. The population of incarcerated women include elderly women, grieving women, and women presenting with mental health issues. The present review showcases a variety of references discussing art therapy, prison rehabilitation, and the intersectionality of both.

The present literature review is divided into five categories to discuss the topic from its simplest to its fullest effect. The categories include: *The Art of Art Therapy, Prison Rehabilitation, Art Therapy in Prison Rehabilitation: Individual and Collective Benefits, Women's Mental Health, Effects of Art Therapy on Female Prison Rehabilitation* and the *Battle of the Sexes*. Section I outlines the functions and approaches of art therapy, regardless of where it takes place and who provides the space (i.e., therapists, counselors, psychologists, psychiatrists, social workers, and even physicians.) This section lays the foundation for what art therapy is and how can it be practiced. Section II explains how prison rehabilitation works, and the roles and benefits of mental health professionals in the prison system. It also mentions ways to use rehabilitation as an intervention, and how they can produce a deep healing process within incarcerated populations when integrated with other techniques. Both section I and II explain what each concept means individually, which serves as a helpful guide for the reader.

Section III examines the benefits of both art therapy and prison rehabilitation, creating a space for healing, a sense of self, creativity, and self-discovery; allowing individuals to separate themselves from their inmate identity. This section explores the benefits of art therapy on both an individual and collective level. Section IV provides insights on women's mental health and the conditions under which it can decline. It also describes which therapy approaches are not effective in prison settings. It focuses on how art therapy is a tool that can make a difference in incarcerated women's lives, in a more effective way than traditional approaches can. The last two categories show the intersection among art therapy, prison rehabilitation and incarcerated women. Section V summarizes the main differences between how art therapy impacts the different genders; it also addresses the effectiveness of this practice in women, highlighting how great improvements in this population are possible. This literature review seeks to explore the effectiveness of art therapy as a medium for prison rehabilitation, focusing on women and their responses to the treatment.

## THE ART OF ART THERAPY AS A PRACTICE

A common theme in psychology and literature discusses how Art Therapy is a creative medium to convey emotions. Art Therapy functions through a variety of approaches and populations, with "not only therapists, but with counselors, psychologists, psychiatrists, social workers, and even physicians who use art expression for therapy (Malchiodi, 2003)." With more mental health professionals employing art therapy to aid their patients, art therapy has appeared to be an important and efficacious tool for connecting with patients and for patients to connect with their emotions. This practice is based on the idea that the creative process of art making is healing and life-enhancing and is a form of nonverbal communication of thoughts and feelings (American Art Therapy Association, 1996, as cited in Malchiodi, 2003). This way, patients with different feelings and in some cases, with mental health conditions, can freely express an array of emotions.

Besides clinical approaches, art therapy has two distinct practice approaches. Edwards (2004) describes these approaches as "two parallel strands: art as therapy and art psychotherapy" (Waller, 1993, as cited in Edwards, 2004). Although these strands focus on slightly different aspects of therapy, creativity is still an important part of emotion-evoking therapeutic moments.

Art therapy emphasizes the healing potential of art, by using art to reflect emotions more freely, connect with oneself and to treat a variety of conditions such as Post-Traumatic Stress Disorder (PTSD), Attention Deficit Hyperactivity Disorder (ADHD) and Anxiety. This approach can also be applied in group settings. Meanwhile, art psychotherapy stresses the importance of the therapeutic relationship established between the art therapist, the client and the artwork (Edwards, 2004). In *Art Therapy* literature by David Edwards, it illustrates a diagram (figure 1) that shows the various directions in which art therapy can work, meaning that it is a non-linear mental health approach. This is known as the triangular relationship of art therapy approaches.

*Figure 1. Diagram*

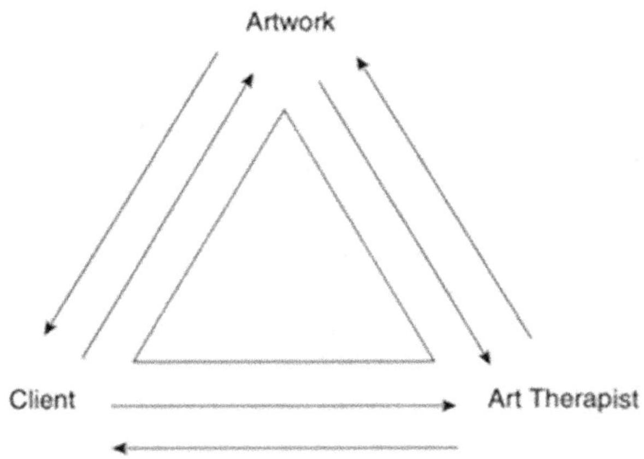


Within the variations of art therapy practices, there are a variety of clinical approaches. Yet, regardless of the clinical approach, art therapy involves both the process and products of image making -from crude scribbling to more sophisticated forms of symbolic expression- and the provision of a therapeutic relationship (Edwards, 2004). As Malchiodi (2003) mentions, the approaches include: psychodynamic, humanistic, learning and developmental, family therapy and other approaches.

- Psychodynamic: Images of the unconscious to display transference and defense mechanisms of the individual, having the therapist as a support figure.
- Humanistic: Sharing an optimistic view of human nature and of the human condition; seeing people in a process of growth and development, with the potential to take responsibility for their fate (Rubin, 1987/2001, as cited in Malchiodi, 2003).
- Learning and developmental: Art therapy as a tool to work with populations such as children with disabilities, whether physical or emotional, fostering cognitive development.
- Family therapy and other approaches: The incorporation and adaptability of art therapy in different approaches such as transpersonal practices, marriage and family therapy, and spiritual concepts.

With these clinical approaches, the client has the ability to delve into all sorts of feelings and emotions. Depending on their needs, specific or various approaches can be implemented to understand who they are as an individual and how their surroundings can cause them discomfort and distress. Having different approaches enables the treatment to be more tailored and more meaningful for inmates.

## PRISON REHABILITATION

In prison rehabilitation, specifically in women's prisons, psychologists play an important role, but there is always a downside. As discussed by Benson (2003), when there's a lack of funding and strict sentencing guidelines, it is harder for inmates to get rehabilitated. However, he highlights the benefits of mental health professionals in the prison system who provide mental health services to the prison population. This type of support is crucial since inmates suffer rates of mental illness at least three times higher than the national average (Benson, 2003). Although prison rehabilitation is not new, it's importance has diminished. As Benson (2003) pointed out, until the mid-1970's, rehabilitation was a key part of the U.S. prison policy. Prisoners were encouraged to develop occupational skills and to resolve psychological problems such as substance abuse or aggression that might interfere with their reintegration into society.

Prison rehabilitation has changed; the system has been supplemented with different approaches for support, but rehabilitation took a back-seat due to states getting tougher on crimes. These states saw punishment as the prison's main function rather than rehabilitating individuals to re-enter society (Benson, 2003). This approach created an unstable situation in the prison system. In contrast to punishment being the principal purpose of prison, Benson (2003) noted that individual-centered approaches to crime prevention need to be complemented by community-based approaches. This direction will help individuals in every way, leading to a more effective individual-based approach. That said, van der Meulen and Omstead (2021) suggest that without attention to broader systemic barriers, social injustices, and neo-liberal contexts, prison arts programs can perpetuate and uphold simplistic and individualized understandings of criminal justice involvement. In other words, art programs and approaches can do the opposite of what they're intended to accomplish if art therapy is the only form of rehabilitation that inmates are receiving. Using diverse approaches to heal is important but they should be accompanied by justice and proper procedures in the criminal system, to fairly represent and aid the inmates.

It is important to note that Prison Rehabilitation or Criminal Rehabilitation are terms used "without clear referent, and in ways that are consistent with widely divergent conceptions (Forsberg and Douglas, 2020)." It is for this reason that it is important to have a clear definition of what prison/criminal rehabilitation is and does. This leads to a better understanding of rehabilitation and may allow society to better appraise moral objections to rehabilitation and rehabilitative theories of criminal justice (Forsberg and Douglas, 2020). Prison and criminal rehabilitation can help inmates connect with their emotions and grow; this can be done through emotional connection while being removed from the environment that triggers negative emotions, negative behaviors, and discomfort. Rehabilitation is a matter of restoring the inmates' social or moral standing in society, their social or moral relations with others, and/or fostering the capacities needed for such restoration (Forsberg and Douglas, 2020).

Based on this definition, Forsberg and Douglas (2020) offer us a better understanding of rehabilitation. The aforementioned definition helps us determine the extent to which rehabilitation theories are capable of overcoming other significant concerns that caused them to fall out of favor. Yet, it is important to note that rehabilitation as described above, is not the same as reform. The differences are outlined, as follows: reform seeks to alter character traits, motivations, or dispositions while rehabilitation aims to improve skills, capacities, and opportunities (Forsberg and Douglas, 2020). Put simply, the key difference between the two concepts involves altering character traits rather than improving skills. Additionally, Forsberg and Douglas (2020) mentioned two ways to use rehabilitation as an intervention: for anti-recidivism and harm-reduction. Anti-recidivism refers to an intervention by the criminal justice system that reduces the possibilities of future offenses. This intervention prepares inmates with the necessary tools according to their needs, for their transition out of prison. Harm-reduction refers to an intervention by the criminal justice system to prevent harmful conduct by the inmate. This intervention works with inmates to address their behaviors through safe practices and treatment plans, to improve their overall health. This way, rehabilitation, if joined with other techniques, such as art therapy, will allow for deeper healing. For example, according to Keehan (2015), a repeated theme in the discourse on theater practice in prisons over the last 20 years (in Canada) can be summarized as follows: theater and drama projects have a positive effect on those who are incarcerated and may contribute toward rehabilitation (van der Meulen & Omstead, 2021). Furthermore, supporting the notion of a positive effect as a part of art programing, van der Meulen and Omstead (2021) state that many artists who facilitate prison programs have aligned their work with the distancing theory of crime, a theory that states that a reduction in recidivism results from a changes in lifestyle, related in particular to an individual's maturation or growing up and out of time.

Although the van der Meulen and Omstead (2021) study was conducted in Canada, it nevertheless provides insight into crime rehabilitation and how it relates to practices put in place. However, it reminds the reader that although prison shouldn't be the place where people are placed to heal from trauma, the resources can and should be used for the benefit of mental health reformation. In their study, rehabilitation was not the ultimate goal of the arts program, but rather it focused on the participants' experiences, such as community building and artistic engagement (van der Meulen and Omstead, 2021). Their study took place at a women's federal prison with a weekly arts program, consisting of activities and workshops using a variety of artistic tools, that proved to be successful, especially for the purpose of community building (van der Meulen and Omstead, 2021).

## ART THERAPY IN PRISON REHABILITATION: INDIVIDUAL AND COLLECTIVE BENEFITS

Art Therapy and Prison Rehabilitation as separate entities have their own benefits, but when art therapy is added to a general prison rehabilitation program, a new possibility of healing is created. Gussak (2016) reinforces the importance of art therapy in prison environments. There are many societal beliefs that inmates do not need emotional support; however, the author explains that mental health support and art therapy are the types of help that this population needs, since they have had their "identity stripped away" by imprisonment.

Moreover, the author explains that generalizing and stereotyping the prison population is damaging for inmates, especially inmates with mental health conditions. This generalization can prevent inmates from greatly benefiting from art therapy practices. For example, the author mentions that a common and uneducated notion is that such inmates do not deserve such support and attention because they are criminals, they have 'broken societal laws' and 'therefore do not deserve the support of the system' (Gussak, 2016). These notions are and can continue to be harmful, not only for the rehabilitation of an individual but for collective rehabilitation, as well. Individuals may fail to recognize that those who are in prison, are a mirror of the society from which they've emerged (Gussak, 2016). Recognizing this, Gussak (2016) suggests that the first act of true social justice is to give imprisoned folks a voice, a new label, a sense of self, and to help them rise above their current situation and confront their emotions. Art therapy, in such a restricted environment, creates an opportunity in prison rehabilitation for inmates to express themselves through a non-verbal activity, giving them this one-on-one personal time with themselves; helping them gain a healthier sense of self, separate from their inmate identity (Gussak, 2016). Art therapy can truly be a vessel for humanizing those who have been previously dehumanized, (Gussak, 2016). Creating these spaces where developing a sense of self and belonging is encouraged through art therapy and art psychotherapy, allows the inmates to be in touch with their identity and emotions.

Brewster (2014) brings to light the importance of art therapy, through a 12-week art program study. The participants were inmates from a variety of state prisons, who reported on their behavior in a pre and post program survey. Results of the surveys show the impact of said programs on the inmates, and their lack of ability to regulate emotions and to reduce disciplinary actions before the healing practices were put into place. The author reiterates how the benefit of this program goes beyond the inmate, since it also allows for their families, society, and the prison environment to enjoy positive outcomes due to the arts program. Individuals reconnecting to society through art, was among the benefits of arts in prisons, according to Brewster. Research and experience suggest that prison arts programs have significant benefits and positive outcomes for the incarcerated, their families, the prison environment, and society (Brewster, 2014). Brewster (2014) notes that research shows that people of any age can feel a sense of emotional satisfaction when involved in the creative process. This satisfaction comes from having control over art materials, or a musical instrument, the use of words in writing, or lines memorized and acted out in a play, since all of these methods lead to self-expression and creativity (Brewster, 2014).

Art therapy is arguably making a 'comeback' in the prison rehabilitation programs, since it is a staple and is a wonderful tool for creativity and expression. Regardless, the prison art programs in the United States declined sharply in the 1980s, likely due to demands by political leaders and the public for prisons to cease providing prisoners with what were thought to be unwarranted privileges and amenities (Johnson, 2007). However, art therapy had prevailed through time as a form of rehabilitation, due to research that has shown great improvements in the mental health of those who use it in programs. Art therapy offers a mode of judgement-free expression, that can be used to treat incarcerated clients who suffer from substance abuse issues, mental illnesses and disabilities, physical impairments, child abuse and other victimization issues. Issues of grief and loss, in addition to help in identifying those who may be potentially harmful to themselves, are further boons to Art Therapy (Johnson, 2007). Although individual benefits of art therapy are seen more frequently, collective benefits are also an important part of art therapy in prison rehabilitation, such as in group and family therapy. Art can help improve and maintain relationships between inmates and their families. The artwork can convey thoughts and feelings to family members, that are difficult to express verbally, as well as a way to provide them with gifts (Johnson, 2007). This is not possible though, if harsh conditions affect the outcomes of rehabilitation. Johnson's (2007) study found the following:

*Prisoners who become distressed by, or adapt to, this environment are not being equipped for cooperative relationships and achieving personal growth during the stay, or for re-entry and re-integration into the community. Humanizing the prison environment would reduce the "prisonization" of incarcerated persons, reducing potential barriers to rehabilitation. Art programs help humanize the prison environment. (p. 77).*

## WOMEN'S MENTAL HEALTH: EFFECTS OF ART THERAPY ON WOMEN'S PRISON REHABILITATION

The intersection of art therapy and women's prison rehabilitation includes a range of populations, such as grieving women, and women who have a variety of mental health conditions. Women in prison have a diverse range of mental health conditions, including trauma such as PTSD (post-traumatic stress disorder). Additionally, those who are incarcerated (Erikson, 2008) have limited access to mental health treatment. Traditional therapies, like cognitive behavioral therapy and exposure therapy, which require intense and individual counseling, are unfortunately not practical in a prison setting. Many therapists agree that since memories of trauma are stored in a *visual form*, it is a natural and effective practice to encourage visual representation of the memories before a verbal disclosure of them (Rubin, 2001 and Gladding, 2005, as cited in Erickson, 2008).

A study by Erickson (2008) examined how effective art therapy can be as an intervention for decreasing symptoms of trauma and psychological distress in incarcerated women. The study was carried out in six sessions of art therapy, where a two-part (pre/post) survey was distributed at different jails across the southeast of the United States. Additional data was collected through observation; the study was limited with only 26 participants. Regardless, positive feedback was displayed on the post-study survey for individual treatment. In contrast, the overall scores on the surveys did not have significance regarding the symptoms being measured, but participants were able to experience decreased psychological distress and symptoms of trauma after the art therapy was completed. Similarly, in a more recent study, Nambiar and Joy (2020) explored how emotional wellness can improve the situation for incarcerated women. This study employed art therapy practices to determine how women with poor emotional wellness, reacted to this treatment. Poor emotional wellness was used as an umbrella term for women who had experienced trauma from being separated from their families, long conviction times, and more (Nambiar and Joy, 2020). The study engaged 60 participants from two different prisons; the study used Tanjore, a major art form from classical South Indian paintings with vivid colors, as the art therapy tool. This medium was used as a way for the participants to channel their emotions and use their imagination and creativity while creating artwork. The use of vivid colors helped ease their minds to be more present with their feelings and focus on the art. Art therapy with this art form, was a means of catharsis for them. Nambiar and Joy (2020) assumed that art therapy can be an intervention for incarcerated women to cope with adversities and allow them to live their lives fully by being authentic about their emotions.

Another group of women who have been in art therapy studies are women who have experienced the death of a loved one. Ferszt et al. (2004) showcases a study on incarcerated women who are grieving. The study had a duration of eight weeks with one-hour sessions. With eight participants -all incarcerated women- the study reinforced the practice and implementation of art therapy as a medium to improve mental health in prisons. The researchers (Ferszt et al., 2004) used the following participation criteria: the participant had experienced the death of a significant person during imprisonment, the participant had the ability to speak and read English, and the participant had no major medical or psychiatric health issues that would interfere with the ability to participate in the study.

Furthermore, throughout the duration of the study, the participants had clinical staff available upon request and were also made aware that their information was confidential unless they were in imminent danger. The results of this study revealed that art therapy was, in fact, an effective tool for processing internalized and repressed emotions, etc. The participants' testimonies were positive overall; they were able to share how art therapy helped them look inward and discover positive aspects of themselves. It was reported that some of the participants even kept the art they created as a reminder of their journey, creative ability, and competence.

Studies with art practices and women who are aging, have been crucial in the understanding of wellness and healing. Many studies have indicated that older adults benefit from wellness programs and health initiatives that are well-rounded and inclusive of all their needs (Wahidin, 2004, as cited in Hongo, et al., 2015). Hongo, et al. (2015) shine a light on the aging female prison population, for which the prison setting is not typically designed. Hongo, et al. (2015), examined how different themes in art therapy can be used in a creative way for aging women in prison, since this modality can perhaps reduce the number of visits to the mental health unit and the need for costly medication. The art therapy themes included: the potential to dream, feeling connected, mutual understanding, releasing of feelings and unselfish concern.

Hongo et al. (2015) engaged 20 participants who were women between the ages of 50 and 76; most were survivors of domestic violence and/or other traumatic experiences. Most hailed from different backgrounds, which created a very diverse sample of participants. The art workshops for aging female prisoners, consisted of six art expression workshops to encourage the practice of freely expressing their feelings in a nonjudgmental and relaxed environment. The "healing squad," a group of interns from a variety of mental health specializing schools (including social work and marriage & family therapy) led the one-hour workshops. These workshops helped the inmates be in touch with their emotions, connect with others and challenge themselves. It was a way to foster a supportive community, allowing them to reconnect with their identity. According to Hongo, et al. (2015), the results indicated that art therapy groups encourage support between members by offering creative ideas and positive outcomes, and by soliciting healing connections with others.

Similarly, a study described by Santamaría (2019) explores the use of different art therapy practices such a visual art and collaborative poetry among incarcerated women in a medium security prison. The participants were all women with serious mental illness and histories of trauma who participated in a two-hour session. The participants hailed from diverse backgrounds and were all diagnosed with PTSD, in addition to other diagnoses such as depressions and personality disorders. The women's ages ranged from 31 to 58 and they were white cisgender women, with one participant presenting with gender dysphoria. The participants showed progress during the art therapy intervention encouraging the connection between art therapy and healing trauma for incarcerated women. This connection consisted of creating deep emotional bonds with other participants and the facilitators, that enabled the expression of complex feelings and emotions within themselves and around others. Materials such as watercolors, chalk, oil pastels, crayons, and markers, were used for the two art therapy sessions. Both sessions had the same structure: brief check in, warm up, art making, group discussion and closure. The results showed that the participants responded favorably to both sessions and to their various methods of art therapy, helping them demonstrate self-awareness, ability to work with others and improvements in behaviors. The participants remained active and engaged throughout the group session, even with non-mandatory attendance. No distance or negative feelings were observed nor communicated throughout the sessions (Santamaría, 2019). All of these studies show evidence that incarcerated women with varying trauma histories and mental health conditions benefit from art therapy as a healing modality. It is hoped that the prison system continues to aid in the healing of women in the system.

## BATTLE OF THE SEXES

Another notable aspect of art therapy in prison rehabilitation is the discrepancy between men and women. Gussak (2014) examined the impact of art therapy on male and female inmates and how it affected their mood and locus of control, based on gender. The results showed that females presented with higher levels of depression, an external locus of control, and more antisocial tendencies, prior to the study, compared to men. The women in the study also showed greater improvement in mood and locus of control, or feelings of empowerment, after the art therapy programs were over. Gussak (2014) noted that diverse approaches may cause different reactions toward inmates, depending on gender. Group art therapy appeared helpful for both females and males, although their journey to get there (into therapy) was different. The author grouped them into three general categories:

- Female inmates who exhibited higher levels of depression than their male counterparts at the outset of the study.
- Female inmates who exhibited a more external locus of control than their male counterparts at the start of the study.
- The men and women ended with similar scores on depression and locus of control. Were female inmates more susceptible to art therapy interventions?

These differences in Gussak's (2014) study show how using the same practices within art therapy in different groups, could result in diverse outcomes. Additionally, in an earlier article, Gussak (2009) examines the difference of gender in art therapy on inmates. In this study, the focus was to determine how art therapy impacts female and male inmates with depression. The researcher used a pre-test/post-test control group design, with two hypotheses addressing how effective art therapy is in prison inmates. The participants were from medium to maximum adult correctional facilities and were assigned to either a control or experimental group, with three measurement tools. Despite the results of the Formal Elements Art Therapy Scale (FEATS), the overall results indicated that art therapy was in fact effective, and the results from both the Beck Depression Inventory-Short Form (BDI-II) and Adult Nowicki-Strickland Locus of Control Scale (ANS) supported the assumption that art therapy was effective in reducing depression and improving locus of control in adult male and female inmates. Though Gussak (2009) noted an important distinction - a trend indicated that female inmates showed a greater improvement in mood and internal locus of control than their fellow male inmates. This may be further evidence that while both genders can benefit from art therapy while incarcerated, women's mental health may be significantly improved with art.

## CONCLUSION

The research gathered for the intersection of art therapy and prison rehabilitation demonstrate art therapy's effectiveness with this specific demographic. Different themes were identified through the articles: women's mental health, aging women, grieving inmates and women versus men. Through these themes, it was confirmed that art therapy is effective with incarcerated women, yielding similar or better results than in incarcerated men. The results indicate that art therapy or arts programs in the themes identified above, are successful across the board, even when met with more difficulties such as complex trauma diagnoses. Overall, art therapy appears to be an effective modality for nonverbal therapy in different settings, using different approaches such as: psychodynamic, humanistic, learning and development, and family therapy, along with other approaches. Additionally, although a number of studies support the notion of rehabilitation through the arts in incarcerated women and it has been shown to work, not much literature can be found on this matter, let alone on specific groups of women. Regardless, incarcerated women with suppressed emotions and or memories could benefit the most from art therapy, since it is a creative and nonverbal way to effectively communicate how they feel.

## FUTURE DIRECTIONS

As mentioned earlier, the work on art therapy as a form of prison rehabilitation on incarcerated woman is limited. With this obstacle, current researchers have a harder time gathering information about the topic. The studies in this chapter engaged the prison population of women; further research is recommended to gather a wide array of data for varying populations of women. For future research on this topic, it would be beneficial not only to have more access to research in this area, but to also have studies about art therapy rehabilitation and its specific impact on women of color and women with diverse backgrounds. These would not only reveal if art therapy is effective across all groups of incarcerated women, but how to optimally implement it across groups. At the time of this research, almost no articles about the impact of art therapy in women of color were either accessible or in existence. If this gap can be filled with sufficient research on woman of color undergoing art therapy as rehabilitation in prison, it would ensure a more diverse pool of participants and accurate findings.

## REFERENCES

Benson, E. (2003). Rehabilitate or Punishment? *American Psychological Association*. https://www.apa.org/monitor/julaug03/rehab

Brewster, L. (2014). The Impact of Prison Arts Programs on Inmate Attitudes and Behavior: A Quantitative Evaluation. *Justice Policy Journal*, *11*(2), 1–28.

Edwards, D. (2004). *Art therapy*. Sage Publications.

Erickson, B. (2008). *Art Therapy Treatment with Incarcerated Women*. [Doctoral Dissertation, University of Central Florida]. STARS.

Ferszt, G., Hayes, P. M., DeFedele, S., & Horn, L. (2004). Art Therapy with Incarcerated Women Who Have Experienced the Death of a Loved One. *Art Therapy: Journal of the American Art Therapy Association, 21*(4), 191–199. doi:10.1080/07421656.2004.10129695

Forsberg, L., & Douglas, T. (2020). What is Criminal Rehabilitation? *Criminal Law and Philosophy*, 1–24. doi:10.100711572-020-09547-4 PMID:35530429

Gussak, D. (2009). Comparing the effectiveness of art therapy on depression and locus of control of male and female inmates. *The Arts in Psychotherapy*, *36*(4), 202–207. doi:10.1016/j.aip.2009.02.004

Gussak, D. (2009). The effects of art therapy on male and female inmates: Advancing the research base. *The Arts in Psychotherapy*, *36*(1), 5–12. doi:10.1016/j.aip.2008.10.002

Gussak, D. (2014). The Distinction Between Male and Female Inmates in Art Therapy. *Psychology Today*. https://www.psychologytoday.com/us/blog/art-trial/201401/the-distinctions-between-and-inmates-in-art-therapy

Gussak, D. (2016). Art Therapy in Prison Is Social Justice. *Psychology Today*. www.psychologytoday.com/gb/blog/art-trial/201602/art-therapy-in-prison-is-social-justice

Hongo, A., Katz, A., & Valenti, K. (2015). Art: Trauma to Therapy for Aging Female Prisoners. *Traumatology*, *21*(3), 201–207. https://www.researchgate.net/publication/281537684_Art_Trauma_to_Therapy_for_Aging_Female_Prisoners. doi:10.1037/trm0000042

Johnson, L. M. (2007). Jail Wall Drawings and Jail Art Programs: Invaluable Tools for Corrections. *International Journal of Criminal Justice*, *2*(2), 66–84. https://www.sascv.org/ijcjs/jhonsonijcjsjuly2007.pdf

Malchiodi, C. (2003). *Handbook of art therapy*. The Guilford Press.

Nambiar, N., & Joy, M. (2020). Impact of Art Therapy on Emotional Wellness among Incarcerated Women. *International Journal for Research in Engineering Application & Management*, *6*(3), 1–6.

Santamaría, M. L. (2019). *Creating Connection: Group Expressive Arts Therapy with Incarcerated Women.* [Capstone Thesis, Graduate School of Arts and Social Sciences]. Expressive Therapies Capstone Theses.

Schouten, K. A., de Niet, G. J., Knipscheer, J. W., Kleber, R. J., & Hutschemaekers, G. J. M. (2015). The Effectiveness of Art Therapy in the Treatment of Traumatized Adults: A Systematic Review on Art Therapy and Trauma. *Trauma, Violence & Abuse, 16*(2), 220–228. doi:10.1177/1524838014555032 PMID:25403446

van der Meulen, E., & Omstead, J. (2021). The Limits of Rehabilitation and Recidivism Reduction: Rethinking the Evaluation of Arts Programming in Prisons. *The Prison Journal, 101*(1), 102–122. doi:10.1177/0032885520978477

## KEY TERMS AND DEFINITIONS

**Art therapy:** integrated mental health and form of psychotherapy that involves encouragement and self-expression through art such as painting, drawing and more.

**Cognitive behavioral therapy:** CBT is a type of psychotherapeutic treatment that helps people learn how to identify and change destructive or disturbing thought patters that have a negative influence on behavior and emotions.

**External locus of control:** the person generally believes that their successes or failures result from external factors beyond their control.

**Internal locus of control:** when people believe that their success or failure is a result of the effort and hard work they invested in their education.

**Prison rehabilitation:** the process of helping inmates grow and change, allowing them to separate themselves from the environmental factors that made them commit a crime in the first place.

**Psychotherapy:** the treatment of mental health disorders by psychological rather than medical means.

**PTSD:** short for post-traumatic stress disorder, is an anxiety disorder that develops in reaction to physical injury and/or severe mental or emotional distress.

**Recidivism:** the tendency of a convicted criminal to reoffend.

# Chapter 5
# History of Art Therapy as an Effective Treatment for Cognitive Deficit and Disorders With Psychotic Features

**Emmalynne Knuth**
*Marymount Manhattan College, USA*

## ABSTRACT

*The lasting positive impact of Art Therapy on clients is expansive and widely understood, however there has been little research done to quantify this data. The research found that the data that is available shows a significant, positive impact on clients who attend art therapy as a means of treatment for personality, mood, and psychotic disorders as well as those with disorders characterized by varying levels of cognitive deficit. This review analyzes the effects of taking part in an art therapy program on the aforementioned groups and addresses the issue of accessibility to care, weighing the ethics of experiential, self-directed art therapy.*

## INTRODUCTION

In the contemporary world, the need for access to mental health care has grown significantly and with it the variety of services clinicians can offer has also grown, from more standard talk therapies to now more creative treatment options. These innovative programs have expanded to include practices such as dance, art, music,

DOI: 10.4018/978-1-6684-7856-1.ch005

drama, and equine therapy. While these forms of therapy are relatively new, art therapy is one form of treatment that has grown in popularity due to its more accessible nature in terms of materials and individualized to one's personal artistic ability. The effects of exploring the self and emotions through creating and interpreting visual imagery have significantly and positively impacted those who attend art therapy. As the research shows in this review, art therapy can be a successful modality in treating a wide variety of disorders as well as in aiding clients in the general direction of growing a sense of identity and developing the ability for free expression.

## Fundamentals of Art Therapy

Art therapy's acceptance into the public domain as a valid therapeutic approach was a contemporary movement, taking place simultaneously between primarily Europe and America in the mid-20th century. The words "art therapy" were first used in 1940s England by artists and patients of sanatoriums, who discovered that making art was a beneficial way to experience freedom and a constructive way to process emotions about the time. The term rose in popularity post World War II and mental health care providers including psychologists, psychiatrists, and social workers began to utilize these creative outlets as forms of treatment.

As the movement grew, Malchiodi (2012) explains that two American psychologists were at the forefront of this movement, Edith Kramer and Margaret Naumburg. Margaret Naumburg is often thought of as the "mother of art therapy" since she is considered the main founder of the American art therapy movement, which gained momentum in the 1960s and 70s, making way for some of the first organized research in the area.

## Margaret Naumburg

Naumburg is primarily credited with her expansion on the theory that children develop better when they can express themselves creatively and pursue subjects that are aligned with their own specific interests. Naumburg was heavily influenced by theories involving the psychoanalytic approach to therapy and she viewed visual language and art-making processes as tools to receive clearer communication about one's unconscious thoughts and emotions.

Her personal treatment approach consisted of trying to take the visual experience of her client's mind and combine it with verbal communication to achieve a true level of healing, believing that this goal was entirely possible through art therapy sessions. She would go on to author several publications and books that have stood the test of time and have become staple pieces of literature in the art therapy world and are still useful resources today.

## Edith Kramer

Edith Kramer was another giant in the field of art therapy and was able to build from the foundations that Margaret Naumburg set by focusing her work on the sublimation aspect of art therapy. She believed that sublimation was the key to the success of the therapy and focused heavily on the principle of making something productive out of any negative emotions that may arise during the session. Kramer and Naumburg helped to pave the way for the development of innovative ideas on the use of creativity to heal.

## Contemporary Methods and Materials

Today, art therapists operate on expanded Naumburg and Kramer theories and use various methodologies to conduct their sessions toward the direction of free thinking and expression. As seen through case studies provided by Case & Dalley (2014*)*, an art therapy session can consist of a variety of projects like painting, drawing, sculpture, collage or even using textiles; these sessions can also use any kind of medium such as oil paint, charcoal, ink, graphite, markers, crayons, or truly anything that would be necessary to create art since the supplies are simply modes to get the emotions out.

These case studies also indicate that art therapy is an effective resource for individuals of various ages and abilities, so the necessary methods and mediums for art-making are highly client-specific and can change as necessary because what works for one client/group will not always work for the other. Since materials and methods of art-making can vary so widely depending on the client, it is important to also assess the types of approaches: psychoanalytic, cognitive-behavioral, humanistic, and multimodal.

# TYPES OF THERAPEUTIC APPROACHES

## Psychoanalytic Model

Rubin (2015) was able to discuss the main goals of the psychoanalytic approach to treatment which includes a focus on the client's inner world. Art therapists who work under this model are often concerned with the correction of developmental tasks and working to create an environment where growth is driven by the freedom of self-expression, wherein the therapist guides the sessions based on client needs. Interpretation of the final products is also largely important to this model of treatment.

### Cognitive-Behavioral Model

Cognitive-behavioral models of art therapy as suggested by Rosal (2018) are mostly reliant on behavioral modification through the development of healthy coping mechanisms and the rewiring of thought processes. This model teaches clients how to recognize and disengage from harmful behavior by exploring core beliefs that are best explained through visual constructs and using that to redirect behavior. Cognitive Behavioral Therapy (CBT) is one of the most common therapies used to treat disorders characterized by behavioral issues and negative rumination since it aims to change the client's destructive patterns and to replace them with healthier coping strategies.

### Humanistic and Multimodal Models

The humanistic approach contrasts with the cognitive-behavioral and psychoanalytic models since it operates from a place of helping clients focus on strengthening their will to live and working to develop a more optimistic outlook. As Garai (1984) described, humanistic methods of art therapy tend to follow a holistic personality integration direction by helping the clients to find identity and meaning in their lives through the freedom of expression. Finally, because of the nature of freedom within the practice of art therapy, many clinicians choose to employ multimodal approaches that are dependent on the client.

## EFFECTS OF ART THERAPY ON MOOD DISORDER SYMPTOMS

### Common Therapeutic Approaches

In patients with mood disorders and disorders characterized with psychotic effects, the most common approach to art therapy is Cognitive-Behavioral Therapy. In a case study by Lefebvre (2008), the results yielded by the study correlated to symptom reduction in behaviorally troubled adolescents who are typically treatment resistant. The clinician developed the ability to identify manic episodes before they occurred by looking for cues in the adolescent's artwork and reactions to work; in doing so, the therapist was able to build rapport with the client and the client found it easier to express his feelings visually rather than verbally with the therapist.

The therapist in this case also indicated that a multimodal approach may be helpful since it was also noted that after forging a working relationship, the adolescent became more engaged with the therapist since he was allowed to direct sessions toward his own specific hobbies and interests, which followed a more psychoanalytic approach.

## Bipolar Disorder

This multimodal approach was also described by Henley (2007) wherein the case studies demonstrated that art therapy can be valuable in treating pediatric populations diagnosed with early forms of bipolar disorder and other comorbid conditions, especially when it is difficult to find other effective methods of treatment. The study consisted of the vignettes of four children and young adolescents who took part in over 184 sessions with sixteen children over the course of 2-1/2 years. The cases selected for the report were representative of these sixteen cases involving children ages nine to fifteen who received thirty-two trials of art therapy with an emphasis on encouraging healthy sublimation of impulses and proper integration of one's sense of self for client autonomy to minimize any dichotomy.

The researcher was able to conclude that there was some level of progress made with each of the cases to varying degrees. Each of the clients mentioned in the brief vignettes saw a general reduction of symptoms and were able to express their current mental state to the clinician through the visual picture plane. Some children with more mixed-type bipolar symptoms had an easier time creating structures for ideas and feelings, while those with more manic symptoms were able to use their time to create art that helped them understand constant flows of emotion.

After reviewing these case studies, the consensus seems to be that art therapy is a helpful intervention tool for individuals with bipolar disorder and even for those with pediatric forms of the disorder. Research does suggest that younger patients typically have a better response to creative arts therapy since adult clients may be wary of having such freedom and tend to be reserved and unsure. In a relevant experiment conducted by Petrillo, Winner (2005), the findings suggest that after viewing a series of traumatic images, the group that performed art making as a means of catharsis and redirection saw a greater range of improved mood while the group that was asked to put together a word puzzle, did not experience an improved mood. These findings suggest that more psychically expressive means of redirection and catharsis can help clients process traumatic images and increase the pleasure dimension of mood.

One can also hypothesize from these findings that expressive arts therapies may be particularly helpful to those with mood disorders, who have also been victims of traumatic experiences. This research provided a significant clue as to why art therapy can be a highly effective supplemental tool in the treatment of mood disorders, including for bipolar disorder. The article briefly mentions that there were only five instances where the interventions were not completely successful and precipitated the splitting in clients between "good" and "bad" ideologies. Aside from the generalizations that these clients all had acute illness and the intervention was not accurately presented or explained by the facilitator, there is not a detailed explanation as to why these interventions were not successful and further research is warranted.

## Schizophrenia and Schizoaffective

The study conducted by Ruddy and Milnes (2005) noted via correlation that among the patients with schizophrenia, the patients assigned to the art therapy group were more likely to fully complete their allocated therapy sessions whereas those assigned to the standard group/talk therapy were less likely on average to fully complete the full number of sessions allocated to them. This and the additional data provided in the study allow us to make the inference that patients assigned to the art therapy group saw the most improvement in terms of general mental state. With the general mental state of these patients improving, we can begin to examine our broadened understanding of the potential main motivations for using art therapy in lieu of traditional practices. The authors state that they believe one possible explanation for this improvement in this population is that art therapy offers certain freedoms, allowing the patients to express their mental state in a way that is safe and offers a direct visual explanation of their inner world more so than perhaps a spoken statement. The data from the study showed a small but significant difference that favored the art therapy groups, but because of the general lack of studies in this particular field, further research is necessary to conclude this with certainty. However, this study did bring attention to the fact that art therapy may only be effective in cases of psychotic disorders if it is performed in a more structured environment under close supervision by a clinician and if the art therapy is supplemental to a regular medication regimen as the first line of treatment.

## Role of Psychotic Symptoms in Treatment

Killick and Schaverien (1997) argue this same theory that art therapy is best practiced under the close supervision of a clinician who can offer several helpful observations about the sessions. When working, it is the job of the art therapist to provide an environment built on trust that allows artwork to be made, seen, and evaluated with trained eyes for it to be most effective; this is especially important with those who are developmentally sensitive. It is mentioned that when working with clients who have psychotic tendencies, there need to be boundaries in which the imagination can have the freedom to be expressed but also enough structure to promote healing and acceptance. The case studies explored here offer better insights into this theory and explain that individuals with psychotic illnesses will always utilize some level of psychotic defense mechanisms, structured art therapy also allows these clients to build more mature defense mechanisms that allow them to better function in relation to their psychotic disorders. Many of these theories were influenced by Edith Kramer and by Freudian ideologies.

Additionally, the case study by Hanevik, Hestad, Lien, Teglbjaerg, and Danbolt (2013) suggests that while the exact mechanisms that cause art therapy to be efficacious are still relatively unknown, there is great value in the use of creative therapy techniques in patients who suffer from psychosis. The clients in this study self-reported improvements in their ability to differentiate between reality and delusions through semi-structured interviews. This case study also included human spirituality and religion, which are often absent from more quantitative research. It should be noted that clients also had a better understanding of existential perception and their experience of spirituality after art therapy. Possible limitations of this study include the studied population, since it was only women and a small sample size.

## EFFECTS OF ART THERAPY ON PERSONALITY DISORDER SYMPTOMS

### Improvements in Behavior and Mood

Like mood and psychotic disorders, Fonagy (2012) and Haeyen, Chakhssi, Van Hooren (2020) explored several theories in relation to clients who were diagnosed with a personality disorder and their growth progress through art therapy. The readings suggest that while art therapy is under-researched as a whole, it has been a particularly therapeutic tool for individuals with personality disorders. Art therapy seems particularly helpful in connecting with others and creating pathways for communication that may otherwise be difficult for those with a personality disorder.

Research suggests that art making is inherently human and that may be why art therapy is so effective for its clientele. In addition, the research suggests that a great number of clients with personality disorders say improvements due to art therapy programs. It is suggested, however, that the benefit increases over time and clients who were able to associate more meaningful expression in the work they created, derived the most benefit. These articles, like the Killick and Schaverien (1997) text, suggested that clients with personality disorders do best in a structured environment that offers a judgment free zone, adequate freedom to create, and an empathic practitioner who takes them seriously.

### Effects on Acute Psychotic Symptoms

Preliminary research reported by Montag, Haase, Seidel, Bayerl, Gallinat and Herrmann, (2014) offers a generally positive outcome of art therapy for patients with characteristics that are attributed to borderline personality disorder, who experience acute psychotic symptoms. The research showed a correlation between art therapy and a reduction of positive and negative symptoms and an improved level of psychosocial functioning. In the group that received art therapy, the patients demonstrated a greater sense of emotional awareness, especially in their ability to show empathy for others. The report does mention that this is one of the first studies of its kind, but the results indicated that further research would be helpful in gathering more substantiation for the results of this study.

## EFFECTS OF ART THERAPY ON INDIVIDUALS WITH COGNITIVE IMPAIRMENT

### Alzheimer's and Dementia

Through the previous research discussed, it has been established that art therapy offers benefits for improving symptoms of various other disorders, it has also been helpful with disorders that are characterized by cognitive impairment like Alzheimer's and other forms of Dementia. Chancellor, Duncan, and Chatterjee (2014) discovered in their research that patients with Alzheimer's Disease and other forms of Dementia can make, view, and appreciate the visual arts. Research studies suggest that art therapy may improve their symptoms as well as their self-image, thus benefiting and aiding in improving social behavior.

This information can be further supplemented by a neurological study conducted by Lusebrink (2004) that discovered correlations between stimulation associated with expressive therapies and activation of specific areas within the brain that process that sensory input. Knowing that there is specific brain activation in relation to visual and tactile stimulation when making art as a method of therapy demonstrates to the reader that art therapy has the potential to assist in healing/acceptance on a neurologic level and could help establish better neuroplasticity. This may help to explain why creative and expressive therapies are so effective in communities with forms of dementia.

## Autism Spectrum Disorder and ADHD

Disorders like ASD (autism spectrum disorder) and ADHD/ADD (attention deficit hyperactivity disorder/ attention deficit disorder) are also characterized by forms of developmental delay and cognitive deficit in terms of social relationships, attention/ decision making, and issues in the acquisition and learning of various forms of information. While there is paucity of research with this population, an experiment by Schwiezer, Knorth, Van Yperen, Spreen (2020) reported that Expressive Art Therapies may benefit and act as an intervention tool in improving the social behavior and mood of children with autism spectrum disorders (ASD).

The researchers observed and maintained data for an art therapy group of eight to twelve year old children with ASD who had concerning behaviors and needed intervention. Over the course of the program, all children were scored through teacher, therapist, parent, and a self-reported self-image scale. By the end of the program, all the children were reportedly much happier and several of them saw significant improvements in their behavior. These findings suggest that art therapy is a helpful intervention tool for children with ASD and potentially for other developmental disorders like ADHD and ADD, as well.

The research conducted by Habib and Ali (2015) also reflects this idea that expressive arts therapies are of particular benefit to children with various kinds of cognitive impairments, specifically ADHD that is comorbid with other intellectual disabilities. The study was created from an experimental design which included data collection from different schools specializing in students with special needs. The sample included 14 children from a middle socioeconomic status background with ADHD, with comorbid intellectual disability and ranging in age between six to 12 years from 2011-2013.

The sample was divided into a treatment and control group, the treatment group received art therapy sessions while the control group received regular classroom-based activities. After several hours of observation, the children were scored on a series of tests and statistics, leading the researchers to find that art as therapy is a seemingly effective tool in the reduction of impulsive behaviors in children with ADHD and other comorbid disabilities. The findings of this research study have implications for researchers and practitioners alike, offering room for further research and implementation of art therapies as interventions in children with symptoms of cognitive deficit through schools and private therapy sessions.

## ISSUES OF ACCESSIBILITY AND ETHICS OF SELF-DIRECTED ART THERAPY

### Creative Arts Therapy use With Disabled Populations

The discussion about disorders Like ADHD/ADD and ASD prompt discussions about the importance of art therapy in populations with disabilities. Being diagnosed with a disability or chronic illness can instill feelings of fear and can make it difficult for a patient to separate him or herself from their diagnosis, thus causing issues with self-esteem and identity. Many often report feelings of isolation and being trapped, which is precisely why creative, expressive arts therapy is a workable solution to those populations who experience those thoughts and feelings.

All of the research that has been discussed in this review has established that art therapy has proven to specifically strengthen self-esteem, to assist in creating an integrated view of individual identity, and to assist with neuroplasticity, especially in cases of trauma. The wide variety of materials and methods used to create work in sessions makes it a strong choice for individuals with both intellectual and physical disabilities since it reinforces that there is an approach and method that will be able to cater to their specific needs.

Additionally, creative arts therapy offers an abundance of opportunities for clients who may not have a disability, but who may struggle with communicating their emotions verbally, which would be central to more standard forms of talk therapy. Art therapy builds confidence in clients until they either become more comfortable speaking/expressing their emotions verbally or can constructively communicate/organize their emotions through their work more efficiently.

Art therapy connects individuals from varying backgrounds and ages because it is based on the human nature of a desire to create. Unfortunately, limitations of this service do exist, creating issues with accessibility, affordability, and available research.

### Accessibility and Affordability

In America, accessibility to services like art therapy is limited for a variety of reasons. One of the biggest issues facing those trying to take advantage of these programs is that of affordability and availability. Often clients will have trouble finding a practitioner who has openings in their client list and is within budget as many insurance companies either do not cover those types of therapies or there are restrictions on who is allowed to provide care if they do pay for part of the visit. This severely limits the number of providers they can choose from.

Another issue of accessibility is having providers from a variety of cultures and backgrounds who can serve their respective communities. People of color typically feel safer seeking care from providers of a similar background as racial bias in mental health care has posed issues in providing care in some instances. A lack of trust between communities of color and the general medical care field have caused communities of color to be historically underserved.

Issues of accessibility also arise from a lack of reputable clinics in the immediate area, with individuals who are seeking care needing to travel out of their way to receive care. This is not always possible, especially for working-class families who depend on being able to go to work every day. For single working parents with young children, this also poses issues since they may not always be able to find someone to watch their children while they receive care.

### Limitations of Self-Directed Art Therapy

As a result of these issues of accessibility and affordability, many who cannot afford or do not have access to art therapy through a clinical setting, choose to practice a form of self -directed experiential art making to achieve a level of catharsis. While having a creative outlet does seem to be helpful for many, Killick and Schaverien (1997) and Haeyen, Chakhssi, and Van Hooren (2020) suggest that art therapy will serve the client best if conducted in an environment where there is supervision and assistance in processing the emotions and the work itself.

Structure appears to be just as important as the freedom art therapy sessions offer since it provides a point of evaluation for growth. Providing better public information about how people can use art creation to better connect with themselves and as a mindfulness practice would be beneficial and may help those who do not have care available to them. This would offer a level of helpful structure to their self-directed projects.

## FUTURE DIRECTIONS

After discussing the limitations of this type of care, this field still needs to progress to reach its full potential as a therapeutic service. First and foremost, with the modern age, technology has become a valuable tool which can be developed to aid in issues of accessibility. It's widely available and even in families where it is not the most affordable, it is commonplace for schools to provide devices to aid in student learning; this means that it is entirely possible for schools to find ways to keep students connected to resources like school counselors or their art therapists.

Video call visits rather than in-person visits may also help affordability. The field is ever-changing and while it is still a contemporary concept, it is central to human nature and community, so it's likely that other issues of accessibility will be corrected over time, with the increased inclusion of community-based practitioners from diverse backgrounds.

The creative nature of this field could allow for creative opportunities to transport basic mental health care to these historically underserved communities. It would be fascinating to see community building initiatives based on art therapy techniques or even the mobilization of care providers so they can help members of the community who could not leave to seek care. A bit more unlikely, issues with insurance should also be resolved and reformed to allow for greater access to a selection of providers as well as to ease some of the financial burden that can come with receiving mental health care.

Lastly, more studies need to be conducted on the efficacy of art therapy, using larger samples. The field is still expanding, and the preliminary research is promising, but it is necessary to continue the research. Most of the information available to researchers and therapists alike includes mostly small case studies and it would be highly beneficial to see the development of studies and experiments regarding the neuroscience of art therapy, the effectiveness of art therapy across different ethnicities, the effectiveness of art therapy across different genders, and similar studies that would work to expand the framework of what we know.

## CONCLUSION

The articles and findings presented in this literature review sought to organize and compile a general overview of the effectiveness of art therapy across multiple demographics and mental health conditions. It also aimed to lightly address topics that affect the way vulnerable communities receive care and what limitations the field still encounters today. In conclusion, the research literature supports the overall success of art therapy in practice. Research has found that practices of art therapy techniques are effective for patients with a variety of disorders and cognitive challenges, including, but not limited to: Bipolar Disorder, Schizophrenia and Schizophrenia-like disorders, acute psychotic symptoms, personality disorders, ADHD, ASD, and ADD.

As for limitations, art therapy in theory knows no bounds but in practice must have some structure for it to be the most efficient and helpful to the client. The literature reviewed in this chapter shows that art therapy provides the ability to teach clients social skills, improves social behavior, increases self-esteem and confidence, and teaches clients about identifying and expressing their emotions in a way that is more comfortable. While the practices of art therapy can be further researched and expanded upon, it is a helpful tool for many therapists and clinicians and will remain that way in the foreseeable future.

## REFERENCES

Case, C., & Dalley, T. (2014). *The Handbook of Art Therapy*. Routledge. doi:10.4324/9781315779799

Chancellor, B., Duncan, A., & Chatterjee, A. (2014). Art Therapy for Alzheimer's Disease and Other Dementias. *Journal of Alzheimer's Disease*, *39*(01), 1–11. doi:10.3233/JAD-131295 PMID:24121964

*Effects of Art Therapy* 20. Petrillo, L. & Winner, E. (2005) Does Art Improve Mood? A Test of a Key Assumption Underlying Art Therapy. *Art Therapy, 22*(4), 205-212, doi:10.1080/07421656.2005.10129521

Fonagy, P. (2012) Art Therapy and Personality Disorder. *International Journal of Art Therapy, 17*(3), 90. doi:10.1080/17454832.2012.740866

Garai, J. (1984). New Horizons of Holistic Healing through Creative Expression. *Art Therapy: Journal of the American Art Therapy Association*, *1*(2), 76–82. doi:10.1080/07421656.1984.10758751

Habib, H. A., & Ali, U. (2015). Efficacy of Art Therapy in the Reduction of Impulsive Behaviors of Children with ADHD Co-Morbid Intellectual Disability. *Pakistan Journal of Psychology*, *46*(2). http://pjpku.com/index.php/pjp/article/view/72

Haeyen, S., Chakhssi, F., & Van Hooren, S. (2020). Benefits of Art Therapy in People Diagnosed With Personality Disorders: A Quantitative Survey. *Frontiers in Psychology*, *11*, 686. https://doi.org/https://doi.org/10.3389/fpsyg.2020.00686. doi:10.3389/fpsyg.2020.00686 PMID:32351431

Hanevik, H., Hestad, K. A., Lien, L., Teglbjaerg, H. S., & Danbolt, L. J. (2013) Expressive art therapy for psychosis: A multiple case study. *The Arts in Psychotherapy, 40*(3), 312- 321. doi:10.1016/j.aip.2013.05.011

Henley, D. (2007). Naming the Enemy: An Art Therapy Intervention for Children with Bipolar and Comorbid Disorders. *Art Therapy: Journal of the American Art Therapy Association*, *24*(3), 104–110. doi:10.1080/07421656.2007.10129421

Killick, K., & Schaverien, J. (1997). *Art, Psychotherapy, and Psychosis*. Routledge.

Lefebvre, A. D. (2008). *Art Therapy Interventions with an Adolescent with Bipolar Disorder.* [Thesis, Ohio]. OhioLINK Electronic Theses and Dissertations Center. https://rave.ohiolink.edu/etdc/view?acc_num=urs1210794791

Lusebrink, V. (2004). Art Therapy and the Brain: An Attempt to Understand the Underlying Processes of Art Expression in Therapy. *Art Therapy: Journal of the American Art Therapy Association, 21*(3), 125–135. doi:10.1080/07421656.2004.10129496

Malchiodi, C. A. (2012). *Handbook of Art Therapy*. The Guilford Press.

Montag, C., Haase, L., Seidel, D., Bayerl, M., Gallinat, J., Herrmann, U., & Dannecker, K. (2014). A pilot RCT of psychodynamic group art therapy for patients in acute psychotic episodes: Feasibility, impact on symptoms and mentalizing capacity. *PLoS One*, *9*(11), e112348. doi:10.1371/journal.pone.0112348 PMID:25393414

Rosal, M. L. (2018). *Cognitive Behavioral Art Therapy from Behaviorism to the Third Wave. Routledge, Taylor &amp.* Francis Group. doi:10.4324/9781315459257

Rubin, J. A. (2015). Psychoanalytic Art Therapy. In D. E. Gussak & M. L. Rosal (Eds.), *The Wiley Handbook of Art Therapy*., doi:10.1002/9781118306543.ch3

Ruddy, R., & Milnes, D. (2005). Art therapy for schizophrenia or schizophrenia-like illnesses. *Cochrane Database of Systematic Reviews*, (4), CD003728. Advance online publication. doi:10.1002/14651858.CD003728.pub2 PMID:16235338

Schwiezer, C., Knorth, E. J., Van Yperen, T. A., & Spreen, M. A. (2020). Evaluation of "Images of Self," an art therapy program for children diagnosed with autism spectrum disorders (ASD). *Children and Youth Services Review*, *116*, 105207. https://doi.org/10.1016/j.childyouth.2020.105207. doi:10.1016/j.childyouth.2020.105207


## KEY TERMS & DEFINITIONS

**Accessibility:** The practice of making information, activities, and/or environments sensible, meaningful, and usable for as many people as possible.

**Cognitive Deficit:** Impairment in an individual's mental processes that lead to the acquisition of information and knowledge.

**Comorbid:** The simultaneous presence of two or more diseases or medical conditions in a patient.

**Existential:** Concerned with existence, especially human existence as viewed in the theories of existentialism.

**Neuroplasticity:** The ability of the nervous system to change its activity in response to intrinsic or extrinsic stimuli by reorganizing its structure, functions, or connections after injuries.

**Pediatric:** Medical term meaning in relation to children and adolescents.

**Psychosocial:** Relating to the interrelation of social factors and individual thought and behavior.

**Psychotic Features:** A collection of symptoms that affect the mind, where there has been some loss of contact with reality.

**Sublimation:** The channeling of socially unacceptable behaviors into socially acceptable ones.

**Transference:** The act of the client unknowingly transferring feelings about someone from their past onto the therapist.

# Chapter 6
# The Impact of Art Therapy on the Elderly Population

**Shira Davis**
*Marymount Manhattan College, USA*

## ABSTRACT

*In the past century, the creative arts therapy sphere has exploded, specifically art therapy. Art therapy is now offered in many clinics, schools, and hospitals. The popularity of this therapy can be attributed to its success in helping individuals express themselves and build mastery and confidence. Although art therapy is beneficial for everyone, this paper will examine the substantial benefits of art therapy on the elderly population. The evolution of art therapy from its beginning to the present will be reviewed. Different subgroups will also be discussed, such as those incarcerated or suffering from depression and dementia. The various techniques and their effects will be analyzed as well.*

## INTRODUCTION: A HISTORY OF ART THERAPY

Art therapy is the oldest form of creative arts therapy. Although it was discovered in America in the early 1900s, art therapy even has roots in the Paleolithic Era. Those religious cave paintings expressed the emotions of the painters who hoped for salvation from the gods. Years later, Plato was the first to recognize that art can influence emotions (Packard, 1980, pp. 10). However, even so, it was not until thousands of years later that modern art therapy was discovered and established.

Modern art therapy is first rooted in the work of early nineteenth-century American philosopher John Dewey. Like Plato, he recognized that art could soothe a troubled soul. However, more than that, Dewey taught that children must be allowed to

DOI: 10.4018/978-1-6684-7856-1.ch006

express themselves freely. He encouraged the child to produce art freely, without the restrictions of a teacher and lessons. Similarly, educator Frank Cizek of Vienna urged teachers to support children from afar to offer them free reign to express themselves as they wished through their art.

In truth, Dewey's perspective was based on the teachings of Sigmund Freud, a contemporary of Dewey. Freud is known as the "Father of Psychology," particularly for his psychoanalytic modality. He discussed the unconscious mind established in young childhood that set the course for the rest of life. Psychological issues arose due to the pull between the id and the ego, the lower and higher parts of the self. Freud prescribed catharsis as the cure as it would unleash the unconscious mind from the tyranny of the conscious. Although Freud, himself, was not a proponent of art therapy, the idea behind it, of releasing the unconscious, emerged from his perspective.

Hans Prinzhorn, a German psychiatrist, had quite a different perspective on art and psychology. At that time, people believed that the scribbles drawn by psychiatric residents were no more than just another symptom of their madness. He saw them as the residents' form of communication to the outside world. Unlike Freud, he did not see any psychoanalytic function within the art. Instead, it was the need for a creative outlet and communication for people, usually those with schizophrenia, who could not easily express themselves. Through Prinzhorn's writings, the value of expressive art became more recognized.

Margaret Naumburg was a twentieth-century American psychologist and artist who took art therapy to the next level. She began as an art teacher at the school she started, the Walden School. Like John Dewey, she taught that art was a form of free expression for children, as essential as free speech. Later, she developed this as a part of psychotherapy and called it "Analytically Oriented Art Therapy." The patient sat at an easel and drew or painted. Afterward, the patient would free associate and discover parts of themselves that they may not have had the courage or insight to express verbally. Because of Naumburg and her writings and lectures, art therapy has become widely accepted and practiced today.

The last art therapy pioneer was Edith Kramer. Like Naumburg, she began as an art teacher at the Wiltwyck School for Boys. However, her opinion was that art therapy is a kind of catharsis in that the act of drawing or painting healed the unconscious. In her words, "Through the creative act, the patient is able to graphically pictoralize inner sensations, desires, etc., and experience feelings which will become satisfactory and desired substitutes for their earlier more destructive feelings… It is an area where experience can be chosen, varied and repeated at will. In the creative act, conflict is re-experienced, resolved and integrated. . ." (Kramer, 1958, p. 6). Her writings, along with Margaret Naumberg's, were the first to be published in *The Bulletin of Art Therapy,* later renamed *The American Journal of Art Therapy.*

From there, art therapy only grew and expanded. In 1969, the AATA, or the American Art Therapy Association was founded. At the same time, the first graduate training program was opened at the Hahnemann Medical College and Hospital. As of January 1, 2021, there are over 4,000 members of AATA, who define art therapy as "a mental health profession that enriches the lives of individuals, families, and communities through active art-making, the creative process, applied psychological theory, and human experience within a psychotherapeutic relationship" (AATA National Office, 2021). Their mission is to advance art therapy as a mental health profession and build a community of art therapists so that all can access art therapy for a better quality of life.

Although art therapy is beneficial for individuals of diverse backgrounds, this chapter will focus on the effects of art therapy on elderly people. This is especially important today since the population worldwide is getting older (Vespa, 2021). In Japan, a quarter of the population is over 65. Europe's population is getting older as well, even older than the American one in the case of Germany, France, Italy, and Spain. In 2018, fifteen percent of Americans were over 65 but that percentage is growing rapidly. By 2060, it will jump to twenty-five percent. This means that the medical and psychological world must prepare for this possibility, including researching more alternative forms of therapy.

## ART THERAPY FOR INDIVIDUALS WITH COGNITIVE IMPAIRMENTS

Cognitive performance is one of the most common areas researchers examine in the elderly. The effects of late-stage cognitive decline can be devastating for the quality of life for the patient and the individuals around them. Eventually, cognitive decline can lead to Alzheimer's Disease, which is fatal. But if mild cognitive impairment is caught early enough and treated, it may be reversible in about 40% of cases (Larrieu et al., 2002). However, since this is the most important and relevant topic for the elderly population, we will discuss this topic from a few different perspectives.

### Early Intervention for Individuals With Cognitive Impairments

One way that older adults can improve their cognition is by self-monitoring their own progress and by building confidence in their learning and memory skills (Dunlosky et al., 2007). Studies show that patients with higher confidence in these areas make fewer errors than those with lower confidence (Bandura, 1993). This is because memory is not as factual and unwavering as we think. As researcher Chai Tyng and his colleagues (2017) put it, emotions have a powerful impact on memory processing and vice versa. In one study, those who believed that their memory was getting worse had more memory errors and less cognitive functioning six years later (Potter et al., 2009). In other words, their belief that their memory was deteriorating caused their memory to worsen. This ties in with core cognitive psychology beliefs about the connection between learning and our thoughts and beliefs. Our thoughts and beliefs affect our motivation, which in turn affects attention and information processing.

An important concept related to cognitive performance is cognitive training. Cognitive training is the process used to enhance cognitive performance through education (Sitzer, Twamley, & Jeste, 2006). Thanks to research and brain imaging, scientists are able to see the neurogenesis or the creation of new neural pathways that continue even after full maturity (Linden, 2006). Education, in general, can be used for cognitive training since new information and activities will trigger more neural pathways and better cell interconnectivity. Art education specifically can boost cognitive performance in three areas: verbal/episodic memory, inductive reasoning, and visual search and identification. Episodic memory is one of the seven types of memory that is responsible for remembering times, places, events, and emotions (Tulving, 2002). When artwork is examined, the objects within it are named and discussed in relation to their placement. This usage of both verbal and episodic memory keeps them in working order (Arkin, 2007). Inductive reasoning is the ability to observe patterns and make conclusions based on those patterns (Boron et al, 2007). It is part of executive functioning and is one of the first indicators of cognitive decline. But with art creation and education, inductive reasoning and problem-solving skills are used and are therefore retained (Hass-Cohen & Carr, 2008). There are also health benefits that derive from the creativity involved in art, such as better information processing (Chamorro-Premuzic, & Furnham, 2005) and healthy cortical thickness (Jung et al., 2009). Lastly, the process of visual learning and process can improve cognitive performance, as well. Participants are asked to study and interpret the designs which means using their processing and memory skills. Additionally, many people are visual learners and are therefore more likely to engage and succeed.

In an experiment conducted by Alders (2011), 24 Latin participants were given the opportunity to receive art therapy to determine if it would improve their cognitive performance (2011). Alders (2011) gave them three forms. The first form asked them for their demographic information, such as their age and education level. The second form was the Cognitive Failures Questionnaire (CFQ), which asked them to report the number of lapses in their cognitive performances while doing average activities. The last form was the Clock Drawing Test (CDT), the most universal test for cognitive functioning. They then could attend weekly two-hour art sessions for the next ten weeks. Those who attended zero or one class were the de facto control group and those who attended two or more classes were the de facto experimental group. After ten weeks of sessions, the participants were given the CFQ and the CDT again. The results showed that those who participated in the art sessions demonstrated improved cognitive performance.

## A Blend of Neuroscience and Art Therapy for Individuals With Dementia

Even though it may not be obvious at first, a blend of art therapy and neuroscience can help answer this prevalent problem. According to the Alzheimer's Association, 6.5 million Americans aged 65 or older or were diagnosed with dementia in 2022. The numbers jump to 46.3% of all people over the age of 75. Dementia is actually not a specific disease but an umbrella term for the many diseases that all share similar symptoms. According to American Psychiatric Association's Diagnostic and Statistical Manual of Mental Disorders (2017), these symptoms include memory impairment and cognitive disturbances in at least one other area of functioning. Usually, these symptoms worsen until they interfere with everyday activities.

The most diagnosed subtype of dementia is Alzheimer's Disease, which accounts for 60-70% of all dementia cases (World Health Organization, 2022). Alzheimer's is characterized by clusters of misshapen proteins both inside and outside the neurons. Amyloid beta proteins are usually found in the spaces between the cells, but clump together in deposits called amyloid plaques. Inside the neuron, the tau proteins also clump together in misshapen knots called neurofibrillary tangles. Both of these deformed proteins cause the death of synapses (the connections between the cells) (Davis and Luddington, 1999).

Alzheimer's includes four stages. During Stage I, the patient has some memory loss and shows some confusion and disorientation. Processing information and concentration also start to decline in this stage which can last from two to five years. Stage II is characterized by more disorientation, poor judgment, and withdrawal from social situations, likely because of the confusion present. Some patients with Stage II Alzheimer's exhibit paranoia and aggression towards those around them, often claiming that their caregivers are stealing from them. Stage II can last from three to 12 years. Patients with Stage III Alzheimer's have extreme difficulty with both expressive and receptive communication. Many cannot perform basic living skills like dressing and bathing. Their aggression and agitation may worsen with this further loss of independence and dignity. The last stage, Stage IV, is marked by major physical decline. The patient can no longer walk or talk or recognize family members. They progressively worsen to a vegetative state and then finally pass away, usually from infection or organ failure.

After Alzheimer's, the second most commonly diagnosed cognitive-based disorder is vascular dementia. Vascular dementia is when the brain undergoes a number of mini strokes that block smaller arteries. There are also a few rare, reversible types of dementia caused by psychological disorders, infections, and medications. However, they are unfortunately a lot less common than the more severe types of dementia.

Art therapy can provide an opportunity for self-expression for patients who lose their ability to communicate normally. Although individuals with dementia can lose their ability to speak relatively early, they still feel the range of emotions that they felt before they were diagnosed. In one case study, the participant had dementia that led to expressive aphasia in which she was unable to communicate, but could understand language (Khan-Denis, 1997). Without any encouragement, she drew a face and showed it to her therapist to convey her sadness. The therapist told the participant's daughter, who then took her mother to the doctor. The participant was suffering from an infection but was unable to tell anyone verbally.

Art can also be used as a diagnostic tool for cognitive functioning. One of the most famous neuropsychological evaluations is the Clock Drawing Test (CDT) (see Figure 1). The drawing of an analog clock pointing to a specific time is difficult for those with any kind of cognitive deficiency, as seen below. The Formal Elements Art Therapy Scale (FEATS) Assessment, which was developed by Gannt and Anderson (2009), evaluates cognitive functions based on the participant's drawing of a person picking an apple from a tree. The premise is that diagnoses can be made from the manner in which the drawing is drawn and not based on what the drawing is. Although patients with severe dementia found this specific drawing too difficult, the FEATS did provide insight into the disease progression and general cognitive functioning.

Art therapy can be a cathartic tool, especially for those struggling with negative memories from their past. In an aforementioned study, the researchers examined the impact of an art therapy method called, "life review" on patients' mental health (Ilali et al, 2018). They discovered that drawing and discussing depictions of the different stages of their life greatly improved the participants' mental health. Researcher and art therapist Ellen Greene Stewart found similar results with Catherine, a 90-year-old patient with dementia (2004). Always a natural worrier, Catherine's anxiety shot up when she could no longer recognize the people around her or her settings. However, through the process of making collages with her art therapist, Catherine worked through her anxiety and even her depression over a secret miscarriage in her youth.

Art therapy can help reduce the severity of the symptoms of dementia and can improve the quality of life. Dementia usually attacks the temporal and parietal lobes first, which is why skills such as language are the first to be affected. However, the frontal lobe, which is responsible for personality and emotional control, is usually only affected in the later stages (Gardner, 1974). Instead of the losses one has come to expect with aging, it can actually be a time for self-expression and discovery of new skills and relationships that had not been explored earlier.

## ART THERAPY FOR INDIVIDUALS WITH DEPRESSION

Depression has been on the rise in the past decade for individuals of all ages and ethnicities. In 2020, one out of every ten people in America was depressed (Goodwin et al, 2022). Elderly people are not an exception to this trend either. Studies have shown that 10.3% of the older population are depressed worldwide but that number is doubled for those in developed countries, such as the United States (Barua, Ghosh, Kar, & Basilio, 2010). Depression can lead to a number of health conditions if left untreated. There is a higher risk of suicide, especially in countries where there is still stigma around mental health. Their quality of life is compromised and the body is weakened by psychological stress. Elderly individuals with depression are three times more likely to develop high blood pressure and are more vulnerable to heart attacks, hip fractures, pneumonia, and other infections (Vakilabad, Fallahi Khoshknab, Madah, & Hosseini, 2013). Thus, depression in elderly people is an issue that must be addressed.

Art therapy can be extremely beneficial for elderly individuals with depression. It can help them explore themselves and their feelings in a non-threatening and enjoyable way. This can also help elderly people develop more effective and innovative problem-solving skills. It can also boost their creativity and sensory stimulation (Blomdahl, Gunnarsson, Guregård, &

Bjorklund, 2013). As aforementioned, one method that was particularly successful was the life review through art therapy. Life review is a process where the person undergoing therapy creates artwork representing different stages of their lives. This can be therapeutic for participants since they can relive their experiences in a safe environment (Haber, 2006).

In Iran, researchers Ehteram Sadat Ilali, Farzaneh Mokhtary, Nouraddin Mousavinasab, and Abdul Hakim Tirgari (2018) tested this method of life review through art therapy on older participants. They selected 60 adults over the age of 60 to participate in the study from an old age home. The participants were given the Abbreviated Mental Test or the AMT first which screened for dementia and other mental impairments. They were also given the Geriatric Depression Scale (GDS). The sixty participants were then divided into control and experimental groups. The control group continued with their daily schedule that was already part of the center's curriculum. For six weeks, the experimental group attended an art therapy session once a week. They were asked to draw themselves or representations of themselves at various points in their lives, as well as their regrets, accomplishments, and opinions. The last session was dedicated to understanding and processing their drawings with a psychologist and then sharing them with the other members. The researchers then reevaluated the participants' mental health using the GDS again and compared them to the previous scores. The results confirmed that art therapy and life review decreased the elderly participants' depression. They had discovered a way to live and honor their memories and experiences without being pulled down by them. They also enjoyed the simple pleasure of making art, just like many people of other ages. Lastly, the sessions provided an opportunity for social interaction, that was lacking.

## ART THERAPY FOR THE INDIVIDUALS WHO ARE INCARCERATED

As a general rule, the elderly population can at times be forgotten about and relegated to the back of the public's mind, overtaken by the more contentious issues. However, the elderly individuals, who are most forgotten about, are those who are incarcerated in prisons. According to the Federal Bureau of Prisons (2023), almost 20% of inmates are over age 50. Obviously, these individuals have different physical, mental, and emotional needs than the younger inmates. However, even elderly individuals, who are not incarcerated, report higher levels of loneliness and depression which negatively impacts their overall health (Luanaigh and Lawlor, 2008). In a prison setting, the loneliness and depression are worse, due to the inmates' separation from their family and friends. Thus, the impact of incarceration on their mental and physical health can be that much more detrimental compared to the general elderly population.

Besides the separation from their friends and family, those incarcerated in prisons can obviously no longer work at their jobs. This can lead to feelings of loss of purpose and meaning, which is essential for self-actualization and esteem. Self-actualization and esteem are the two levels above love and belonging on Maslow's (1943) Hierarchy of Needs. The younger inmates can usually fill this void with physical activity such as working out at the gym, but that level of physical activity is often not as possible for older inmates. Hence, there is a need for an activity that older inmates can master and gain that feeling of accomplishment.

De Guzman (2010) conducted a study in the Phillipines in order to learn more about the effect of traditional Filipino art therapy on elderly inmates. He selected five participants whose ages ranged from 54 to 70. Only one of the participants finished high school. Most suffered from some kind of chronic illness and rarely had any visitors. The researchers interviewed the participants about their life in prison and evaluated their mental health, specifically their self-esteem. The participants were also asked to draw and then explain representations of themselves before and after their imprisonment. They then attended Puni-making class and were given the materials for making more afterward. Puni is a traditional Filipino art of creating objects from dried palm leaves. The researchers then conducted the second round of interviews and drawings. The gains from the art therapy were multifold. Practically speaking, the inmates were able to sell their creations and create a source of income, which meant better food and medical care for them. However, beyond the impact of finances, the inmates felt they had something to fill their days and it gave them a sense of accomplishment.

## ART THERAPY TECHNIQUES FOR THE ELDERLY POPULATION

### Collage Therapy for Elderly Individuals

One method of art therapy is the creation of collages or using pieces of pre-made art together to make a whole innovative design. Collage-making can be a good option especially for the elderly population. Some may have lost their ability to use their fingers precisely due to age-related diseases, like arthritis. Others may have never had a special affinity for drawing and painting and may feel embarrassed about trying more typical versions of art therapy. Selecting pictures can also give the participants the feelings of control and independence that they are sorely lacking.

A study was conducted by Stallings (2010) to test the impact of collage-making on older adults with dementia. The researcher had three participants make collages from precut images from magazines, write what the people in the pictures might be thinking or saying, name each picture from a pile as good or bad, and describe the situation transpiring in the picture. The participants thoroughly appreciated the opportunity to express themselves beyond their verbal and cognitive abilities. They also enjoyed indulging in enjoyable recollections of their pasts.

### Mask-Making Therapy for Elderly Individuals

One of the more unusual forms of art therapy is the creation of masks. They can be made using tissue paper, clay, or paper mâché (Nash, 2022). Mask-making may not be the best option for elderly individuals with more advanced physical deterioration, but it has many benefits for those who are able to do it. It can express the different ways people behave in different relationships and situations. This can be especially relevant for older adults who are still adjusting to their physical and cognitive decline. Mask-making can also represent the strengths and qualities inside the person (Chilton and Wilkinson, 2016).

### Group Art Therapy for Elderly Individuals

Many forms of art therapy are conducted in groups rather than through individual sessions. This can be very beneficial for elderly individuals who may not have the same social opportunities as their younger counterparts. Many older people report feelings of loneliness and isolation, especially after the death of their loved ones. Group art therapy can provide an opportunity for them to socialize more with their peers. A study was conducted by Kim, Kim, and Nomura (2016) on the effects of group art therapy on older Korean adults with neurocognitive disorders. Fourteen participants attended 36 group art therapy sessions that each lasted approximately 45 minutes. The researchers provided a large number of sessions in order to build the relationships among the participants in order for more friendships to form. The participants had lower depression and higher self-expression because they had an audience with which to share their thoughts and accomplishments. The sessions themselves helped the patients develop a sense of pride in their work and a sense of friendship with the other group members. Eventually, the participants were able to build long-lasting friendships, which positively impacted their mental and consequently physical health.

## Cultural Art Therapy for Elderly Individuals

Cultural art is any form of art that is based on a certain nation or group of people. As aforementioned, one example is the Puni-making classes in the Filipino prison (de Guzman et al, 2010). Another example is the clay dolls and wet pulp masks made in the Korean group art therapy sessions (Kim et al., 2016). Researchers found that participants were more willing to engage when presented with traditional materials from their culture. This may be because it brought back positive memories for the participants and connected them to their heritage.

# CONCLUSION

There has been much research and progress made in the past century in the art therapy world, as shown above. Art therapy has come a long way since the times of Margaret Naumburg and Edith Kramer. It can be used to strengthen the brain's neuroplasticity and processing, build confidence and mastery skills, and provide an enjoyable pastime for elderly individuals. However, there is still more work to be done. Many of the studies conducted have been case studies, which are not as generalizable as studies with larger sample sizes. Additionally, art therapy is not always easily accessible, especially for those of a lower socio-economic status. With so much change needed in the world, art therapy is not always at the top of the list. Yet art therapy has proven to improve quality of life at a relatively low cost. The American Art Therapy Association's vision resonates - a world where everyone has access to professional art therapy for improved mental health and well-being (AATA, 2021).

## REFERENCES

AATA National Office. (2021, February 10). *About our members: AATA at a glance 2021*. American Art Therapy Association. https://arttherapy.org/news-member-infographic/

Alders, A. (2011). Perceived self-efficacy and its role in education-related cognitive performance in Latino American elderly. *Journal of Latinos and Education*, *10*(4), 299–319. doi:10.1080/15348431.2011.605680

Alzheimer's Association. (2022). *Alzheimer's disease facts and figures*. Alzheimer's Disease and Dementia. https://www.alz.org/alzheimers-dementia/facts-figures

Arkin, S. (2007). Language-enriched exercise plus socialization slows cognitive decline in alzheimer's disease. *American Journal of Alzheimer's Disease and Other Dementias*, *22*(1), 62–77. doi:10.1177/1533317506295377 PMID:17534004

Bandura, A. (1993). Perceived self-efficacy in cognitive development and functioning. *Educational Psychologist*, *28*(2), 117–148. doi:10.120715326985ep2802_3

Barua, A., Ghosh, M. K., Kar, N., & Basilio, M. A. (2010). Distribution of depressive disorders in the elderly. *Journal of Neurosciences in Rural Practice*, *01*(02), 067–073. doi:10.4103/0976-3147.71719

Blomdahl, C., Gunnarsson, A. B., Guregård, S., & Björklund, A. (2013). A realist review of art therapy for clients with depression. *The Arts in Psychotherapy*, *40*(3), 322–330. doi:10.1016/j.aip.2013.05.009

Boron, J. B., Turiano, N. A., Willis, S. L., & Schaie, K. W. (2007). Effects of cognitive training on change in accuracy in inductive reasoning ability. *The Journals of Gerontology. Series B, Psychological Sciences and Social Sciences*, *62*(3), P179–P186. doi:10.1093/geronb/62.3.P179 PMID:17507586

Chilton, G., & Wilkinson, R. (2016, January 6). *Exploring strengths through masks: Art therapy from a positive psychology perspective*. Retrieved from https://arttherapy.org/exploring-strengths-masks-art-therapy-positive-psychology-perspective/

Cook, R. (1994). *An historical and psychological context for the phenomenon of art therapy* [Thesis, Edith Cohen University].

Davis, K. L. (1999). Alzheimer's disease: Seeking new ways to preserve brain function. Interview by Alice V. Luddington. *Geriatrics*, *54*(2), 42–48. PMID:10024872

de Guzman, A. B., Santos, J. I., Santos, M. L., Santos, M. T., Sarmiento, V. V., Sarnillo, E. J., & Sarsagat, J. M. (2010). Traditional Filipino arts in enhancing older people's self-esteem in a penal institution. *Educational Gerontology*, *36*(12), 1065–1085. doi:10.1080/03601270903534713

Dunlosky, J., Cavallini, E., Roth, H., McGuire, C. L., Vecchi, T., & Hertzog, C. (2007). Do self-monitoring interventions improve older adult learning? *The Journals of Gerontology: Series B*, *62*(Special_Issue_1), 70–76. doi:10.1093/geronb/62.special_issue_1.70

Federal Bureau of Prisons. (2023, February 25). *BOP Statistics: Average Inmate Age*. Federal Bureau of Prisons. https://www.bop.gov/about/statistics/statistics_inmate_age.jsp

Gantt, L. M., & Anderson, F. (2009). The formal elements art therapy scale: A measurement system for global variables in art. *Art Therapy: Journal of the American Art Therapy Association*, *26*(3), 124–129. doi:10.1080/07421656.2009.10129372

Gardner, H. (1974). *The shattered mind*. Vintage Books.

Goodwin, R. D., Dierker, L. C., Wu, M., Galea, S., Hoven, C. W., & Weinberger, A. H. (2022). Trends in U.S. depression prevalence from 2015 to 2020: The widening treatment gap. *American Journal of Preventive Medicine*, *63*(5), 726–733. doi:10.1016/j.amepre.2022.05.014 PMID:36272761

Haber, D. (2006). Life review: Implementation, theory, research, and therapy. *International Journal of Aging & Human Development*, *63*(2), 153–171. doi:10.2190/DA9G-RHK5-N9JP-T6CC PMID:17137032

Hass-Cohen, N., & Carr, R. (Eds.). (2008). *Art therapy and clinical neuroscience*. Jessica Kingsley.

Ilali, E. S., Mokhtary, F., Mousavinasab, N., & Tirgari, A. H. (2018). Impact of art-based life review on depression symptoms among older adults. *Art Therapy: Journal of the American Art Therapy Association*, *35*(3), 148–155. doi:10.1080/07421656.2018.1531276

Kahn-Denis, K. B. (1997). Art therapy with geriatric dementia clients. *Art Therapy: Journal of the American Art Therapy Association*, *14*(3), 194–199. doi:10.1080/07421656.1987.10759281

Kim, H.-K., Kim, K. M., & Nomura, S. (2016). The effect of group art therapy on older Korean adults with neurocognitive disorders. *The Arts in Psychotherapy*, *47*, 48–54. doi:10.1016/j.aip.2015.11.002

Kramer, E. (1958). *Art therapy in a children's community: A study of the function of art therapy in the treatment program of Wiltwyck School for Boys*. Charles C Thomas Publisher.

Larrieu, S., Letenneur, L., Orgogozo, J. M., Fabrigoule, C., Amieva, H., Le Carret, N., Barberger-Gateau, P., & Dartigues, J. F. (2002). Incidence and outcome of mild cognitive impairment in a population-based prospective cohort. *Neurology*, *59*(10), 1594–1599. doi:10.1212/01.WNL.0000034176.07159.F8 PMID:12451203

Linden, D. E. (2006). How psychotherapy changes the brain – the contribution of functional neuroimaging. *Molecular Psychiatry*, *11*(6), 528–538. doi:10.1038j.mp.4001816 PMID:16520823

Luanaigh, C. Ó., & Lawlor, B. A. (2008). Loneliness and the health of older people. *International Journal of Geriatric Psychiatry*, *23*(12), 1213–1221. doi:10.1002/gps.2054 PMID:18537197

Maslow, A. H. (1943). A theory of human motivation. *Psychological Review*, *50*(4), 370–396. doi:10.1037/h0054346

Murman, D. (2015). The impact of age on cognition. *Seminars in Hearing*, *36*(03), 111–121. doi:10.1055-0035-1555115 PMID:27516712

Nash, J. (2022, October 16). *Expressive arts therapy: 15 Creative Activities and Techniques*. PositivePsychology.com. https://positivepsychology.com/expressive-arts-therapy/

Packard, S. (1980). The history of art therapy education. *Art Education*, *33*(4), 10–13. doi:10.2307/3192416

Potter, L. M., Grealy, M. A., & O'Connor, R. C. (2009). Healthy ageing, perceived motor-efficacy, and performance on cognitively demanding action tasks. *British Journal of Psychology*, *100*(1), 49–70. doi:10.1348/000712608X304478 PMID:18447971

APA. (2017). *Diagnostic and statistical manual of mental disorders: Dsm-5*. CBS Publishers & Distributors, Pvt. Ltd

Sarokhani, D., Parvareh, M., Hasanpour Dehkordi, A., Sayehmiri, K., & Moghimbeigi, A. (2018). Prevalence of Depression among Iranian Elderly: Systematic Review and Meta-Analysis. *Iranian Journal of Psychiatry*, *13*(1), 55–64. PMID:29892318

Sitzer, D. I., Twamley, E. W., & Jeste, D. V. (2006). Cognitive training in alzheimer's disease: A meta-analysis of the literature. *Acta Psychiatrica Scandinavica, 114*(2), 75–90. doi:10.1111/j.1600-0447.2006.00789.x PMID:16836595

Souillard-Mandar, W., Davis, R., Rudin, C., Au, R., Libon, D. J., Swenson, R., Price, C. C., Lamar, M., & Penney, D. L. (2015). Learning classification models of cognitive conditions from subtle behaviors in the digital clock drawing test. *Machine Learning, 102*(3), 393–441. doi:10.100710994-015-5529-5 PMID:27057085

Stewart, E. G. (2004). Art therapy and neuroscience blend: Working with patients who have dementia. *Art Therapy: Journal of the American Art Therapy Association, 21*(3), 148–155. doi:10.1080/07421656.2004.10129499

Tulving, E. (2002). Episodic memory: From mind to brain. *Annual Review of Psychology, 53*(1), 1–25. doi:10.1146/annurev.psych.53.100901.135114 PMID:11752477

Tyng, C. M., Amin, H. U., Saad, M. N., & Malik, A. S. (2017). The influences of emotion on learning and memory. *Frontiers in Psychology, 8*, 1454. doi:10.3389/fpsyg.2017.01454 PMID:28883804

Vespa, J. (2021, October 9). *The U.S. joins other countries with large aging populations*. Census.gov. https://www.census.gov/library/stories/2018/03/graying-america.html

World Health Organization. (2022, September 20). *Dementia*. World Health Organization. https://www.who.int/news-room/fact-sheets/detail/dementia

## KEY TERMS AND DEFINITIONS

**Alzheimer's Disease:** The most common form of dementia that affects memory, thinking, and behavior in a progressive and degenerative manner.

**Art therapy:** A mental health profession that enriches the lives of individuals, families, and communities through active art-making, creative process, applied psychological theory, and human experience within a psychotherapeutic relationship.

**Clock Drawing Test (CDT):** A screening tool to differentiate normal individuals from those with cognitive impairment, and has proven useful in helping to diagnose cognitive dysfunction associated with neurological disorders such as Alzheimer's disease, Parkinson's disease, and other dementias and conditions.

**Cognitive training:** A process used to enhance cognitive performance through education.

**Dementia:** An umbrella term for the many diseases that all share similar symptoms including memory impairment and cognitive disturbances in at least one other area of functioning.

**Episodic memory:** One of the seven types of memory that is responsible for remembering times, places, events, and emotions.

**Formal Elements Art Therapy Scale (FEATS):** An assessment that evaluates cognitive functions based on the participant's drawing of a person picking an apple from a tree.

**Inductive reasoning:** The ability to observe patterns and make conclusions based on those patterns.

**Life review:** A process where the person undergoing the therapy creates artwork representing different stages of their lives.

**Vascular dementia:** A disease in which the brain undergoes a number of mini strokes that block smaller arteries.

# Section 2

# Benefits of Diverse Creative Arts Therapies

# Chapter 7
# Improve Through Improv:
## An Examination of the Art and Science of Improv

**Marisa Tamar Cohen**
*Embracing Change Marriage and Family Therapy, PLLC, USA*

## ABSTRACT

*This chapter examines improv, or the art of skillfully, spontaneously, and collaboratively building a scene in the present moment. Improv as an art form, and its governing principles will be discussed, as well as the application of this craft to business, education, and medical settings, with special focus on the use of improv in therapeutic practice. Exploring improv as a science, the research centering on how it can affect well-being, enhance creativity and divergent thinking, and strengthen social connections will be detailed. Additionally, the connection between improv exercises and psychological principles will be highlighted through the presentation of activities that can be applied to any group setting.*

## INTRODUCTION

A group of people walk confidently onto the stage. One solicits a suggestion for a scene from the audience, and then it begins…the improv show. You may be acquainted with improv from television programs such as *Whose Line Is It Anyway?* (Leveson & Patterson, 1998) or from visiting a local performance arts center or comedy club in your city or town. Some people put improv in the same category as theater, and others associate it with comedy, however it is in a category of its own.

DOI: 10.4018/978-1-6684-7856-1.ch007

Improv requires players, or improvisers, to be spontaneous, creative, and present. These skills lead to the creation of a collaborative scene that can delight both the audience and the improvisers themselves. Beyond the enjoyment associated with this art form, improv has also been shown to enhance inter- and intrapersonal skills. As such, it has been used within business, education, and healthcare settings.

This chapter will examine the principles governing the creation and building of an improv scene with others, as well as the psychological principles associated with this art form. Additionally, this chapter will delve into research surrounding the multitude of benefits conferred to those engaging in improv. Finally, the connection between improv and therapeutic practice will be highlighted and a series of group activities will be presented, connecting the theory and research to applied practice.

## What Is Improv?

Improv is the art of building a scene around audience suggestions (Poissant, 2018). The characters, story, and narrative are created spontaneously by the players on stage (Schwenke et al., 2021). For the improvisers, it involves getting on stage without fully planning or preparing the specific scene as it is made up in the moment (Halpern et al., 1994). Improv isn't about telling jokes or even being funny but requires people to create connections among the different characters on stage, the components of story being told, and with the audience (Dohe & Pappas, 2015).

This art form falls under the larger category of creativity and involves the process of generating something new over time. The main distinction between creativity and improv is that improv is spontaneous, and as such, there is no time for preparation or space for correction (Lewis & Lovatt, 2013). As no preplanning is involved, neither the players nor the audience know in advance what will happen. However, this does not mean that improv is completely a free-for-all. Rather, it is has a particular structure in which new components build upon what has already been introduced (Lemons, 2005).

The birth of improv is often attributed to commedia del-arte, a theatrical style made popular in Italy in the 17$^{th}$ century (Cole, 2016). In this form of art, comedic troupes would perform plays that were made up on the spot. Similar to improv there were no scripts, however a carefully curated scenario was practiced before each performance and masked actors would depict a particular character and stay in the character for the duration of the play. These actors would also rehearse to perfect their embodiment of the character they commonly depicted. In the early 1900s Jacob Moreno developed the Theater of Spontaneity which put on the first fully unscripted theater performance (Cole, 2016).

In the United States, Viola Spolin is considered to be the mother of modern-day improv (Cole, 2016). Her work became popular in the 1930s and was aimed at engaging children in community theater. In her influential text, *Improvisation for The Theater* (Spolin, 1963), she notes that players, or those engaging in improv must eagerly adapt and respond to many simultaneous suggestions and scenarios. Her work has been adapted and referenced in business, education, therapy, as well as other industries.

There are two main forms of improv: short- and long-form. Shows such as *Whose Line Is It Anyway?* (Leveson & Patterson, 1998), and much of what you see comedy troupes perform is short form (Cole, 2016). This form of improv involves a series of games, each lasting a few minutes (Cole, 2016). These games are often initiated by a suggestion from the audience and there isn't necessarily a theme tying them together. Long-form improv is cohesive and involves storylines, in which there are call backs to earlier components throughout (Cole, 2016).

## Why Improv?

In their book *Life Unscripted,* Katzman and O'Connor (2018) note that improv helps people to become more present and engaged. They share that improv enables people to break out of their patterned way of thinking and helps them to create something new and spontaneous. These skills can prepare people to be better suited to everyday life, as there are always moments that require adjustment and adaptability (Katzman & O'Connor, 2018). People are often used to following routines as patterns help make sense of the world and may offer a sense of comfort. However, becoming aware of these patterns, and changing them when possible, makes way for new adventures (Katzman & O'Connor, 2018).

Engaging in improv can enhance mental health and well-being. As an effective tool for self-care, it can lead to improvements within one's own life, as well as enhance interpersonal connections. Improv also helps people to hone their collaboration and communication skills, tap into their divergent thinking abilities, and strengthen their active listening skills. It also assists with embracing imperfection and getting comfortable existing in the present moment. As a result, improv not only leads to benefits interpersonally, but intrapersonally as well.

## Skills Used During and Developed Through Improv

Improv requires adaptability, as well as the ability to accept the influence of others. That, in turn, involves cognitive flexibility and vulnerability. This can be a challenge, as many people operate based on schemas, or the mental organizational maps which they hold for situations. Events or occurrences that don't neatly fit into our existing schemas are often avoided altogether, since existing in that space could lead to discomfort and lack of control. This is because schemas enable people to predict, plan, and understand the world, and are built as a result of convergent thinking, in which there is one solution to a problem (Walton, 2003).

When improvising, participants break away from set patterns of thinking so that they can access alternative solutions (Lewis & Lovatt, 2013). Lemons (2005) shares that improv can improve communication, collaboration, and lead to the ability to take risks. Additionally, it can enhance self-expression and joy, lead to feelings of safety, and assist in moving toward self-actualization.

Improv also requires people to stretch their active listening muscles and to be present. It is quite common for people to know what they want to say and steer the conversation with the purpose of communicating that point. This often occurs at the expense of fully listening to and engaging with other conversation partner(s). Dohe and Pappas (2015) share that we must step outside of our comfort zone and not simply repeat ourselves without considering our circumstances, as "[t]here is a difference between talking *at* and talking *with*, especially if the subject has been covered before" (p. 5). In that respect, improv requires us to go beyond just listening, to actually hearing, understanding, and affirming those with whom we engage.

## THE PRINCIPLES OF IMPROV AND PSYCHOLOGICAL UNDERPINNINGS

As previously noted, improvisers rely on a set of rules or principles when on stage. These rules are not meant to confine or interrupt the creative process, but rather to give players something to lean on and build upon. To connect the art and science of improv, the most common rules will be presented along with the accompanying psychological principles.

### Be Present

Improv requires players/participants to be fully present and engaged. They must actively listen to their teammates or for the audience suggestion, without preplanning their next move. Working without a predetermined plan requires people to let go of their expectations and engage with in-the-moment thinking (Lemons, 2005).

For many, including this author, improv is an effective way to practice mindfulness. Mindfulness, or mindful awareness, enables people to become better acquainted with their emotions, and more deeply in touch with their experiences. As with mindful awareness, there is no preparation for improv performances and thus no ability to plan out all possible scenarios (and how they may potentially go wrong). It's just the players, their peers, and their non-judgmental presence that creates the scene.

One of the first mistakes new improv students make is focusing on the witty line they want to land (Chin, 2020). This prevents them from fully listening to their partners and being able to build upon what others have offered up. By being present, improvisers are able to pivot from focusing solely on their own thoughts to gathering information from their surroundings (Cole, 2016).

### Psychological Connection

Being completely present on stage or in an improv group also shares similarities with Csikszentmihalyi's concept of flow. Flow, or complete engagement with a task, is often associated with a focus on the task itself and the loss of the sense of space and time (Csikszentmihalyi, 1990). The task is neither too challenging nor too easy, but keeps a person optimally engaged. Additionally, when participating in a group with others, a state of flow can facilitate higher levels of engagement and achievement (Csikszentmihalyi, 1990).

Bermant (2013) notes that the metaphor of working without a net can be used to describe how improvisers perform without a script. He emphasizes that while there is preparation involved, it's at the beginning, a time in which you are learning the craft and form. The actual scene itself is impromptu, creative, and spontaneous. This requires attention and a present focus.

## "Yes, and"/Accepting Influence

"Yes, and" is considered by many to be the guiding principle of improv. A player will accept (the "yes") and then add onto the suggestion of another player (the "and"). For example, if a performer were to come onto the stage and say, "What a lovely day it is at the zoo," the other improviser would try to take it further, and perhaps say, "Yes, it is! I'm so glad we decided to come. Look at the elk!" This helps to build connections (and trust) between those on stage. If, on the other hand, the improviser rejected the offer and said, "No, it's not. It's cold, raining, and I want to go home," the scene ends, and the speaker will feel dejected. This prevents any opportunities for forward movement or growth.

"Yes, and" enables the players in the scene to be on the same page and accept the reality being offered by one another. This can present a challenge as it is often easy to default to a no pattern or shoot down someone else's suggestions, opting instead to follow the pre-planned path already on their mind. "Yes, and" requires people to suspend these plans and surrender to the moment, rely on their partner, and trust the process.

When you employ "Yes, and," you keep the scene moving and keep everyone playing the same game (Drinko, 2021). Researcher and improviser Clay Drinko, the author of *Play Your Way Sane* also notes that "Yes, and" doesn't literally mean always saying "yes," but rather going along with someone else's ideas (Drinko, 2021). This is because agreement between partners in and of itself has no forward movement (Dohe & Pappas, 2015). Rather, by using the principle of "Yes, and," you build on the previous idea, move the group forward, and continue to develop the scene.

### Psychological Connection

This important rule connects with emotional bids, which are requests for connection between partners and involve a verbal or nonverbal message. Bids are attempts made by one partner to get attention or receive affection or affirmation (Brittle, 2015). By responding to a partner's bid, the receiving person is emotionally attuned to them and is turning toward, rather than away from them. An example of a verbal bid would be a person explicitly asking their partner to spend time with them. An example of nonverbal bid would be a person making a move to hold their partner's hand.

"Yes, and" also connects to the constructs of affirmation and validation. While closely related, these two terms should not be used interchangeably. Affirmation, similar to "Yes, and" is when one person agrees with the other. Validation, on the other hand, is acknowledgement. To validate someone involves accepting their feelings, thoughts, beliefs, and experience (Linehan, 1997). Both affirmation and validation are involved when creating a scene and accepting the influence of the other players.

Finally, the principle "Yes, and" shares many similarities with the Rogerian concept of unconditional positive regard (UPR), which is often discussed in relation to therapeutic practice. By practicing UPR, a clinician does not discriminate against clients or view them as more or less worthy (Rogers, 1959). An individual is valued even if the therapist does not agree with them or their actions. This is a state of total acceptance, which in turn can lead to personal growth and well-being.

## Make Bold Choices

When arriving on stage, it is important for an improviser to make choices, such as who they are, what their objective is, what their relationship to the other players is, and what type of environment they are in (Katzman, & O'Connor, 2018). This creates the scene and, by using "Yes, and," other players can continue to build onto it and make the vision come to life.

Making bold choices requires a person to be comfortable and confident in their ability to make a selection and stick with it. A person must be a risk taker as opposed to waffling while rife with self-judgment. This can be a challenging task, as it is easy for a person to get in their own head and talk themselves out of decisions.

Exposure to improv assists in overcoming the fear of making a choice by helping a person become more resolute in trusting their instincts. Additionally, the next principle, in which mistakes are seen as gifts, can also assist by removing the feared negative consequences of what a person may view as a wrong choice.

### Psychological Connection

The principle of making bold choices relates to the idea of the spotlight effect in which people tend to overestimate how much others are aware of their appearance or behaviors (Myers, 2015). This phenomenon can create a great deal of anxiety for people, as they feel self-conscious in social situations and are more likely to stay in the background. Relating this to improv, exposure to an environment in which choices are encouraged and mistakes are viewed as gifts leads to an increase in self-confidence and the ability to trust one's instincts. Additionally, the unconditional support of a player's fellow team members helps them bolster their ability to make a bold choice.

## There Are No Mistakes/Mistakes Are Gifts

In improv, there is no such thing as a mistake since anything that a player offers is a good and relevant suggestion. When there is a focus on what may initially be seen as a mistake, it is important to reframe the mistake as a gift. By doing this, what the participants feel is a mistake is acknowledged, and they are given the space and grace to make them. Also, by reframing a mistake as a gift, or opportunity for a creative course correction, the power and ability to induce anxiety amongst people may be taken away. Improv gives people permission to make mistakes, all within the comfort of a supportive atmosphere.

### Psychological Connection

The fear of making a mistake is heightened when people are plagued by self-doubt or problematic, distorted thought patterns. Cognitive distortions, or irrational thoughts, lead to inaccurate perceptions of reality. Distortions, originally conceived of by psychiatrist Aaron Beck (1963), can instill anxiety and fear amongst those who hold them. Furthermore, these thoughts often reinforce negative thinking (cognitions) and emotions. Research supports this in that negative events and information receive more attention and more thorough cognitive processing than do positively valenced events and information (Baumeister et al., 2001). Taken together, this means that the focus is often on the negative.

Examples of common cognitive distortions are "should" statements, personalization, labeling, and filtering. "Should" statements are those in which people tell themselves that things *should* be the way they imagined them, such as "I *should* be able to come up with a wittier response in this improv scene." Personalization is when a person attributes negative occurrences to themselves. An example would be a person blaming themselves if a friend didn't call them back. Labeling is when a person identifies with their shortcomings. For example, a person may label themselves as lazy, which in turn affects how they view themselves and how they interact with others. Filtering is when a person focuses on the negative and filters, or potentially blocks out the positive aspects of a situation. This focus on the negative can cause a person to fixate and may alter their view of whatever they are thinking about.

Improv helps people make a choice, trust their instincts, and move on without perseverating on the negative. It also teaches improvisers to look at what they may perceive of as a mistake as an opportunity for growth, rather than an indication of failure. Additionally, improv assists with reframing negative situations, thereby highlighting the positive aspects of them.

## Collaboration is Key/Making Your Partner Look Good

Improv is inherently a collaborative process. Each participant, or player, along with their partner creates a scene in response to a suggestion. To do so, they must fully engage with one another (Cole, 2016). Therefore, to fully embrace the experience, improvisers surrender their own plan and follow the scene being co-created by the improv group and the audience.

Making your partner look good involves considering what you can add to the scene, rather than detracting from it. You can do this by affirming them (you "Yes, and" them), and supporting what they are doing. For example, if one player is doing the breaststroke, you would not walk up and ask them, "Why are you running around the track?" Rather, you would start to swim along and perhaps comment on how good the water feels on this hot, sunny day.

### Psychological Connection

Bermant (2013) notes that an important feature of improv is the cooperation involved. It is called "group mind" when a person forgoes their ego and focuses on the other players. He shares that this is often evidenced in the activity Mind Meld, in which players will rapidly free associate to the point in which they produce the same word simultaneously.

An individual's personal goal is to give to their partner, and their partner's goal is hopefully the same. Players/improv teammates are out for one another, rather than focusing on the self. With each player on the team acting accordingly, they are inherently involved in a collaborative process.

Additionally, this connects with the aforementioned idea of emotional bids. Improvisers are going beyond affirmation (the "Yes, and") to validation, by making their teammates look good.

## APPLIED IMPROV

### The Current State of the Application of Improv

Improv is now moving beyond the theaters to the general public, and into classroom and business settings. Siliezar (2019) shares that the "…skills performers learn in improv- teamwork, collaboration, listening, communication, and the ability to adapt and problem-solve- can translate to social and professional skills sought after in many workplaces" (para. 7). Improv is also being applied to organizational settings to promote behaviors and traits that enable people to flourish (Cole, 2016).

The Second City Theater in Chicago has an 8-week Improv for Anxiety course which includes an hour of improv exercises and an hour of group therapy lead by clinicians with backgrounds in improv (Chillag, 2019). The Improv Therapy Group has classes for a wide variety of students, including therapists, with the goal of teaching clinicians to incorporate improv skills and exercises into their own therapeutic work (Improv Therapy Group, 2022). Their courses also aim to instill empathy and emotional intelligence, improve communication, assist people in embracing imperfection, and helping them to practice important life skills (Improv Therapy Group, 2022).

The Applied Improvisation Network (AIN), formed in 2002 with 30 members, now has a global community of over 8,000 participants (Applied Improvisation Network, 2022). The members are focused on cultivating a sense of community and professional excellence by applying the principles of improv across fields and in a diverse array of settings and global contexts (Applied Improvisation Network, 2022). The network is comprised of practitioners who use improv in their practice with the goal of building collaborative opportunities amongst them, as well as promoting best practices in the field.

### Improv in the Workplace

There is a need for individuals skilled in improvisation in the workplace. This is because organizations often require people to make quick decisions, adapt easily, work independently, and develop creative and innovative solutions to problems (Cole, 2016).

Improv has traditionally made its way into the corporate sector in the form of teambuilding activities, since it assists with spontaneity and trust (Cole, 2016). Moving beyond this, improv can help instill and strengthen valuable skills for those in the workplace, such as the ability to actively listen to colleagues, quickly process information, and creatively solve problems. It has also been shown to improve communication and collaboration (Cole, 2016). Taken together, these skills can boost morale, enhance employee engagement, and increase workplace satisfaction.

## Improv in Education

Improv has also made its way into educational settings. While role-playing has long been used in the classroom, improv differs in that there is no pre-planned script or agenda. Rather, the participants engage in collaborative storytelling and co-creation through a series of engaging exercises (Gao et al., 2019).

Dohe and Pappas (2017) created a workshop for librarians based on the principles of improv for the purpose of tackling some of the challenges of collaboration that are commonly faced by libraries in higher education. They note that the principles of improv assist with fostering collaboration, communication, and increasing resilience amongst staff, which is important as a major responsibility of libraries is interdisciplinary collaboration.

The researchers note that each workshop is generative in nature in that the participants are free to create and shape the conversation (Dohe & Pappas, 2017). Throughout the process, they have found five themes of improv central to their discussion. This first is Listen, De-Center, and Check Your Ego at the Door, which involves focusing on and actively listening to other people. The second is Build Your Ensemble, Support Your Team, in which ideas are accepted as the collective property of the group. The third is, Bring More than Yes, which is when the reflexive response becomes yes, and agreement (and addition) is the expectation. The fourth is Learn to Speak a Different Language, in which you are engaged, spontaneous, and willing to accept suggestions. Fifth and finally is: Fearless Failure is the Source of Creation, in which failures are viewed as opportunities. Rather than focusing on what went wrong, people learn to look for ways to learn, adapt, and grow. These principles stimulate collaborative discussion and lead to meaningful change.

## Improv in Medicine

Improv has been used successfully in medicine and in the training of medical students. Headspace Theater, a program designed for students to learn about psychiatric conditions, involves role-play and is a useful tool in helping learners understand what patients may encounter and experience. It is different from a traditional role-play in that learners are assigned an experience that turns out to be different from the real role they play. Specifically, the main character is led to believe that they are a doctor interviewing a patient. However, this character is in fact a person with psychosis and the other actors/group members help to create an atmosphere of paranoia (Ballon et al., 2007). Essentially, the main characters must interact with their peers and make meaning of the situation in real time without a script. This is tied to improv in that the participants are experiencing and acting within the scene as it develops. It is important to note that the one major difference between Headspace Theater and improv is that in improv all players are working together to build the same scene, whereas in Headspace Theater one person is operating based on a different perception of reality (the role they thought they were assigned).

Ballon et al. (2007) note that there are several goals of Headspace Theater which involve increasing the empathy of clinicians toward their patients, teaching the students the skills needed for role-play, promoting the synthesis and retention of new skills, and reflection about the experience. Dr. Ballon ran a series of these workshops at the University of Toronto, which consist of 10-minute role play exercises followed by discussion. These exercises were followed by a debriefing activity in which students processed the experience and their feelings around it. Specifically, a discussion was had about the main character's experience, the experience of the other players and the audience, as well as a general discussion. The workshops received favorable evaluations by participants, who noted that they were engaged and had a greater understanding of the material. They also reported feeling a greater level of empathy for those suffering from mental health conditions; they wanted to continue the learning exercises.

## RESEARCH ON THE BENEFITS OF IMPROV

### Enhancement of Learning and Pedagogy

Improv has been used in educational settings to assist students in better understanding their course material and to assist them in engaging with others about their course content. Lavik (2020) used improv techniques to teach a graduate level thermodynamics seminar for the purpose of fostering discussion and building community. Lavik (2020) noticed that students were having difficulty making connections between their research and the concepts being taught in class and wanted to trigger deeper, more meaningful conversations. She split her class of 16 students into two groups, one that just began with the typical seminar discussion, and the other which started with brief improv exercises. At the end of the semester, she gave her students a survey to assess their experience. While a small sample, the researcher reported that improv improved her class discussions. She noted that those exposed to improv were more likely to participate. Specifically, 50% of those who didn't experience improv spoke during class, whereas all of those who had participated in improv contributed to the discussions. She also noted that that improv created a more connected environment in which students were more willing to ask questions.

Improv can also be used to enhance specific skills within the classroom setting. DeMichele (2015) found that improv affects and improves the writing fluency of students. Two quasi-experimental action research studies were conducted to examine students' word and sentence usage after being exposed to the improv concept of "Yes, and." The study took place at an inner-city high school in New Jersey during a six-week summer program and consisted of one experimental class and two comparison classes. Students in the experimental class were taught improv games by the researcher, who was both a social studies teacher and professional improv actor, along with a substitute teacher who was pursuing teacher certification. In total, over the six weeks of schooling, those in the experimental class were exposed to 9.5 hours of shortform improv games. Results revealed a 101% increase in word usage and a 131% increase in sentence usage of those in the experimental group, compared to those in the control group.

DeMichele (2015) conducted a second quasi-experimental study between September and December 2004 in a 9th grade World History class and a 10th grade American Studies class. Students engaged in their regular work during the pre-assessment phase from September through November, and were then instructed for eight days in December on a sequence of improv games, including the concept of "Yes, and." After this, they engaged in three days of journal writing, used as a post assessment. Results demonstrated that after eight days of improv games, the 9th grade students showed a 34% increase in word usage and 51% increase in sentence usage. The 10th graders demonstrated a 55% increase in word usage and a 112% increase in sentence usage post intervention. Overall, improv games increased writing fluency, demonstrating that it is a beneficial educational intervention. The reason this intervention was helpful is likely because the students internalized the concept of "Yes, and" which assisted them in adding on/building consecutive thoughts.

Not only is improv effective for those in the primary and secondary grades but can assist adult learners as well. "Medical improv" is a growing field that focuses on the connection of improv to instruction in the health professions. Gao et al. (2019) reviewed seven studies on medical improv and found several key curriculum components. These include having facilitators with both clinical and theater expertise, a low stakes learning environment, and time for debriefing in which clinical relevance is highlighted. The researchers also shared that the benefits of improv are far reaching, including, but not limited to, comfort with uncertainty, team management, self-reflection, active listening, non-verbal communication, trust, resilience, and confidence (Gao et al, 2019).

Beyond just helping students, improv also assists educators. Seppänen et al. (2020) conducted a study to examine the impact of improv on student teachers' stress responses, as well as the influence of interpersonal confidence (IC), which is the belief of ones' ability in social interactions, concerning their response to stress. Previous work by Seppänen and colleagues, (2019, as cited in Seppänen et al., 2020) demonstrated that improvisation interventions had been particularly useful for those low in IC, who found social situations more stressful.

In the current study, participants were split into two groups, the intervention group (19 participants), who received seven weeks of improv training for 2.5 hours once a week at the University of Helsinki and the control group (16 participants). All received the Trier Social Stress Test (TSST). It involves an impromptu speech and math test taken in front of others, which elevates stress levels.

Results demonstrated that the improv group exhibited less stress when compared to the control group. Additionally, interpersonal confidence also reduced stress responses. Overall, the researchers found that improv interventions may reduce pre-performance stress, and that repetition of a challenging tasks leads to habituation, especially amongst those with low IC.

Seppänen et al. (2020) share that the improv training helped to cultivate a mindset that allowed for connection and communication, which enhanced the student teachers' ability to tune in to their social environments.

## Uncertainty Tolerance

Another major benefit of improv is its ability to help participants tolerate uncertainty. Spolin (1963), in her influential text in which she introduces improvisation for the theater notes that through spontaneity

*...personal freedom is released, and the total person, physically, intellectually, and intuitively, is awakened. This causes enough excitation for the student to transcend himself- he is freed to go out into the environment, to explore, adventure, and face all dangers he meets unafraid (p. 6).*

While engaging in improv may feel uncomfortable at first, embracing the process can lead to numerous benefits. Uncertainty is a part of our everyday lives and also influences how people navigate their environment and adapt to change. Hillen et al. (2017) examined uncertainty in relation to the healthcare system. The researchers note that uncertainty in this domain involves many unknowns, including if a patient will develop a condition, the prognosis of the condition, which treatment to seek, and whether or not the patient is receiving the appropriate care. Such uncertainty can lead to avoidance, anxiety, and fear, and can create a situation in which a person feels disempowered and unable to get the information they need to make informed decisions (Hillen et al., 2017).

Many factors contribute to the uncertainty faced such as the source of the uncertainty, traits of the patient, and larger societal factors such as the resources and structures in place within the healthcare settings. Additionally, the uncertainty can arise from the ambiguity and complexity of the information presented. Uncertainty is unlikely to be eliminated entirely, so being able to practice acceptance of it may make it less uncomfortable and less anxiety-inducing. The researchers found that improv serves as a type of exposure therapy, in that repeated experiences with uncertainty may desensitize a person to the experience of anxiety often associated with it. This can in turn lead to a decrease in the tendency to disengage from situations that lead to distress.

## Communication Enhancement

Improv gets to the core of how people communicate and has been shown to increase confidence and interpersonal connections. Clinicians can benefit from being able to listen to their patients and clearly communicate with them in a way that engenders trust and empathy. Additionally, improv enables clinicians to make strong and bold choices and strengthen the conviction to advocate for vulnerable populations and patients at risk. In addition, the skills gained through improv give clinicians the confidence to steer their organizations in the direction of social change (Chin, 2020).

By using the principles of "Yes, and," staying present, and fostering collaboration, clinicians trained in improv are uniquely positioned not only to hear their patients, but to understand them, work with them, and advocate on their behalf. They are also more likely to employ the assistance of and work within a cross collaborative team to find the best approach in treating or managing the health issue(s).

## Well-Being and Connection

Improv has also been shown to enhance overall well-being. Lindquist et al. (2021) conducted a study to see how improv would affect those living in a long-term care facility. Specifically, they wanted to examine how an 8-week improv course would affect well-being, self-efficacy, socialization, isolation, emotional distress, anxiety, and perceived stress (Lindquist et al., 2021). Sixteen residents with a mean age of 83.6 years at a continuing care retirement community (CCRC) in Chicago took part in the study. The course, Humor Doesn't Retire (HDR), was held in-person from September through November 2019.

Results, comparing baseline measures to 1-month post course measurements, demonstrated significant changes in social isolation and perceived stress. Improvement was also shown for positive affect and well-being, self-efficacy for managing emotions and managing social interactions, as well as a reduction in emotional distress. Residents reported that the course made them feel more positive and attentive. They also reported meeting other residents through the course and felt better prepared to socialize with others. Additionally, they noted that it helped with their communication and made them feel better able to be spontaneous and handle situations as they arose. Importantly, they noted that the course was fun.

The specific skills required of improvisers, such as spontaneity, also affect well-being. Kipper and Shemer (2006) conducted a study to examine the Revised Spontaneity Assessment Inventory. This measure assesses six features of spontaneous behavior, which include novelty, immediacy, appropriateness, effortlessness, engagement, and level of control (Kipper & Shemer, 2006). Their research focused on 105 adults in San Diego, California and found that spontaneity was positively related to well-being and negatively related to stress. Therefore, the spontaneity used and developed in improv can have far-reaching psychological effects.

Specific improv activities can also increase connection. Cohen and Miller (2009) conducted a study with 21 clinicians-in-training, with a mean age of 26 years, in graduate school at an urban university to evaluate the effect of mindfulness training on mental health professionals. Participants engaged in a 6-week interpersonal mindfulness training (IMT) program, modeled after the manualized mindfulness stress-based reduction program (MSBR), with a focus on relational awareness. The experiment followed a pre and posttest design, and the intervention consisted of a series of mindfulness exercises, one of which was the "mindful mirror" in which partners took turns mimicking the moves of the other. This mirror exercise is also commonly used in improv training. Participants were given a series of measures such as the Mindful Attention Awareness Scale, Satisfaction with Life Scale, Perceived Stress Scale, and the Meaning in Life Questionnaire, as well as tests for anxiety, depression, and emotional intelligence. Results showed that participants experienced enhanced connection, increased mindfulness, decreased anxiety, and enhanced well-being. While the study focused on mindfulness, the use of an improv activity as an intervention is noteworthy.

Improv can also affect self-efficacy and esteem. Schwenke et al. (2021) conducted a study in a school setting with 30 participants in the intervention group and 28 in a control group. Those in the intervention group took part in a 6-week group-based improv training program, with a total of two hours of improv per week. Participants were an average of 26.55 years old, with a majority being female. While the improv program did not demonstrate a significant effect on mindfulness or tolerance of uncertainty in this experiment, a beneficial effect of improv on self-esteem and self-efficacy was shown. Schwenke et al. (2021) note that the findings

*...indicate that improv helps to develop a mindset that welcomes and embraces possible failures or shortcomings and enhances an attitude toward self-respect and self-acceptance...Improv most of all provides a positive atmosphere of openness and trust fostered by group coherence and mutual support (p. 41).*

## Creativity and Divergent Thinking

As previously noted, improv enables people to break out of their pre-existing patterned responses, employ creativity, and act with flexibility (Lewis & Lovatt, 2013). As improv has been linked to innovative thinking and personal growth, it has been applied to a variety of fields (Lemons, 2005).

Lemons (2005) interviewed seven individuals from diverse disciplines who incorporated improv into their work to examine the common elements of improv that may lead to creative thinking as a way to examine how the elements of improv parallel the components of creativity. All seven participants were previously known by the researcher through their publications or presentations that focused on connecting improv to their respective work. The themes that emerged from the interviews were communication, community/teamwork, risk/challenge, safety, honest emotional expression, self-actualization, and joy (Lemons, 2005).

For the theme of communication, players noted that they must hear and respond to others. For community/teamwork, they noted that improv is a cooperative effort. With regards to honest emotional expression, improviser interviewees shared that they stay in the moment and don't have a chance to plan. With regards to risk/challenge those interviewed noted that improv requires emotional risks to both think and act spontaneously. For the theme of safety, it was noted that there is a need to create a safe environment in which people can take the risks involved in improv. Improv also leads to self-actualization, in which people have an opportunity to grow and develop; and joy, which involves the fun found in the process of engaging in improv (Lemons, 2005).

In further exploring the improv-creativity connection, Kudrowitz (2010) conducted a study with the goal of finding new ways to improve upon the idea generation process of employees. The researcher's specific goal was to assist designers and engineers in becoming creative idea generators.

A total 84 participants, with a mean age of 28 (52 of whom were male), consisting of students, professional designers, and improv comedians took part in the study. Participants were split into four groups: 24 product designers, 21 improvisational comedians, 26 MIT students, and 13 labeled "other." Participants took part in a cartoon caption test and a brainstorming task in which they were told to develop as many innovative ideas as possible around a given product.

It was shown that the ability to generate many ideas was highly correlated to producing promising creative ideas. Kudrowitz (2010) noted that those who produce a lot of creative ideas may be better at divergent thinking, which is a related thought process, or that as more associations are made, the probability of producing a creative one increases. Additionally, those who are uninhibited may be editing their thoughts less, and, as a result, are more creative. The improvisational comedians produced on average 20% more product ideas and 25% more creative product ideas than professional product designers.

In order to examine how improv affects idea generation, a workshop based on short-form improv exercises was created (Kudrowitz, 2010). The improv workshop lasts a total of 60-90 minutes, depending on how long it takes to complete all exercises, and consists of a series of games intended to stimulate associative thinking. Eleven MIT students participated in this workshop, and it was shown that they generated 37% more ideas during a subsequent brainstorming session, compared to the 26 MIT students from the previous study. This demonstrates that improv can foster creativity.

Improv has also been shown to increase divergent thinking, which is the ability to explore multiple scenarios or solutions to problems. Divergent thinking involves the intellectual abilities that contribute to generating a variety of ideas, such as fluency, flexibility, originality, and elaboration (Walton, 2003).

Felsman et al. (2020) conducted two experiments to examine the effect of improv on divergent thinking, uncertainty tolerance, and affective well-being. In their first study, Felsman et al. (2020) examined 74 undergraduates with a mean age of 18.83 from a midwestern university. Participants were assigned to an improv group and exposed to short improv exercises, or to a control group, which was exposed to a similarly structured social interaction. Both groups were given pre and posttests and participated in a series of social interaction tasks. The improv exercises consisted of 7 warm-up activities that took a total of 20 minutes.

Results demonstrated that in both groups affect and uncertainty tolerance increased from pre to posttest, but the change did not differ by the group participants were assigned to. Divergent thinking did improve, with a difference between groups, in that the improv group demonstrated gains in fluency and originality compared to the control group.

In the second study, the researchers further amplified the differences between the treatments, by being sure that the improv activity involved performance without planning or preparation. A total of 131 undergraduates with a mean age of 18.92 participated in this experiment. Results from this study demonstrated that there was an increase from pre to posttest in affect, with a significant difference between the groups. Self-reported affect increased for the improv group relative to the control group. Uncertainty tolerance scores also increased for the improv group relative to the control condition. A difference was also shown between groups for divergent thinking, specifically in fluency, flexibility, and elaboration. Overall, this was one of the first studies that experimentally demonstrated that improv improves well-being and positive affect relative to a social interaction control (Felsman et al., 2020).

Felsman et al. (2020) posit that the reason some studies find no differences or marginal differences when it comes to improv in relation to divergent thinking, is that the benefits may be eclipsed by the inherent need to engage in novel situations during the course of social interactions often used in control conditions. This study is important in that only a 20-minute engagement in improv exercises was shown to have an effect, which has profound clinical implications.

Lewis and Lovatt (2013) also studied improv in relation to creativity, and specifically focused on divergent thinking. They note that improv requires the ability to create something spontaneously and flexibly, which relies on the ability to think divergently (Lewis & Lovatt, 2013). Forty-one psychology undergraduates from a university in the UK participated in their first experiment, a majority of whom were female with a mean age of 22 years. Twenty-one were in the experimental group, who experienced 20 minutes of improvisation, and 20 were in the control condition, who took part in 20 minutes of verbal discussion. Those in the improv condition engaged in a series of activities in which they had to produce a speech that could not be preplanned. Those in the control condition were given lists to recite and spoke with others in a way that involved minimal spontaneous creation.

Participants then spent three minutes writing down all of the unusual uses for a common item as per the instructions of the Alternative Uses Task (AUT; Guilford, 1967). This allowed the researchers to examine fluency, which involves the number of responses created; originality, which looks at how unique the answer given is; elaboration, which involves the level of detail given in an answer; and flexibility, or the number of distinct categories a response falls into (Lewis & Lovatt, 2013).

Results showed an increase in fluency, originality, and flexibility on the AUT for those in the improv condition. This suggests that improv helps people to break away from their patterned thinking, thus enhancing the ability to think divergently (Lewis & Lovatt, 2013).

The researchers conducted a second experiment in which they replicated the previous study, this time using non-verbal treatment conditions. A total of 36 participants took part and were either assigned to 20-minutes of musical improvisation tasks or 20-minutes of music practice. Results replicated those in experiment 1, in that AUT fluency, originality, and flexibility scores significantly increased post improvisation when compared to the control condition.

## Stress Reduction and Mental Health

Improv is a type of low intensity intervention, which often involves workshops or psychoeducational series, in which participants are provided with cost-effective and evidence-based treatments for mild to moderate mental health problems, such as stress and anxiety (Acosta, 2021). Beginning improvisers are exposed to a safe environment which serves as a way to help people combat their anxiety, stress, and potential insecurities (Acosta, 2021).

To examine college students' feelings regarding an improv-based intervention, the "Improv(e) Your Life Workshop," as well as their perception of the therapeutic benefits of such a workshop, Acosta (2021) conducted an exploratory study. Additionally, the researcher examined participants' reported level of stress and anxiety (Acosta, 2021). A total of 144 undergraduates from the University of Hartford participated in this study with a mean age of 18.88 years, a majority of whom were female.

Participants were given scales to measure their stress and anxiety and read a vignette about a highly stressed, moderately anxious college student, as well as information about an improv-based intervention. The participants were also shown four videos of proposed improv interventions that would be included in a hypothetical workshop. The four units they observed were, "Yes, &!;" Surrendering to the ensemble; Making mistakes and being bold; Identifying emotions in self and others; and, Approaching life with flexibility and resilience. Finally, participants were given modified versions of the Treatment Acceptability Questionnaire (TAQ), which assesses the acceptability of psychological treatments for adult and child populations to gauge their perceptions of the interventions they witnessed.

The majority of participants gave treatment acceptability appraisals in the neutral to high range when considering the use of the hypothetical workshop for the person mentioned in the vignette, as well as for themselves. Participants also held moderately positive opinions about the workshop in helping the person in the vignette with interpersonal concerns, as well as moderately positive opinions about the workshop being able to help the participants themselves in moving toward self-improvement, joy, and interpersonal communication (Acosta, 2021). Overall, the study suggests that people view improv as a viable and acceptable treatment option for those who experience mild to moderate stress or anxiety.

Qualitative studies have also demonstrated participants' positive perceptions of improv. Reid-Wisdom and Perera-Delcourt (2020) conducted semi-structured interviews of nine British participants (6 male, 3 female), with a mean age of 41 years, to understand the benefits of improv for mental health. All participants had at least two years of experience in improv. The researchers found several themes from their work. The first: Improv's activities and values support growth in the participants' outlook, means that participants benefit from increased tolerance of uncertainty and challenges to their thought patterns and their fear of failure. The second; Improv contributes to a change in attentional focus, enabling people to shift from a focus on the self to be more attentive to others. The third, and final theme: The internal effects of improv have external consequences, leading to improved social confidence and the ability to take risks off stage (Reid-Wisdom & Perera-Delcourt, 2020).

Overall, improv was shown to enhance confidence, connection, and self-awareness, as well as to improve focus, attention, and listening skills. Reid-Wisdom and Perera-Delcourt (2022) shared that the mechanisms by which improv enhances mental health surpass acceptance and non-judgmental awareness which are the principles often promoted in mindfulness. Improv, instead, goes a step beyond, and includes a celebration of what the other person offers in interpersonal engagements.

Improv also confers benefits to elderly adults. Morse et al. (2018) conducted a study to examine the benefits offered by the Humor Doesn't Retire Course, a class taught by Second City, a Chicago-based improv theater to participants 55 and older. Qualitative analysis was used to extract common themes from the surveys of 10 participants, who had a mean age of 71.6 years. Participants chose to take the course due to an interest in improv, for self-development, and to experience fun.

Participants reported increased positivity and a sense of comfort with the unexpected, as well as an enhancement in self-awareness. Another theme was participants' reports of acceptance by their social group. Participants also noted that the benefits enhanced their problem-solving abilities and their social lives (Morse et al., 2018). Overall, this study has implications for using improv to help provide opportunities for self-development and social connection, which can enhance the process of aging. Additionally, the changes that occurred as a result of the improv program underscore the potential for improv to assist seniors in asserting their agency and to live in a way that they find fulfilling and meaningful. (Morse et al., 2018).

## Neurobiological Outcomes and Treatment of Psychological Disorders

Beyond mental health, improv has implications for neurobiological development. DeMichele and Kuenneke (2021) conducted a study with adolescents who were diagnosed with complex developmental trauma (CDT), which is a result of prolonged exposure to traumatic events in early life and leads to the breakdown of neurobiological integration. This can cause a person to live in a constant state of hyperarousal in which a fear response is continuously being triggered.

The study was a quasi-experimental pretest-posttest design. A total of 28 individuals between the ages of 15 and 18, a majority of whom were female, participated. The intervention, One Rule Improv, involved 20-minutes of short-form improv games.

Participants had a qEEG scan to measure brainwaves prior to the intervention, played the games while wearing a qEEG cap, and had another qEEG scan after the session.

Results demonstrated that the improv intervention affected functional connectivity changes, meaning that it enhanced the relationship between the different brain regions. This moves individuals from a state of survival to a state of connection to others (DeMichele & Kuenneke, 2021). Just one 20-minute improv session led to changes in the nervous system, which shows how powerful this art form can be.

Improv has also been shown to be effective in reducing the symptoms associated with certain psychological disorders, such as social anxiety disorder. Phillips Sheesly et al. (2016) discuss comedic improv therapy (CIT), which is a model inspired by improv for the treatment of social anxiety disorder (SAD). The program incorporates the therapeutic elements of group cohesiveness, play, exposure, and humor. This form of therapy exposes participants to anxiety-inducing scenarios in which they perform without a script. During this time, and by being in a supportive environment, CIT can provide them with a corrective emotional experience (Phillips Sheesly et al., 2016).

## IMPROV IN THE GROUP THERAPEUTIC SETTING

Improv can be used with clients in one-on-one therapeutic settings and in couples counseling. Additionally, it can be extremely beneficial when incorporated into a group format, both allowing members to engage in the activities and process their feelings and reactions to them. Improv can lead to personal growth and development, and as such it is often used by mental health professionals for both group therapy and in the treatment of psychological issues (Phillips Sheesly et al., 2016).

It is important to note that while improv can be used as a therapeutic aid, it is not intended to be a standalone mental health intervention. As such, it should not be the sole approach for those seeking treatment for anxiety or other mental health conditions. What improv in a therapeutic setting does is provide participants with the ability to engage in games as a form of self-care, learn the principles and apply them to their lives, as well as to interact with others in a safe and supportive space.

Debriefing sessions after each of the activities are strongly encouraged since these sessions have been shown to be an essential instructional design element (Ballon et al., 2007; Gao et al., 2019). This is because the post-improv discussion assists in helping participants/improvisers apply the experiences to their lives, as well as in connecting the activities to the underlying psychological principles and learning goals. Finally, debriefing enables the participants to build self-awareness and enhance self-reflection, and aids with personal and professional growth.

Below are some considerations for incorporating improv into group therapeutic practice, as well as in-depth descriptions of activities that work well both in virtual and in-person settings.

## Group Settings

The author had the honor of facilitating several Improv for Self-Care groups in a virtual format during the course of the Covid-19 pandemic. While there is a certain energy in the room that may be diminished when in a virtual format, many of the activities were effectively adapted for those who are socially distanced.

### Special Considerations for Virtual Settings

In the virtual format, a unique challenge is having everyone fully attuned to the conversations and focused on the same person. To facilitate this, all members should change their display to gallery view (if possible), allowing them to see all members participating. The person hosting the group can assign numbers next to each person's virtual square and request that members rearrange their grid so that the boxes appear in numerical order. To evaluate the effectiveness of this, you can instruct everyone to look at, and physically turn toward, box #1, then box #2, and so on. The group members should be instructed to be aware of how their body shifts and how their posture changes when focusing on different members.

In the virtual setting, since there is a short delay between the audio and video, there are times in which people talk over one another, or in which an individual member may not be heard. This is to be expected and is okay. By managing the expectations of the group members, they will be less likely to disengage if they accidently speak over one another or if their audio was not picked up.

### Introduction for Members

At the beginning of the sessions, it is helpful to frame the purpose of engaging in improv activities for the participants, as well as to clarify the connection between the activities and underlying psychological connections. You may consider:

*Some of the skills that we will hone over the course of our time together are accepting influence/suggestions from others; turning towards our partners and acknowledging their bids; creating shared spaces/joint experiences; enhancing active engagement in an activity; and boosting our tendency to be seen and feel heard when in conversations. Additionally, we will practice mirroring the emotions of others and building empathy; working on our affect regulation and awareness;*

*getting immersed in character(s) which may enable us to express our wishes/needs. We will be present and mindful, accept imperfections and abandon pre-conceived notions of "what ifs" and "shoulds" as all choices are wonderful group offerings.*

*Please note that the games presented are used in a variety of improv schools. They have been adapted both for a virtual setting and to meet the needs of a self-care group. As these games are an amalgamation of games commonly played in the improv world, many of which do not have a clear origin, citations are only presented for the components that have a clear source. Additionally, the activities are presented in first person since this section can be used as a manual for a therapeutic group improv setting.

## GROUP IMPROV ACTIVITIES

### 1. **Angry Alphabet**

This activity begins by getting everyone comfortable with speaking aloud and in the group. First, if in a virtual setting, have group members take turns using their assigned numbers as a guide, each person saying one letter of the alphabet (in alphabetical order). If a person were to skip a letter, and for example go from A to D, the next person would pick up at E, rather than correcting the previous person. Remember, that there is no such thing as a mistake. You should go around the group from A to Z several times, each time, quickening the pace. This is a great warm-up activity and an effective way to get people comfortable with their numerical order.

After this, have any group participant call out an emotion, such as happy or sad. This person would start at the beginning of the alphabet, saying "A" embodying the emotion with their voice and mannerisms. Moving to the next number in the virtual setting, or clockwise if in person, the next participant will say B, using that same emotion. After Z, a new emotion can be chosen. Beyond emotions, you can also embody adjectives, such as "tired" or "sloppy." All choices are good choices.

Once you have cycled through a few iterations of the alphabet with different emotions, wrap up by having participants discuss their reactions to the game and their expressions of the emotions.

**Important note:** Tell participants to "take it to a 10," meaning that they should fully and freely embody the emotion. The stronger they embody it, the better.

This activity requires participants to access their emotions and mirror the emotions expressed by others, enabling them to create a joint experience through a simple and fun recitation of the alphabet.

## 2. This Emotion is For You

This activity builds off of the previous Angry Alphabet game, but takes it a step further, by allowing participants to further embody the emotions using their facial expressions and vocal intonation. In this particular game, the first player starts by making a face. Allow participants to get creative and see what they produce. After settling into the facial expression that they feel best embodies the emotion they selected they will say, "This emotion is for you." The next participant will copy their mannerisms and intonation and say, "Thank you." They will then move from mimicking the previous face to selecting another facial expression that embodies a different emotion and pass this on to the next member by saying, "This emotion is for you." You will continue to go around the circle, or if virtual, in numerical order, accepting the emotions in the manner in which they were given and choosing another expression to share with the next person.

Once you have gone through a few rounds, you can have a debriefing discussion in which people share how they felt about embodying the emotions, sharing them, and receiving them. Additionally, you may want to discuss if people were always aware of the emotion they were being sent, or if they just did their best to mimic the person they received it from, even if not knowing exactly what it was.

**Important note:** Tell participants not to preplan any emotions/faces, but to focus on accepting the offering given in the moment. The same emotion can be shared multiple times since there are no wrong choices. As in the previous game, you may consider having participants use facial expressions and mannerisms that go beyond emotions to attributes, such as tired, lazy, or punctual.

This activity requires participants to access their own emotions and those of others. Additionally, it relies on active listening skills and the ability to turn toward their partners, staying in the moment.

## 3. Categories!

You may notice that this game has an exclamation point at the end. That is intentional. People really enjoy this game! The premise is simple; pick a category and name items in that category. If in a group setting, have people stand around a circle and ask for a suggestion. Moving clockwise if in person or to the next number if virtual, the group member following the individual who named the category is the first to name an item that belongs in the category. Continue to move around the circle in a clockwise direction after this. To switch things up and keep people on their toes, the facilitator can change the direction at random points throughout the game. If in a virtual group, just continue to go in numerical order.

The facilitator will jump in at random intervals to change the category in between participants. This helps to keep participants present and less likely to recite any preplanned list of items they may have for the current category. The facilitator can name the new category themselves, or just break the chain and have the person who was about to name the next item select the new category. Sample categories for your consideration may be nail polish colors, names of yoga poses, the next great American novel, the world's scariest horror film, and flavors of gum.

After several rounds, debrief with your group by discussing how they felt about the exercise. You may want to solicit responses to find out if they liked categories in which they knew several members/items, or those in which they were unfamiliar with relevant items. While some participants may like to have a familiar reference point, others may enjoy the lack of constraints that exist when creating items for categories they are not familiar with.

**Important note:** Participants may start with items that are real, and part of the categories. This is fine. For example, if you say brands of water and start with "Dasani," "Poland Spring," etc., that's great. Those are certainly brands of water. However, there are no wrong answers. "Unicorn tears," "Icy blue," and "Tomato" are perfectly wonderful choices as well.

This activity requires participants to actively employ their active listening skills, be comfortable in the moment, and abandon ideas of the "perfect" item for each category, thereby embracing imperfection and avoiding the tendency to move toward self-judgement.

4. **Yes, but…**

**Disclaimer:** The next two games go together. They will help to highlight the principle of "Yes, and" as well as allow participants to compare and contrast the way they felt in changing "Yes, but…" to "Yes, and…."

This game is to be played by two people at a time. If in person, you may want to have two people stand in the center of the circle or at the front of the group. If virtual, you may want to spotlight, or focus on, the two people engaging in the activity and/or have the other participants turn their cameras off.

Person A will begin by saying, "Let's go to the _______ so we _______." They may choose to say, "Let's go to the zoo so we set all of the zebras free." Or, "Let's go to DMV to take my written driving test." The more specific the better, since this helps to create a scene for both participants to become part of. "Let's go to the mall to shop" is a lot less descriptive than "Let's go to the mall to buy a new dress for my sister's upcoming wedding." The second offering sets up what the players are shopping for, why they need it, and what stores they might be in.

Person B will begin each sentence of each turn with, "Yes, but…." Using the first example above, we have:

**Person A:** *"Let's go to the zoo so we can set all of the zebras free."*

**Person B:** *"Yes, but the zoo doesn't have any zebras."*

Person A can resume the conversation by saying anything. Person B must always start with "Yes, but…." It is also important to tell participants to make definitive statements and avoid asking questions.

Each person in the group should have a turn playing person A, the one giving the suggestion and Person B, whose main goal is to "Yes, but…" Person A.

Once done, debrief by asking participants how they felt and if it was easier for them to be Person A or B. You may want to ask them to compare and contrast their experiences, noting the similarities and differences that the group members supply.

**Important note:** People may revert to asking questions or saying that they don't know what to say. The facilitator will want to reassure them that there is no such thing as a mistake so whatever statement they offer up is an excellent choice. The reason questions are not allowed, is because participants must learn to get comfortable with making a definitive choice.

This game tends to touch on the default state for many people, in which they say no to something or set limiting parameters on their choice. Person B often has an easier time, as they are shooting all of the scenarios down (the default for many individuals), whereas Person A must find a way to recover and continue on with the conversation. Comparing this game to the next one will allow the facilitator to highlight the importance of accepting emotional bids.

5. **Yes, and**

Yes, and was initially derived from the principle of improv that was made famous by Victoria Spolin (Spolin, 1963). This game follows the same rules of "Yes, but…" with one major change. Person B begins each sentence with "Yes, and…." Borrowing the example from above, we may have:

**Person A:** *"Let's go to the zoo so we can set all of the zebras free."*

**Person B:** *"Yes, and let's let the lemurs out too!"*

Once everyone in the group has had a chance to participate, both as Person A and

Person B, it is important to debrief. Focus on how this game differed from the previous one and how participants felt about this difference.

**Important note:** Participants may defer back to "Yes, but...," but be sure to reorient them to this game by noting "Yes, and we are now focusing on yes and-ing one another."

This game is integral to the art of improv. Here, players are accepting the suggestion of their partner and building the scene. In conversation this is when there is acknowledgement of the conversation partner, and in relationships this is the acceptance of an emotional bid from a significant other.

### 6. Do You Have a Question for Me?

For this game, either the facilitator or a member of the group will offer a scene suggestion to two participants who will be taking part in the activity. The suggestion should be general, such as "on a lake," allowing the participants engaging in the game to fill in the details. The participants will have a conversation, by taking turns asking questions. That's it; that's the only rule. Questions only.

Once everyone has had a chance to participate, debrief by asking members to describe how they felt and to describe any challenges they encountered.

**Important note:** Participants may say that they cannot think of a question. Give them time and allow them to try. This game can be quite challenging. Do not allow them to offer up a statement. Also, participants may try to fill in details of the scene by creating long run-on questions. The questions should all be short statements, allowing both participants to go back and forth, in a conversational manner, without one dominating the question-conversation.

Additionally, many people will wind up getting stuck on questions about some object present in the scene. For example, if the scene suggestion is people fishing on a lake, you may see:

**Person A:** *Where are we?*

**Person B:** *Is this a boat?*

**Person A:** *How big is this boat?*

**Person B:** *What is the name of this boat?*

Participants need not be constrained by the lake nor the boat, but simply use the scene/setting as a reference point. Players can be two people on a boat pondering the meaning of life, occasionally inserting questions about what fish just swam by. The focus is on the conversation between the partners, not on the boat.

This game requires participants to trust their scene partner and stay in-the-moment. Each must avoid trying to impose a certain narrative on the scene, but rather build it along with their partner. It is easy to notice when a person is trying to control the scene as they begin trying to fit in a lot of details at the beginning of their question.

## 7. Committee of Experts

Divide your group into small subgroups of 3, 4, or 5. Each subgroup will be a panel of experts engaging in conversation about an object. Think of this as a late-night infomercial, in which each subgroup of members will take turns describing an object, discussing it's use, talking about the benefits of owning it, and presenting any exclusive offers associated with it. Any direction players choose is great. They may want to name the object, describe it for those who are not in the same room as their imagined TV, or even get into detail about the origin story and how it made its way to market.

After each group completed its scene, take a break to find out what the experience was like both for the group members and for those listening. What worked well? What might members have noticed about themselves? How well did they work together? What can they improve upon?

**Important note:** This should be an interactive discussion. Avoid a situation in which one person is doing the lion's share of presenting, with the others simply listening or commenting on what that person has offered. The panel should be building on the suggestions of one another and making this object come to life.

This game requires participants to listen to one another and to accept the suggestions of their peers. They also have to flex their mindfulness skills by engaging with the here and now, rather than producing an entire scenario for how they want the panel to take shape and imposing this narrative on their peers.

## 8. Paraphrase and Extend

In this game, all participants will engage in a conversation. The first person starts with a sentence, such as, "I am worried about how long it will take me to get to work, because there is a lot of traffic today." The next person will use their own words to paraphrase any part of what the previous participant said and then extend it by adding on a new component. The participant does not need to paraphrase the entire sentence, but instead restate part of what the previous person said and then add the next piece onto it. For example, the second participant may say "There's a lot of traffic today. I think it's because Oprah Winfrey is in town and a lot of people are going to the city to see her." The following participant may offer up, "I heard that Oprah Winfrey is in the city today. I think that she may be giving out some of the items from her list of favorite things for free."

After each person has had an opportunity to paraphrase and extend the statements of others, take some time to debrief. Discuss any emotions or thoughts that came up, as well as any challenges that participants may have experienced.

**Important note:** Participants only need to paraphrase part of what the previous person said and should add one to two short sentences on. There is sometimes a tendency for participants to add on several run-on sentences, packed with details so that they can share the story they already have in mind. Instead, participants should focus on what the person before them has said, paraphrase, and extend.

This activity requires participants to build off of what others offer, creating a joint experience. This is "Yes, and" in action, as players are affirming and building the story. It also requires participants to listen carefully to what the previous person offered up, instead of solely focusing on what it is they want to say. In psychology, the next-in-line effect describes the situation in which our memory tends to be the weakest for what the person right before us in line said, due to the tendency to focus on what we are about to share (Myers, 2015). This activity is directly combatting that.

### 9. Find the Positive

This activity requires participants to reframe something negative, and instead focus on the positive. The first participant will share something that they dislike. For example, "I dislike traffic." The next participant will then use the following format to reframe what the previous participant shared: "Oh _______! I love ______." Using the previous example, the person may say "Oh traffic! I love having the opportunity to do my makeup and fix my hair in the car in the mornings on the way to work." Then, that person will offer up something that they dislike to the next participant, keeping this chain moving.

Once every participant has had an opportunity to both offer up something they dislike and reframe someone else's negative item, take the time to debrief. You may find that some people like items or scenarios that others dislike, or that the reframes were helpful to those who shared something they didn't like. Find out which reframes were more challenging to produce and which ones came more naturally to participants.

**Important note:** Stick to items or situations that people dislike, rather than hate. We wouldn't want to put a person in the uncomfortable situation of having them reframe sickness or poverty into something positive. We also don't want people to offer up something that they feel strongly negative about. The offerings should be minor dislikes, such as traffic or getting dripped on by an air conditioner.

This activity gives people the opportunity to reframe something negative and take a more optimistic look at it. This can help people practice reframing negative thought patterns, which is a valuable, yet challenging skill.

## 10. **Paperclip Poker**

This game requires a person to produce as many unusual uses of a common everyday item as possible. For example, a paperclip is typically used to hold papers together. Going around the circle or in numerical order in the virtual setting, each person should produce a new use. Using the paperclip example, you may say, a fingernail cleaner, or a poking device.

Once finished, have all members debrief to discuss which items were easier to produce creative alternatives for and which were more challenging. You will find that when working together in a collaborative manner, members are inspired by one another and become more creative. You may also introduce the concept of creativity, or the ability to produce ideas that are both novel and valuable (Myers, 2015). In fact, one such test, the Alternative Uses Task (AUT; Guilford, 1967), used in the aforementioned Lewis and Lovatt (2013) study, relies on the very same rules as this game.

**Important note:** While most games rely on the principle of there being no such thing as a mistake, this particular game requires participants to play in a realm of reality. Therefore, saying that you can use a paperclip as a bungee jumping harness is off the table.

This game flexes divergent thinking and creativity muscles. It also assists in building a collaborative team.

## 11. **Mirror**

This game requires participants to stand in front of one another in teams of two. This can also be done virtually by spotlighting two members at a time, while instructing all others to turn off their cameras. Participants will mirror one another's movements without speaking, also without any explicit instruction as to who is the leader and who is a follower. Instead, both are equals, and will follow one another and create a joint experience.

Once finished, those who participated can share how the experience made them feel. Those observing should also note what they experienced as they watched the two players build their joint connection.

**Important note:** There is a tendency for participants to want to talk or designate a leader. Encourage them to let the process happen nonverbally and organically.

This game relies on mindfulness skills, specifically interpersonal mindfulness, as well as the ability to create a connection. This is also one of the activities used in the aforementioned Cohen and Miller (2009) study.

12. **One Word**

This is a fun and quick game that you can use to end your group sessions. In this game, participants each take a turn offering up one word so that together they can complete a sentence. You can choose to give the sentence a purpose, such as an affirmation or a goal for the week.

**Important note:** It is extremely difficult to stick to one word. If a participant offers two, take just the first one, allowing the next participant to continue on with the sentence. Also, if the sentence comes to a natural end and participants want to keep going, the facilitator can offer the period to cap off the previous sentence.

This game requires participants to actively listen to one another, stay in the moment, relinquish control, and accept the bids of their partners.

## CONCLUSION

The burgeoning research connecting improv to applied fields such as business, education, and mental health is promising. Not only can engaging in improv exercises build connections with others and instill joy, but improv can enhance the ability to problem solve, think creatively and divergently, and enable people to better tolerate distress or uncertainty. It can instill confidence, help sharpen our decision-making skills, and enhance well-being. These valuable skills cut across industries and disciplines and are useful for both intra- and interpersonal development.

Improv exercises have been shown to confer benefits to participants even when engagement is short-term. The activities presented at the end of this chapter can be useful for any group setting, in-person or virtual. They should be presented in a way that enables players to actively participate and learn from the psychoeducational component connecting both the art and science of improv.

## REFERENCES

Acosta, M. A. (2021). *Exploring the acceptability of an improv-based workshop series for college student stress and anxiety.* [Doctoral dissertation, University of Hartford]. ProQuest Dissertations Publishing.

Applied Improvisation Network. (2022). *About*. AIN. https://www.appliedimprovisationnetwork.org/

Ballon, B. C., Silver, I., & Fidler, D. (2007). Headspace theater: An innovative method for experiential learning of psychiatric symptomatology using modified role-playing and improvisational theater techniques. *Academic Psychiatry*, *31*(5), 380–387. doi:10.1176/appi.ap.31.5.380 PMID:17875623

Baumeister, R. F., Bratslavsky, E., Finkenauer, C., & Vohs, K. D. (2001). Bad is stronger than good. *Review of General Psychology*, *5*(4), 323–370. doi:10.1037/1089-2680.5.4.323

Beck, A. T. (1963). Thinking and depression: I. Idiosyncratic content and cognitive distortions. *Archives of General Psychiatry*, *9*(4), 324–333. doi:10.1001/archpsyc.1963.01720160014002 PMID:14045261

Bermant, G. (2013). Working with(out) a net: Improvisational theater and enhanced well-being. *Frontiers in Psychology*, *4*, 1–6. doi:10.3389/fpsyg.2013.00929 PMID:24339820

Brittle, Z. (2015). Turn towards instead of away. *The Gottman Institute Blog*. https://www.gottman.com/blog/turn-toward-instead-of-away/

Chillag, A. (2018, August 20). How an improv class is relieving anxiety. *CNN Health*. https://www.cnn.com/2018/07/05/health/improv-for-anxiety-staying-well/index.html

Chin, M. H. (2020). Lessons from improv comedy to reduce health disparities. *JAMA Internal Medicine*, *180*(1), 5–6. doi:10.1001/jamainternmed.2019.5930 PMID:31816039

Chin, M. H., Clarke, A. R., Nocon, R. S., Casey, A. A., Goddu, A. P., Keesecker, N. M., & Cook, S. C. (2012). A roadmap and best practices for organizations to reduce racial and ethnic disparities in health care. *Journal of General Internal Medicine*, *27*(8), 992–1000. doi:10.100711606-012-2082-9 PMID:22798211

Cohen, J. S., & Miller, L. J. (2009). Interpersonal mindfulness training for well-being: A pilot study with psychology graduate students. *Teachers College Record*, *111*(12), 2760–2774. doi:10.1177/016146810911101202

Cole, J. (2016). *I've got your back: Utilizing improv as a tool to enhance workplace relationships*. [Master's Thesis, University of Pennsylvania]. University of Pennsylvania Scholarly Commons.

Csikszentmihalyi, M. (1990). *Flow: The psychology of optimal experience*. Harper Perennial Modern Classics.

DeMichele, M. (2015). Improv and ink: Increasing individual writing fluency with collaborative improv. *International Journal of Education & the Arts*, *16*(10). http://www.ijea.org/v16n10/

DeMichele, M., & Kuenneke, S. (2021). Short-form, comedy improv affects the functional connectivity in the brain of adolescents with complex developmental trauma as measured by qEEG: A single group pilot study. *NeuroRegulation*, *8*(1), 2–13. doi:10.15540/nr.8.1.2

Dohe, K., & Pappas, E. (2017). Lessons from the field: What improv teaches us about collaboration. *Library Leadership & Management*, *32*(1), 1–16.

Drinko, C. (2021). *Play your way sane*. Simon & Schuster.

Felsman, P., Gunawardena, S., & Seifert, C. M. (2020). Improv experience promotes divergent thinking, uncertainty tolerance, and affective well-being. *Thinking Skills and Creativity*, *35*, 100632. Advance online publication. doi:10.1016/j.tsc.2020.100632

Gao, L., Peranson, J., Nyhof-Young, J., Kapoor, E., & Rezmovitz, J. (2019). The role of "improv" in health professional learning: A scoping review. *Medical Teacher*, *41*(5), 561–568. doi:10.1080/0142159X.2018.1505033 PMID:30428747

Halpern, C., Close, D., & Johnson, K. (1994). *Truth in comedy: The manual of improvisation*. Meriwether Publishing.

Hillen, M. A., Gutheil, C. M., Strout, T. D., Smets, E. M., & Han, P. K. (2017). Tolerance of uncertainty: Conceptual analysis, integrative model, and implications for healthcare. *Social Science & Medicine*, *180*, 62–75. doi:10.1016/j.socscimed.2017.03.024 PMID:28324792

Improv Therapy Group. (2022). *Our mission*. Improv Therapy Group. https://improvtherapygroup.com/empathy-emotional-intelligence/

Katzman, J., & O'Connor, D. (2018). *Life unscripted: Using improv principles to get unstuck, boost confidence and transform your life*. North Atlantic Books.

Kudrowitz, B. M. (2010). *Haha and aha!: Creativity, idea generation, improvisational humor, and product design* (Unpublished doctoral dissertation). Massachusetts Institute of Technology, Massachusetts.

Lavik, E. (2021). Thermo in the Time of COVID-19: Using improvisation to foster discussion and translating the experience to online learning. *Biomedical Engineering Education, 1*(1), 133–138. doi:10.100743683-020-00022-z PMID:35141717

Lemons, G. (2005). When the horse drinks: Enhancing everyday creativity using elements of improvisation. *Creativity Research Journal, 17*(1), 25–36. doi:10.120715326934crj1701_3

Leveson, M., & Patterson, D. (Creators). (1998). Whose line is it anyway? [Television series]. Hollywood, CA: Hat Trick Productions.

Lewis, C., & Lovatt, P. J. (2013). Breaking away from set patterns of thinking: Improvisation and divergent thinking. *Thinking Skills and Creativity, 9*, 46–58. doi:10.1016/j.tsc.2013.03.001

Lindquist, L. A., Liggett, A., Muhammad, R., Seltzer, A., Kim, K. Y. A., Barish, B., & Ramirez-Zohfeld, V. (2021). Effects of improv training on older adults in a long term carefacility. *Gerontology & Geriatric Medicine, 7*. doi:10.1177/23337214211016111 PMID:34104682

Linehan, M. M. (1997). Validation and psychotherapy. In A. C. Bohart & L. S. Greenberg (Eds.), *Empathy reconsidered: New directions in psychotherapy* (pp. 353–392). American Psychological Association. doi:10.1037/10226-016

Morse, L. A., Xiong, L., Ramirez-Zohfeld, V., Anne, S., Barish, B., & Lindquist, L. A. (2018). Humor doesn't retire: Improvisation as a health-promoting intervention for older adults. *Archives of Gerontology and Geriatrics, 75*, 1–5. doi:10.1016/j.archger.2017.10.013 PMID:29156247

Myers, D. G. (2015). Psychology (11th edition in modules). New York: Worth Publishers. .

Phillips Sheesley, A., Pfeffer, M., & Barish, B. (2016). Comedic improv therapy for the treatment of social anxiety disorder. *Journal of Creativity in Mental Health, 11*(2), 157–169.

Poissant, D. (2018). 'Yes, and': Overcoming anxiety with improv. *UCF Forum*, 1-4.

Reid-Wisdom, Z., & Perera-Delcourt, R. (2022). Perceived effects of improv on psychological wellbeing: A qualitative study. *Journal of Creativity in Mental Health, 17*(2), 246–263. doi:10.1080/15401383.2020.1856016

Rogers, C. R. (1959). A theory of therapy, personality, and interpersonal relationships as developed in the client-centered framework. In S. Koch (Ed.), *Psychology: A study of a science. Formulations of the person and the social context* (Vol. 3, pp. 184–256). McGraw-Hill.

Schwenke, D., Dshemuchadse, M., Rasehorn, L., Klarhölter, D., & Scherbaum, S. (2021). Improv to improve: The impact of improvisational theater on creativity, acceptance, and psychological well-being. *Journal of Creativity in Mental Health, 16*(1), 31–48. doi:10.1080/15401383.2020.1754987

Seppänen, S., Toivanen, T., Makkonen, T., Jääskeläinen, I. P., Anttonen, M., & Tiippana, K. (2020). Effects of improvisation training on student teachers' behavioral, neuroendocrine, and psychophysiological responses during the Trier Social Stress Test. *Adaptive Human Behavior and Physiology, 6*(3), 356–380. doi:10.100740750-020-00145-1

Siliezar, J. (2019, May 1). Improv can boost social and professional skills, students find. *The Harvard Gazette*. https://news.harvard.edu/gazette/story/2019/05/improv-skills-can-translate-to-social-and-professional-skills/

Spolin, V. (1963). *Improvisation for the theater*. Northwestern University Press.

Walton, A. P. (2003). The impact of interpersonal factors on creativity. *International Journal of Entrepreneurial Behaviour & Research, 9*(4), 146–162. doi:10.1108/13552550310485120

## KEY TERMS AND DEFINITIONS

**Actors/Players/Participants/Improvisers:** the individuals engaging in improv.

**Applied Improv:** the application of and use of improv in business, therapeutic, and educational settings.

**Be Present/Mindfulness/Mindful Awareness:** orientation to the present, which enables people to become better acquainted with their emotions and more deeply in touch with their experiences.

**Bold Choices:** the definitive choices an improviser makes, which can include who they are, what their objective is, what their relationship is to the other players in their scene, and what type of environment they are in.

**Cognitive Distortions:** irrational thoughts that often lead to inaccurate perceptions of reality.

**Cognitive Flexibility:** the ability to adapt one's thinking in response to the environment.

**Divergent Thinking:** a thought process related to creativity, in which a person is able to create multiple solutions to a problem.

**Filtering:** a cognitive distortion in which a person focuses on the negative and potentially blocks out the positive aspects of a situation.

**Flow:** a state of complete engagement with a task, which is often associated with a focus on the task itself and the loss of the sense of space and time.

**Improv:** the art of skillfully, spontaneously, and collaboratively building a scene in the present moment.

**Labeling:** a cognitive distortion in which a person identifies with their shortcomings, such as viewing themselves as lazy.

**Making Your Partner Look Good:** the ability for an improviser to surrender their own plan and follow the scene being created by the group and the audience in a collaborative manner.

**Mistakes as Gifts:** the view that a mistake is not a failure or shortcoming, but rather an opportunity for a creative course correction.

**Personalization:** a cognitive distortion in which a person attributes negative occurrences to themselves, such as blaming themselves if a friend didn't call them back.

**"Should" statements:** a cognitive distortion in which people tell themselves that things *should* be the way they imagined them.

**Spotlight Effect:** a social psychology phenomenon in which people tend to overestimate how much others are aware of their appearance or behaviors.

**Uncertainty Tolerance:** the ability to manage/be relatively comfortable with the unknown.

**Unconditional Positive Regard (UPR):** a therapeutic practice in which the clinician does not discriminate against a client or view them as more or less worthy. The client/patient is valued and accepted, leading to their personal growth and well-being.

**Yes, and/Accepting Influence:** the guiding principle of improv in which a person accepts (the "yes") and then adds onto the suggestion of another player (the "and").

# Chapter 8
# The History of Trauma Treatment Intervention and the Movement Into Creative Arts Therapy

**Deanna Alyssa Villetto**
*Marymount Manhattan College, USA & School of Social Work, Columbia University, USA*

**Kayla Villetto**
*SUNY New Paltz, USA*

## ABSTRACT

*This chapter focuses on how trauma and post-traumatic stress disorder impact children, adolescents, and adults. It explores the history of trauma treatment as well as the benefits of creative arts therapy as a trauma treatment intervention. Creative arts therapy is crucial in the psychological realm, as it uses the building blocks of evidence-based practices to transform the narrative around healing the brain and body. Within the chapter, trauma and PTSD are explained, along with the history of trauma therapy, the history of creative art therapy around the world, and the rise of creative arts therapy in the United States.*

DOI: 10.4018/978-1-6684-7856-1.ch008

## TRAUMA AND POST-TRAUMATIC STRESS DISORDER EXPLAINED

Trauma is understood as an event, or series of events, that involve a real or perceived threat of death, serious injuries, or physical and sexual assaults. According to the DSM V, trauma does not include intense stressors such as divorce, loss of a job, or other psychosocial factors that may impact the daily functioning of individuals or the collective (American Psychiatric Association, 2013). While these psychosocial factors are important to note when working with clients and it's important to mitigate the scary or stressful events in their lives, the definition of PTSD and trauma is defined as the former, for the purpose of this chapter. The new model of PTSD as delineated by the DSM V redefined trauma as the complex somatic and psychological response to fear or danger in relation to events such as war, death, torture, domestic violence, interpersonal violence, and sexual abuse (Scrine, 2021). Using this new definition, treating individuals with PTSD or trauma exposure includes regulating the sympathetic nervous system, repairing the locus of control and rebuilding post trauma resilience. This will create a balanced view of the world through healing, wellness, and growth (Scrine, 2021). It is evident that many factors of PTSD and trauma are directly linked to societal structures such as racism, sexism, religious biases, and other macro level issues in society.

The impact of trauma can be muti-layered, especially when multiple traumas occur to an individual or a collective. There are many forms of trauma that lead to PTSD, which include chronic, acute, complex, and collective traumas. Chronic trauma is the prolonged exposure to one type of trauma, such as long-term domestic violence; acute trauma is short term exposure, or one trauma, occurring in a short period of time, such as a car accident; complex trauma is when many traumas occur over the course of one's life, such as long term domestic violence, a car accident, and a natural disaster; and collective traumas can impact many groups of people around the world, such as experiencing slavery, poverty, and natural disasters.

The mind, the body, and the essence of the individual who experienced trauma is shifted when they suffer from PTSD. Trauma can lead to lesions on the brain, the hyperarousal of the nervous system, and a shift in perspective of what is deemed safe and unsafe in the world (Rosen Saltzman et al., 2013). This can lead to a shift in thinking due to "the before," "the during" and "the after a trauma" perspective. The human brain has difficulty making sense of how to move forward with life if things can be, or feel, so dangerous (Spiegel et al., 2006). "The before" refers to one's life before the trauma occurs, "the during" refers to how one feels while trauma is occurring, and "the after" is how one feels and behaves after the trauma is over.

Post Traumatic Stress Disorder is a direct result of failure of the brain to process the traumatic event in a healthy way (Spiegel et al., 2006). When a trauma occurs that leads to PTSD, it is generally a shock or something that was not expected; this shock in turn leads to *hyperactivity* in the amygdala, the hippocampus, and the occipital cortex of the brain. The over-activity in the amygdala causes an intense fear response towards the events that are occurring during the time of a trauma; the hippocampus causes memory flooding which leads to one feeling over stimulated with fear related emotions after the trauma; the occipital cortex causes a flood of visual information to be sent and stored in the brain leading to flashbacks and nightmares post trauma. On the other hand, Broca's area of the brain, which is involved in speech and putting words to thoughts or memories, is *underactive* (Spiegel et al., 2006). This is the perfect storm that can lead to an influx of memories and feelings and a lack of words to describe them. This can cause the traumatized individual to feel locked inside his/her own mind. This mimics the feeling of being triggered, after the trauma is over.

When an individual is triggered, one or more of their senses are picking up on sensations that mimic, or are similar, to the time of the trauma. For example, if someone had a mother who was physically abusive and she wore a certain perfume, the scent of the perfume on another person may lead to the individual's central nervous system being overactivated, believing there is danger around them. Being in a constant state of fear is not conducive to wellness. Therapists can expose the knowledge of these triggers to clients, which can then in turn be useful tools in the therapeutic process. However, typical psychotherapy only allows for the verbalization of fears and memories. With the hypoactivity of Broca's area of the brain, many traumatic memories are stored nonverbally, and can only be accessed with stimulation of other senses, such as touch, smell, and body movement (Campbell et al., 2016). Being able to access these memories can expand the world of therapy from just talking, to drawing, dancing, and creating living and moving expressions of art.

## Children and Post-Traumatic Stress Disorder

Trauma impacts individuals differently at various levels of development. This can lead to differing symptomatology. Children are at the earlier stages of development physically and mentally since their brains and bodies are growing and adapting to their environments and to the caregivers around them. When children are exposed to trauma, they may develop the sense that the world is an unsafe place. Children are under the natural assumption that caregivers or parents are going to respond to their crying with soothing rather than punishment. They cling onto adult figures as a way of protection, a very natural instinct for young humans (Wraith, 2000). According to Nader (1995), children who have been through trauma have a feeling of loss, and the desire for things to go back to the way they were before the incident, or before they experienced loss and grief (Wraith, 2000).

When children experience trauma, they have unique symptoms of PTSD that look different than adults and adolescents' responses. Children may regress to earlier years and may suffer from enuresis, involuntary urination, especially at night, or encopresis, fecal incontinence, have a loss of playful behaviors, and may engage in attachment disorder-like behaviors, such as being more clingy or more isolated around caregivers (Wraith, 2000). They may have issues in school, show signs of aggression or develop new behaviors with peers and caregivers. These issues all stem from the attachment theory by Mary Ainsworth and Bowby. When researching the attachment between children and their caregivers, they found very significant impacts on the emotional health of children if they were abandoned physically or psychologically (Howe, 1999). Further research shows that trauma can lead children to feel emotionally or psychologically abandoned if there is parental neglect or abuse, or the child perceives that the parents did not take actions to protect them from a trauma. As these children become adolescents and adults, this can lead to maladaptive patterns of attachment behavior due to the immense stress and may lead to issues with attachment styles in the future (Howe, 1999).

When a child has developed a secure attachment, they feel safe and secure with their caregivers; they feel that their emotional needs are met and they can thrive and move through the world safely, even if a traumatic event were to occur. Children who have developed an anxious or ambivalent attachment style feel that their needs are not being met by caregivers and use behavioral or emotional outbursts to gain the attention of the caregiver. This can look like crying, whining, or throwing a tantrum since these children are depending on the attention they receive from their caregivers to be protective since the care they receive is not consistent. Sometimes children can develop avoidant attachments with caregivers, which stem from the child feeling like the caregiver is controlling, mean and neglectful of their emotional needs. When a child throws a tantrum for attention, a parent in this situation may become angry, volatile and aggressive with the child, leading the child to numb or avoid their emotions to avoid the negative feedback from the parents. Children may also develop a fourth attachment style when they feel their emotional needs are not being met. This is called a disorganized attachment and occurs when the caregiver is generally the trigger for the child to feel threatened or dysregulated; for example, this might occur if the parent is mentally or physically unwell, if there is addiction in the home, or if the caregiver is abusive in any type of way. The child develops a mix of avoidant and anxious responses and may display anger or maladaptive behaviors and generally remain in a state of distress (Howe, 1999). Children with disorganized attachment may try to gain control of their surroundings by using intense aggression, physical violence, or manipulation.

## Adolescents and Post-Traumatic Stress Disorder

Adolescents, or teenagers, in between childhood and adulthood are often exposed to many adult issues while also being expected to respond to authority figures as children do. Adolescents with trauma typically have feelings of mistrust or fear with adults, and they move through the world with uncertainty and growing pains, often finding comfort in other adolescents or peers (Kirk and Madden, 2003). This can lead to healthy attachment with other teens and social groups, or can lead them to bond with other peers who use unhealthy and pervasive coping skills as a way to cope with trauma, such as drugs and alcohol (Kirk and Madden, 2003). During this time of brain and body development, trauma can impact adolescents through adulthood with unhealthy attachment issues and a mistrust of the adult world.

Abuse and mistreatment may lead adolescents to have preconceived notions about themselves regarding being victimized: how they can protect themselves or the lack of protection they feel from caregivers. Natural disasters, war and poverty may lead them to believe that the world is a place where bad things happen, and they may become fearful of moving into adulthood (Campbell et al., 2016). Since adolescents' prefrontal cortexes are still developing during the time of trauma, the brain may be shaped around the fight, flight, freeze, or fawn responses that trauma elicits, and their perception of the world is grimmer. Their brain learns to grow around fear, so they are able to adapt and survive in scary tumultuous situations. This in turn leads to higher central nervous system dysregulation, more pervasive negative coping skills and higher cortisol levels as they age, compared to other children and adolescents (Wraith, 2000).

Post Traumatic Stress Disorder stemming from childhood and adolescent abuse appears to be more pervasive, since trauma in childhood leads to the increased chance of recurring trauma into adulthood. This stems from many reasons such as the "normality" of abuse and violence in one's life, the brain being accustomed and almost addicted to the adrenaline and dopamine rushes from a traumatic event and the resolution. Consequently, the individual feels unable to break the cycle of generational trauma due to poverty, racism, sexism, and consistent family dysfunction (Cloitre et al., 2010). As adolescents advance into adulthood, their negative behavioral and social skills transform from social issues with peers, to social issues with adults. And so it goes: from delinquency in school, to missing work or not being able to hold a job. Then it "progresses" from turbulence with their parents, to toxic or abusive romantic partnerships and from soothing things like video games and junk food, to alcohol and drug use.

As children grow into adolescence, their attachment styles are reflected in their relationships with others and follow them into their teenage years. Adolescents who have developed secure attachments will find themselves going out and exploring the world in a safe way with peers and in romantic relationships. They acknowledge their newly-found independence, but also trust their parents will be there for them if they need support. When adolescents experienced an ambivalent or anxious attachment as a child, they typically experience anxiety when seeking out new relationships, out of fear of getting emotionally injured. They may seek out individuals who make them feel a real or perceived sense of safety and assign a lot of value to these relationships to make up for the anxiety they felt as a child. Adolescents who experienced an avoidant attachment will find themselves avoiding intimate relationships in which they can be hurt emotionally. As a result, when they engage in these relationships, they develop a bond that challenges their sense of emotional safety, and they fear being hurt and tend to leave or run away from even healthy relationships. When a disorganized attachment was developed during childhood, the adolescent tends to have disorganized thoughts, perceptions and relationships with themselves and other people. They tend to fear being emotionally hurt or abandoned, and may become angry, abusive and act out behaviorally when they fear they are being abandoned. Adolescents begin to learn about their own emotions separate from their caregivers and explore the world and the people in it. This is where their attachments are solidified or changed based on the types of relationships they have as teenagers, and whether they are deemed healthy or unhealthy (Brown and Wright, 2001).

## Adults and Post-Traumatic Stress Disorder

When adults experience trauma in adulthood, they have preconceived notions of the world which can change depending on whether they had a trauma-free, or trauma-filled childhood. Trauma can impact the way adults feel about certain risk factors, such as potentially dangerous people, places, and things. However, it may not impact their lifestyle the way it would a child or an adolescent (Campbell et al., 2016). This is based on the way the brain grows and molds; when the prefrontal cortex is fully grown, by the age of 25, the adult is able to adapt to the trauma and mitigate risk factors in the future, such as locating authorities, being able to escape an abusive partner, or drive slower in the snow if there is an accident, based on rational thinking and problem solving skills (Arain et al., 2013). Adults who experienced trauma are more likely to believe the narrative that the world is unsafe and that they are not equipped to keep themselves safe. When healthy adult brains are able to use rationalization skills, they are able to make healthy decisions that keep them safe. However, when a brain is stuck in fight or flight mode, most of the decisions made are highly emotionally driven. Many trauma survivors engage in self-blame and self-doubt due to the fear that was felt during the time of the traumatic event. As a result, most of their life decisions are rooted in fear and in a perception of safety (Rosen Saltzman et al., 2013).

Adult attachment theory has been explored through lifespan research and questionnaires based on childhood experiences and adulthood trauma. Adults who had secure attachments as children typically have secure attachments and relationships as adults. When asked about their childhood and caregivers, they are able to speak freely about positive emotions and situations within their childhood home and surroundings. They are able to evaluate their own emotions and reactions to their childhood and their current life as an adult and are able to regulate unpleasant situations in adulthood. When adults had anxious or ambivalent childhood attachments, they present as confused and angry while thinking back on childhood events and their caregivers. They express confusing or ambivalent feelings of trust and mistrust and hyperfocus on relationships in the past and present to critically evaluate how close they feel to others. When an avoidant attachment was present in their childhood, these adults present as avoidant of emotional or anger-provoking memories and questions about their caregivers. They tend to glaze over or sugarcoat stories and focus on happier or less emotionally charged stories from childhood. Adults who present with a disorganized attachment from childhood present with disorganized thoughts, flashbacks and may lose track of what they are sharing in interviews since they get sucked back into the past. Often, memories are forgotten or blocked out with a numbing response to protect themselves from re-living the past (Howe, 1999). It is more difficult for them to thrive with healthy relationships as an adult, since they typically use control as a way to keep people in their lives.

## History of Trauma Therapy

### Early History

Trauma and PTSD were first recognized as diagnosable conditions in 1980 by the American Psychological Association; however, PTSD was treated before this time. In the 1800's it was recognized as "soldier's fatigue" and "battle exhaustion," characterized by nervous system exhaustion and the "thousand-yard stare." PTSD also became recognized as "railway spine," when members of the railroad crew saw gruesome deaths or experienced physical harm on the railway, leading to symptoms of trauma and hyper-arousal. In the late 1800's and early 1900's, Freud initiating "talking cure" therapy with individuals, which was the beginning of psychotherapy (Green, 2017).

In 1915, the diagnosis of PTSD was called Shell Shock due to the aftermath of bombs, explosions, and gun firing of war. The extreme noises of the war led to the hyperarousal of the nervous system when other loud noises occurred throughout their lives post war. It was found that PTSD was so widespread among the veterans due to the high intensity of the horror and the young age of the soldiers (Kirk & Madden,

2003). Psychotherapy as well as shock therapy was used to treat the symptoms of PTSD during that time (Crocq, 2000). As PTSD and trauma became better understood, new treatment methods began to develop that were more effective than basic psychotherapy, and less invasive than shock therapy. By the 1950's individual and group therapy became more widespread for mental health issues, and psychotropic medications were created and used in mental health settings (Green, 2017).

The 1970's were the trailblazer years for more modern-day trauma treatment interventions as survivors of domestic violence, the Vietnam War, and the Holocaust, suffered from symptoms of PTSD. Psychologists Ann Wolbert Burgess and sociologist Lynda Lytle Holmstrom created the term "Rape Trauma Syndrome" to express the terror and trauma experienced by women who were survivors of domestic violence and sexual assault. This opened the door for women to receive trauma treatment and for research to begin relating to how trauma impacted women's physiological responses, as well (Green, 2017). By 1980, Post Traumatic Stress Disorder was included in the Diagnostic and Statistical Manual of Mental Disorders, and by the 1990's, EMDR treatment, Cognitive Behavioral Therapy, and Debriefing Treatments were used in trauma interventions (Green, 2017).

## Debriefing and CBT

Therapeutic interventions for traumatized individuals began with studies using debriefing and cognitive behavioral therapy methods. Debriefing originated as a group therapy model but was adapted to individual trauma sessions (Ehlers & Clark, 2003). The method of debriefing therapy with traumatized individuals included attending a one-time therapy session to tell the story of the events of the trauma to a licensed practitioner, within the first few days following, but no longer than a month after the trauma occurred (Ehlers & Clark, 2003). During the debriefing session, individuals are encouraged to speak of thoughts and feelings related to the traumatic event, and are given education on the symptoms that may occur in the next week or month. Individuals are then offered coping skills and engage in the "application" stage of these coping skills when the debriefing session is over (Kirk & Madden, 2003). Early research by Bisson et al (1977) included hospitalized adult burn victims, and Mayou et al. (2000) included victims of car accidents in debriefing therapy.

Both of those studies, as well as ones by Bordrow and Porritt 1979; Bunn and Clarke 1979; Conlon et al 1999; Hobbs et al 1996, found that debriefing does not lower the risk or symptoms associated with Post Traumatic Stress Disorder in adults, but may increase their risk of developing symptoms in the future; these risks increased with more debriefing sessions (Ehlers & Clark, 2003). Other researchers such as Mitchell (1989) and Robinson et al (1993) agree that debriefing benefits are less effective the longer the wait time is between the trauma and the debriefing session (Kirk & Madden, 2003). Due to this fact, evidence-based practices such as Cognitive Behavioral Therapy were created.

Cognitive Behavioral Therapy began with individuals who were at risk for long-term PTSD. This theory was developed around the individual speaking of their traumatic event, learning about what trauma is, and reshaping the way they think about the event and the intrusive thoughts or flashbacks that follow (Ehlers & Clark, 2003). This evidence-based treatment model was used to treat the "positive" or externalized, and "negative" or internalized, symptoms of PTSD. Some of the positive symptoms of PTSD include nightmares, hyperarousal, anger, and fear responses; while some of the negative symptoms include intrusive and racing thoughts, feelings of depression and anxiety, and isolation (Spiegel et al., 2006). The process of reshaping thoughts in CBT enhances the individual's ability to see the positive sides of their responses to the trauma (protecting themselves), having a positive view of the future, and feeling in control of their behaviors and thought patterns. An early study by Foa et al (1995) included adult assault victims who were at risk of developing PTSD, or who were diagnosed with acute stress disorder; they attended 4 weeks of two-hour CBT sessions. It was found that individuals who attended these early interventions, about two weeks post-traumatic event, had fewer depressive episodes (a negative symptom) and fewer flashbacks (a positive symptom) than the debriefing and control groups (Ehlers & Clark, 2003). In this light, CBT was more beneficial to trauma survivors than other methods that had been used previously.

Children and adolescents with trauma were also studied using debriefing therapy, and several models were adapted to improve distress tolerance skills; many of these models engaged the children in decreasing positive or externalized behaviors and responses. Debriefing for children is different than with adults; younger individuals need the support of their caregiver through the therapeutic model and need caregivers who are aware of their emotional health and who are emotionally available (Wraith, 2000). Research by Milgram and Toubiana, 1996, found that children who were more resilient and "bounced back" quicker from a trauma had the support of their parents. This research was conducted with 675 students who suffered the loss of peers after a bus accident. The models used, and which will be described, separated children by age groups; one group was under 7 years of age, the next was 7-11 years old, and the final group was 11-13 years old (Wraith, 2000). One model that was used to help children who underwent a collective trauma focused on parental support, trusted peer support, the relationships between all of those involved, and physical touch/ comfort among all of those involved (Wraith, 2000). A number of researchers noted that nonverbal methods of therapy are essential to healing trauma in children; these methods include play, art, and music (MacLean, 1997; Terr, 1989; and Gillis, 1993). A later model of debriefing conformed to engage children in art, play and music therapy in conjunction with the parental support, trusted peer support, and the relationships among those involved. This model was shown to have better outcomes for the children who were involved in traumatic incidents due to the employment of creative arts therapy (Wraith, 2000).

## EMDR and TF-CBT

Later research with adults has shown that Eye Movement Desensitization and Reprocessing (EMDR) and Trauma Focused Cognitive Behavioral Therapy (TF-CBT) were beneficial in reducing internalized and externalized symptoms of PTSD. According to the National Institute for Clinical Excellence (2005), these types of treatments worked best for reducing overall symptoms of PTSD including internalized symptoms such as depressive feelings, when compared to other evidence-based practices of the time (Schouten et al., 2015). EMDR therapy engages the individual's eye movement, back and forth, while thinking and speaking about traumatic memories, as a way to self-soothe during the therapy session. According to Shapiro, 1989, the eye movement bilaterally stimulates the brain, similar to what happens with Rapid Eye Movement during dreams. This allows the brain to reprocess traumatic situations and re-store it in the brain without the fear response. Within EMDR therapy, there are eight phases that the therapist and individual work through together and are labeled as: psychological history taking, preparation for treatment, assessment of the individual and trauma, desensitization from the trauma, installation of the coping skills and a more positive self-belief system, body scanning for somatic healing, closure regarding the trauma, and reevaluation of the impact of the treatment (Oren & Solomon, 2012). This technique also focuses on the past, present, and future belief systems from pre and post trauma. It allows individuals to integrate their lives rather than live in the fragmented reality of before, during and after the trauma. EMDR therapy is relatively consistent among children, adolescents and adults, with naturally child-friendly language in sessions with younger folks.

EMDR therapy allows traumatized individuals to restore the "dysfunctional" thoughts of the trauma and their perception of themselves after the trauma, as a way of feeling safe again (Oren & Solomon, 2012). Research by Aubert-Khalfa, Roques and Blin, 2008, concluded that this type of therapy allows for a decrease in "positive symptoms." It includes a decrease in physiological stimulation, leading to lower heart rate, less physical tension, and slower central nervous system responses. According to the National Institute for Clinical Excellence (2005), Trauma Focused CBT skills enhanced the effects of EMDR therapy.

As aforementioned, CBT skills allow the traumatic event to be spoken about, coping skills to be developed, and thoughts regarding the trauma to be reshaped (Ehlers & Clark, 2003). Trauma-Focused CBT includes the trauma as the focus of the talk therapy and homework. The TF-CBT engages individuals to feel more in control of their thoughts and behaviors, while the bilateral stimulation of the co-occurring EMDR treatments enhance their ability to reprocess the negative or intrusive thoughts from the PTSD. This duality of treatment reduces the "positive," or externalized, symptoms of PTSD, such as nightmares, hyperarousal, and fear. However, the "negative," or internalized symptoms of PTSD, such as emotional numbness, avoidant behaviors and isolation, were not reduced overall with these standard treatment methods. Creative art therapy, while new in the field, has been shown to reduce some of the "negative" symptoms overall for children, adolescents, and adults.

## The Roots of Creative Art Therapy

### Creative Art Therapy Around the World

Creative art therapy is the umbrella term used to describe the creation of expressive forms, in conjunction with therapeutic interventions. These expressive forms include art, music, dance, drama, and expressive writing. Art therapy is the creation of paintings, drawings, sculptures, and other tangible items made through the artist's visual perspective. Music therapy is described as the creation of music, and listening to music for therapeutic purposes; while dance therapy is the use of the body in motion, to process and heal from mental health challenges and trauma. Drama therapy is the acting out of emotional expressions, usually in a group setting; while expressive writing therapy takes form by writing narratives, poetry, and stories (Saltzman, Matic, & Marsden, 2013).

Art therapy has its roots in the 1950s when an educator in Brazil named Paulo Frieire organized a social movement in Latin America that lasted through the 1970s (Kapitan et al., 2011). This movement focused on the collective consciousness and the awakening of community wholeness through art to combat collective trauma, and the oppression of people from the national and international governments. The movement began as social activism as Paulo led people to explore themselves and their communities for internal support rather than relying on external and governmental support that were rooted in oppressing its people. Knowledge, and an internal locus of control, gives individuals back their voice and power; Paulo encouraged folks in Latin America to focus on rebuilding emotional infrastructure and become leaders of internal support to meet the needs of communities that were underprivileged. This form of social activism laid the groundwork for art therapy as it is employed today, by creating connections through traumatized collectives (Kapitan et al., 2011).

People in these countries were suffering the aftermath of war, genocide, natural disasters, illness, and poverty. Paulo and other advocates of this time realized that when psychosocial needs were not being met, the individuals were further underprivileged:

They suffered from a lack of education and knowledge of mental health treatments. Art was used in Latin America, and all around the world soon after, to create a visual of the atrocities that were occurring in these countries. According to Golub (2005), the goal of this art-based social activism was to increase the individual and collective overall wellbeing and increase justice in communities (Kapitan et al., 2011). Lloyd (1999) stated that human rights organizers were able to use art and storytelling as a way to tell the narratives of the individuals who were being impacted, and heal the "damaged social fabric" of the communities (Kapitan et al., 2011). This allowed the individuals who were creating the art to connect through distress and form a collective healing identity.

The understanding of creative art therapy became more widespread when indigenous folks were able to share vignettes about their collective healing process through art and creative art modalities. Culturally, Indigenous individuals take a holistic approach when it comes to healing and feeling connected with oneself. This can be viewed as the macro, meso, and micro levels of being a part of this community; the approach encompasses the spiritual, cultural, social, emotional, mental, and physical parts of each person (Kaimal & Arslenbek, 2020). Some art practices that were and are used to create this holistic healing include painting, knitting, weaving, fabric dying, metal work, woodwork, dancing, storytelling, and drama (Kaimal & Arslenbek, 2020). It is important to also note that these forms of art communication are what keeps the community flourishing. For these indigenous people, many of these creative art forms create important textiles and objects that are needed for daily life. Collective empowerment became the force that tied communities together and brought light and wisdom to the field of therapy and healing practices.

## Creative Art Therapy in The United States

Ginwright (2018) alludes to the fact that trauma work and trauma therapy is not complete and leaves room for growth (Scrine, 2021). Many neglect the fact that trauma can feel very individualized and personal; it is also often forgotten that much of trauma impacts the collective. For example, war-stricken countries contain many traumatized individuals but contend with very collective problems, such as poverty, loss and death, and colonized power. Individuals who have been abused have an individualized trauma in their own life, that stems from the collective roots of disempowerment, gender, age and race. Ginwright (2018) also believes that when trauma work focuses too much on the person who has been traumatized-rightfully-so-the root of the issue is never resolved. The seeds of poverty, domestic violence, sexual abuse and war are not uprooted enough to stop the trauma before it happens (Scrine, 2021).

Through time, expressive art has been an imperative form of social and emotional connection between individuals and communities, and has been used as a form of healing the social collective from trauma. Creative art therapy practices have been adapted from indigenous beginnings, and are an important part of therapy and trauma work done today. Creative art therapists, who are working with diverse cultures and indigenous folks, need to be aware, and culturally sensitive to historical and cultural trauma, oppression, and discrimination. Professionals are encouraged to be aware of how their own biases and worldviews impact the relationship between client and therapist when engaging in any type of therapeutic practice, including art therapy (Kaimal & Arslenbek, 2020).

The origins of modern creative art therapy began in the United States and Europe in the 1900's (Kaimal & Arslanbek, 2020). According to Junge (2010), therapists began using modern art therapy as a way to help World War II veterans heal from PTSD. It also allowed children with special needs to use art as a way to engage in nonverbal communication to express themselves. In the United States, creative art therapy has adapted into a more structured practice, as therapists who use these methods typically need a Master's level degree and training.

Research brought together by the empowerment models and trauma healing models was combined to create the newer-aged model of therapy. This includes human expression such as verbalization in talk therapy, emotional expression through art and music therapy, and physical or somatic expression with drama and dance therapy. Creative arts therapy has a wide range of psychosomatic healing practices that involve the mind and the body. Art, music, dance, and creative writing are all forms of creative arts therapy that are used in the United States and around the world, to aid in the reduction of PTSD symptoms.

## Integration of Creative Art Therapy Into Trauma Work

### Art Therapy

The focus and main goal of art therapy is to reduce the external and internal (positive and negative) symptoms of PTSD and related issues. Most of the evidence-based practices used for treating PTSD focused on the positive symptoms of the diagnosis, such as behavioral issues, anger, depression, and anxiety. However, they are unable to unlock more healing for the negative symptoms such as avoidance, numbing, regression, and interpersonal connectedness. Due to the expressionistic aspect of art (Schouten et al., 2015), Art therapy gives individuals and therapists more opportunity to heal and work on negative symptoms due to the expressionistic aspect of art (Schouten et al., 2015). Many survivors experience a loss of memory or repressed thoughts around parts of the trauma narrative; they are not able to recall the sensory experience or the emotions that were felt in that moment, and verbalize them coherently. Art therapy offers individuals the ability to connect with their bodies, and the creative parts of their minds, to express the somatic aspect of their trauma.

Post Traumatic Stress Disorder was not recognized as an official diagnosis until 1980, but art therapy and art expression have been used in therapeutic interventions since the 1970s (Spiegel et al., 2006). One type of therapy that paved the way for current art therapy was rooted in Adlerian Psychology (Adlerian Therapy) that originated between 1911 and 1937, by a psychologist named Alfred Adler. His psychology practice was one of the first to focus on the community and the dynamics of community-based care and health. Adlerian Therapy became popular in trauma work since it focuses on multiple modalities of the human psyche such as sensory experiences, physical expression, visual dynamics, symbolism, and the verbalization of emotions (Rosen Saltzman et al., 2013). This allows for a client-centered approach with the trauma narrative because it engages individuals in many modalities of expression.

According to Schwartz (1996), art enables the observer to be the witness, allowing the survivor to share and create art; the individual is then able to be seen, heard, and understood through self-expression rather than merely through recounting the events of the trauma (Rosen Saltzman et al., 2013). Art is a place where the trauma narrative and the healing process become one, and art gives interpersonal meaning to the viewers, as well as the creators. When art is used in therapy, the survivor is being asked to trust the process of the intervention, to accept the reaction of the observer or the therapist and to allow for a conversation to occur based on the interpretation of the art being shown. This permits the individual to take a deep dive into their emotions, and the therapist to find the strengths of the individual and the beauty of the work that was created from pain.

Perrin, Smooth, and Yule (2000) noticed that children engage in play with peers, telling stories, and drawing pictures as a way to communicate effectively. Emotions and feelings are typically difficult for children to express since they may not have the capacity to fully verbalize how they are feeling; art therapy has adapted to engage children in the verbalization of their art or play, and the therapists are able to extrapolate and identify the feelings of the children based on what they are observing (Lyshak-Stelzer, 2007). CBT has been useful in therapy and trauma work since it offers goals, homework, and adapts new skills into the individual's life to implement healthy thinking patterns and behaviors after a trauma has occurred (Pifalo, 2006). Art therapy was used to engage children and adolescents in the nonverbal expression of their emotions after abuse had occurred. This type of modality can also allow the young person to engage in age-appropriate behaviors such as drawing, coloring, and sculpting. In the above study, children and adolescents were evaluated with the Trauma Symptom Checklist for Children before and after the treatment;

their symptoms of PTSD decreased compared to other evidence-based practices or CBT alone. Some of the internalized and externalized emotions and behaviors that were reduced include preoccupation with sex, anger, dissociation, anxiety, and depression (Pifalo, 2006).

In a study by Henderson et al. (2007), two groups of adults with PTSD symptoms were given mandala coloring activities for therapeutic art purposes. The control group focused on psychotherapy not related to trauma, and the experimental group focused on psychotherapy related to their trauma narratives. This study's results showed decreased trauma symptoms for both groups of individuals, leading researchers to believe that art therapy in conjunction with other evidence-based practices is an effective therapy model for trauma based healing, even if the psychotherapy did not involve verbal trauma interventions (Henderson et al., 2007). This trial was evidence that art therapy allowed healing of PTSD symptoms through a non-verbal approach. However, it still encourages therapists to use art therapy in conjunction with other evidence-based practices such as psychotherapy, CBT skills and EMDR (Campbell et al., 2016). Art therapy has been found to decrease overall internalized and externalized symptoms of PTSD since it enhances the mind- body connection. Thoughts regarding the trauma are placed into the tangible artwork, aiding in communication (Lyshak-Stelzer et al., 2007).

## Music Therapy

Music therapy engages the cognitive, motor, and speech centers of the brain. The cognitive center of the brain processes thoughts and emotions; the motor center of the brain is used for balance and movement, and the speech center of the brain connects thoughts and verbalizing words. Some of the main goals of music therapy are to engage the brain on many levels, while integrating the creative nature within the person (Heidenreich, 2005). Music therapists give individuals free reign with easy-to-use instruments, to allow judgment free creativity and expression. Music has been an integral part of history and cultural bonding for centuries, ever since the creation of sounds into music. As the sounds traverse the ear, many parts of the brain are engaged that create memory, imagery, and emotional meaning, all part of the science behind the healing of trauma (Tomaino, 2015). It has been found that when enjoyable music is playing, the part of the prefrontal cortex that monitors performance and self-doubt shuts down, while the areas of the cortex that involve spontaneity and autonomy are enhanced (Tomaino, 2015). This means that when the individual is playing, their internal locus of control is enhanced, and negative self-esteem decreases. This can help reverse the negative impact that trauma had on the prefrontal cortex, that lead to disempowerment, irrational thoughts and beliefs, and negative self-esteem. When the individual perceives the music they are creating as emotionally stimulating, the amygdala in the limbic system is activated. The amygdala, in turn, allows emotions to be felt and understood, rather than feared, since it controls the fight or flight response (Tomaino, 2015). Music therapy can reactivate access to emotions when trauma has led to numbness; it can enhance positive emotional flow when flashbacks or nightmares have led to negative feelings and fear.

Many countries such as Afghanistan, Romania, Israel, and India are using music therapy with children for the treatment of PTSD and other mental health conditions (Heidenreich, 2005). Helping organizations, such as UNICEF and War Child, are training therapists in music therapy, in conjunction with psychotherapy, to support children and some adults in war-affected areas around the world. According to research conducted by Gupta (2000), children and adolescents in Sierra Leone and Rwanda exhibited improvements with symptoms of PTSD through evidence-based questionnaires and verbalizing their emotions before and after music therapy (Heidenreich, 2005). This research included 300 children and adolescents ages 8-18 years old, in a four-week program that included music therapy, art therapy, storytelling and psychotherapy. Many reported that they felt a sense of relief when engaging in this program after experiencing war and other types of traumas. This kind of therapy has been shown to decrease positive symptoms of PTSD as well as to improve individual's sleep quality after the music therapy has occurred (Scrine, 2021). Bensimon (2020) suggested that music therapy allows "musical validation," "emotional witnessing through music," "musical witnessing as a self-object," and "attuned music involvement" (Scrine, 2021). This allows for individuals to heal relational mistrust between themselves and others by creating music with others, trusting others in the room where therapy is occurring, and feeling safe while creating. Music has been used for centuries and was used during times of slavery to engage folks in group spirituality, and connectedness to build resilience (Scrine, 2021).

## Dance Therapy

Dance or movement therapy is another functional form of trauma healing, under the creative arts umbrella. This type of therapy incorporates the dance therapist in a group or individual setting, and allows for the connectedness of individuals with their own bodies, and with each other, in a safe space. It focuses on the somatic, or the bodily experiences that are felt by the individual. Early literature and research about somatic psychology began with Alfred Adler, who developed the term expressive movement and by Jourard who established "somatic disclosure and perception of the soma," and "somatic resonance" related to the body in space (Hartley & Hartley, 2004). Rossi (1986) researched the psychological and biological connection of the body and mind relating to an individual's environment, and biological makeup (Hartley & Hartley, 2004). These developments in the history of psychology led to further treatment options for those impacted by trauma but also shed light on person-centered psychology and therapeutic practice.

Dance therapists are trained to aid the somatic release of trauma that can be stored in the body; it encompasses the body as a whole and empowers individuals to take back control of their bodies and their minds, when trauma has taken control away from them (Hartley & Hartley, 2004). Thomas Hanna coined the term "somatics" in the study of the human body through a psychological perspective. Dance therapy allows the individual to see their body as healing itself through movement, and puts space between the dependence on the therapist, and autonomy in the healing process (Hartley & Hartley, 2004). Through this term, individuals are encouraged to see themselves as a whole, and use their bodies to heal their bodies; this begins with grounding skills such as breath work, and leads into practices like dance, yoga and other somatic modalities where complete relaxation and empowerment occur (Hartley & Hartley, 2004).

Dance therapy allows for the awakening of parts of the brain that are under-functioning, or offers a peace to parts of the brain in hyper-arousal. It also enhances attention span, memory of movements, gross and fine motor skills, and creativity (Tomaszewski et al., 2022). Psychological trauma may leave the body in a state of hyper-arousal physically, leading to issues with the cardiovascular system, immune system, metabolism, and internal inflammation. Due to its relaxing nature, dance or movement therapy is very significant in returning the body to homeostasis after trauma has occurred and stimulating the adrenaline or cortisol in a healthy way (Tomaszewski et al., 2022). The more individuals with trauma are able to move their bodies, lower their stress responses, and heal the central nervous system, the better they will feel physically and mentally. When Post Traumatic Stress Disorder leads to the negative symptomatology related to psychological numbing, movement in a therapeutic way can help unlock the endorphins and dopamine the individual needs to begin feeling emotions again.

## Drama Therapy

Psychodrama was founded by Jacob Mareno in 1942. Psychodrama is taken from the root of Greek words psyche meaning spirit, and drama meaning action. Psychodrama is the science behind the "truth," through dramatic methods and acting (Moreno, 1946). Trauma has an impact on an individual's executive functioning and cognitive functioning as a whole; it impacts decision making, social engagements, and rational thinking (Frydman & McLellan, 2014). Drama therapy, like other expressive art therapies, enhances cognitive functioning through making sense of external and internal stimuli and responding accordingly in a healthy way.

In the original psychodrama scheme, there are five important parts including the stage, the patient, the director or the therapist, the staff or therapeutic aides, and the audience to create meaning and purpose behind the trauma healing. Acting on the stage becomes the healing practice behind the therapy work where one can connect to him or herself in spatial orientation, recite words and recalibrate their bodies to feel safe. It became an integrative part of group therapy in which each individual has a role. Drama therapy is a derivative of psychodrama as the roots of both practices use drama to heal trauma; however, drama therapy is more structured in the therapeutic process than the experimental acting of psychodrama (Kedem-Tahar & Felix-Kellerman, 1996). This type of therapeutic process allows individuals to reimagine real life and life on the stage, as well as to reimagine roles and socialization in a creative way (Frydman & McLellan, 2014). When acting, metaphors can be helpful in aiding individuals to express ideas, memories, and somatic feelings. Drama therapy can enhance executive functioning via communication, critical thinking, and the storage of healthy memories in the brain.

In life as well as on the stage, there are roles of the main character or the patient. Landy (2000) created the idea of role theory which examines the individual's life through cultural, biological, social and psychological perspectives (Landy, 2003). According to this theory, balance is sought between the roles, and sometimes things are disrupted with changes or trauma. On the stage with drama therapy, those who are performing are able to seek balance in a therapeutic and cathartic way. There are many types of drama therapy such as psychoanalytic drama therapy, and role theory, but all methods seek to find balance and allow the actor or patient to maintain and find control and harmony among themselves, the stage and the audience (Landy, 2003). These roles can be created via the imagination of the writer (a play) or in a moment of original thought of the actor where they are asked who the main characters are, what situation they are experiencing, and how they feel.

## CONCLUSION

Creative art therapy is a developing field and will continue to blossom over time. Children, adolescents, and adults who suffer from Post Traumatic Stress Disorder can benefit from therapists who work in the field of art, music, dance and drama therapy. This field will continue to bridge the gap where other evidence-based practices have left off. These therapy modalities will encompass the meaning of regaining control again after trauma has taken hold.

There are some missing pieces in the creative arts therapy field that should be explored in the future. Some of these missing pieces, research-wise include differences between the genders, socioeconomic statuses, cultures, and the length of time folks have been suffering from Post Traumatic Stress Disorder. Studies for the future may also incorporate more current forms of art therapy, such as graphic design and photography. This does not take away from the benefits that creative arts therapy has been shown to provide for individuals, and the benefits will continue to blossom throughout time.

## REFERENCES

American Psychiatric Association. (2013). *Diagnostic and statistical manual of mental disorders* (5th ed.). doi:10.1176/appi.books.9780890425596

Arain, M., Haque, M., Johal, L., Mathur, P., Nel, W., Rais, A., ... Sharma, S. (2013). Maturation of the adolescent brain. *Neuropsychiatric Disease and Treatment, 9*, 449. PMID:23579318

Bensimon, M., Amir, D., & Wolf, Y. (2012). A pendulum between trauma and life: Group music therapy with post-traumatized soldiers. *The Arts in Psychotherapy, 39*(4), 223–233. doi:10.1016/j.aip.2012.03.005

Brown, L. S., & Wright, J. (2001). Attachment theory in adolescence and its relevance to developmental psychopathology. *Clinical Psychology & Psychotherapy, 8*(1), 15–32. doi:10.1002/cpp.274

Campbell, M., Decker, K. P., Kruk, K., & Deaver, S. P. (2016). Art therapy and cognitive processing therapy for combat-related PTSD: A randomized controlled trial. *Art Therapy: Journal of the American Art Therapy Association, 33*(4), 169–177. doi:10.1080/07421656.2016.1226643 PMID:29332989

Chapman, L., Morabito, D., Ladakakos, C., Schreier, H., & Knudson, M. M. (2001). The effectiveness of art therapy interventions in reducing post traumatic stress disorder (PTSD) symptoms in pediatric trauma patients. *Art Therapy: Journal of the American Art Therapy Association, 18*(2), 100–104. doi:10.1080/07421656.2001.10129750

Cloitre, M., Stovall-McClough, K. C., Nooner, K., Zorbas, P., Cherry, S., Jackson, C. L., Gan, W., & Petkova, E. (2010). Treatment for PTSD related to childhood abuse: A randomized controlled trial. *The American Journal of Psychiatry, 167*(8), 915–924. doi:10.1176/appi.ajp.2010.09081247 PMID:20595411

Crocq, M., & Crocq, L. (2000). From shell shock and war neurosis to posttraumatic stress disorder: A history of psychotraumatology. *Dialogues in Clinical Neuroscience, 2*(1), 47–55. doi:10.31887/DCNS.2000.2.1/macrocq PMID:22033462

Degges-White, S., & Davis, N. L. (Eds.). (2017). Integrating the expressive arts into counseling practice: Theory-based interventions. Springer Publishing Company.

Eaton, L. G., Doherty, K. L., & Widrick, R. M. (2007). A review of research and methods used to establish art therapy as an effective treatment method for traumatized children. *The Arts in Psychotherapy*, *34*(3), 256–262. doi:10.1016/j.aip.2007.03.001

Ehlers, A., & Clark, D. (2003). Early psychological interventions for adult survivors of trauma: A review. *Biological Psychiatry*, *53*(9), 817–826. doi:10.1016/S0006-3223(02)01812-7 PMID:12725974

Frydman, J. S., & McLellan, L. U. C. Y. (2014). *Complex trauma and executive functioning: envisioning a cognitive-based, trauma-informed approach to drama therapy. In Trauma Informed Drama Therapy: Transforming Clinics, Classrooms, and Communities*. Thomas.

Green, M. (2017, Mrs. 23). The History of Post-Traumatic Stress Disorder and How We Treat it. *Newsweek*.

Hartley, L., & Hartley, L. (2004). *Somatic psychology: Body, mind and meaning*. Whurr.

Heidenreich, V. (2005). Music therapy in war-effected areas. *Intervention*, *3*(2), 129–134.

Henderson, P., Rosen, D., & Mascaro, N. (2007). Empirical study on the healing nature of mandalas. *Psychology of Aesthetics, Creativity, and the Arts*, *1*(3), 148–154. doi:10.1037/1931-3896.1.3.148

Howe, D. (1999). Attachment theory. *Social Work Theories and Methods*, 75.

Junge, M. B. (2010). *The modern history of art therapy in the United States*. Charles C Thomas Publisher.

Kaimal, G., & Arslanbek, A. (2020). Indigenous and traditional visual artistic practices: Implications for art therapy clinical practice and research. *Frontiers in Psychology*, *11*, 1320. doi:10.3389/fpsyg.2020.01320 PMID:32612560

Kapitan, L., Litell, M., & Torres, A. (2011). Creative art therapy in a community's participatory research and social transformation. *Art Therapy: Journal of the American Art Therapy Association*, *28*(2), 64–73. doi:10.1080/07421656.2011.578238

Kedem-Tahar, E., & Felix-Kellermann, P. (1996). Psychodrama and drama therapy: A comparison. *The Arts in Psychotherapy*, *23*(1), 27–36. doi:10.1016/0197-4556(95)00059-3

Kirk, A. B., & Madden, L. L. (2003). Trauma related critical incident debriefing for adolescents. *Child & Adolescent Social Work Journal, 20*(2), 123–134. doi:10.1023/A:1022816731082

Lagorio, R. (1989). Art therapy for battered women. *Advances in Art Therapy*, 92-113.

Landy, R. J. (2003). Drama therapy with adults. *Play Therapy with Adults*, 15-33.

Lyshak-Stelzer, F., Singer, P., Patricia, S. J., & Chemtob, C. M. (2007). Art therapy for adolescents with posttraumatic stress disorder symptoms: A pilot study. *Art Therapy: Journal of the American Art Therapy Association, 24*(4), 163–169. doi:10.1080/07421656.2007.10129474

Malchiodi, C. A. (2003). Art therapy and the brain. Handbook of Art Therapy, 16-24.

Moreno, J. L. (1946). Psychodrama and group psychotherapy. *Sociometry, 9*(2/3), 249–253. doi:10.2307/2785011

Oren, E. M. D. R., & Solomon, R. (2012). EMDR therapy: An overview of its development and mechanisms of action. *European Review of Applied Psychology, 62*(4), 197–203. doi:10.1016/j.erap.2012.08.005

Pifalo, T. (2006). Art therapy with sexually abused children and adolescents: Extended research study. *Art Therapy: Journal of the American Art Therapy Association, 23*(4), 181–185. doi:10.1080/07421656.2006.10129337

Roje, J. (1995). LA '94 earthquake in the eyes of children: Art therapy with elementary school children who were victims of disaster. *Art Therapy: Journal of the American Art Therapy Association, 12*(4), 237–243. doi:10.1080/07421656.1995.10759171

Rosen Saltzman, M., Matic, M., & Marsden, E. (2013). Adlerian Art Therapy with Sexual Abuse and Assault Survivors. *Journal of Individual Psychology, 69*(3).

Schouten, K. A., de Niet, G. J., Knipscheer, J. W., Kleber, R. J., & Hutschemaekers, G. J. (2015). The effectiveness of art therapy in the treatment of traumatized adults: A systematic review on art therapy and trauma. *Trauma, Violence & Abuse, 16*(2), 220–228. doi:10.1177/1524838014555032 PMID:25403446

Scrine, E. (2021). The limits of resilience and the need for resistance: Articulating the role of music therapy with young people within a shifting trauma paradigm. *Frontiers in Psychology, 12*, 26. doi:10.3389/fpsyg.2021.600245 PMID:33584471

Spiegel, D., Malchiodi, C., Backos, A., & Collie, K. (2006). Art therapy for combat-related PTSD: Recommendations for research and practice. *Art Therapy: Journal of the American Art Therapy Association*, *23*(4), 157–164. doi:10.1080/07421656.2006.10129335

Tomaino, C. M. (2015). Music therapy and the brain. *Music Therapy Handbook*, 40-50.

TomaszewskiC.BelotR. A.EssadekA.Onumba-BessonnetH.ClesseC. (2022). Therapeutic impact of dance therapy on adult individuals with psychological trauma: a systematic review. medRxiv. doi:10.1101/2022.10.27.22281614

Wraith, R. (2000). Children and debriefing. *Psychological debriefing: Theory, practice and evidence*, 195.

## KEY TERMS AND DEFINITIONS

**Attachment:** The bond that children develop with their caregivers; the bond that is prolonged throughout adulthood with others.

**Central Nervous System:** The bundle of nerves that controls the movements of the body.

**Cognitive:** Relating to the brain's consciousness, thinking, remembering, using language, etc.

**Creative Arts Therapy:** Incorporating art, music, dance, drama and writing into the therapeutic process to benefit mental health.

**Hyperarousal:** When the body and mind are stuck in the fight or flight mode after a trauma has occurred.

**Physiological:** When the body of an individual is being impacted; the somatic aspect of the person's health.

**Post-Traumatic Stress Disorder:** A diagnosis that may occur when someone has experienced trauma; when the brain copes with the intensity of a trauma and stayed in fight or flight mode to protect the individual.

**Psychological:** Relating to or impacting the mental state of an individual.

**Psychotropic Medications:** Medications that are used to treat mental health conditions.

**Trauma:** Experiencing a scary or life-threatening situation that causes emotional distress.

# Chapter 9
# Dance and Movement Therapy With Children and Developmental Disabilities/Disorders

**Jenna Dawn Rivera**
https://orcid.org/0000-0002-1404-9409
*Marymount Manhattan College, USA*

## ABSTRACT

*Dance and movement therapy has become a quickly growing field in the creative arts therapies, combining psychotherapy and embodiment. Sessions are often available in schools, hospitals, rehabilitation centers, and clinics worldwide. Although dance therapy can be beneficial to individuals of all ages, genders, races, and cultures, the benefit for children is substantial. This chapter will discuss the use of dance and movement therapy with children in the United States and compare it to related practices in other countries. Additionally, approaches and techniques will be analyzed through the lens of best and most practical uses for children. Developmental disorders in children will also be examined to assess the benefits of dance therapy on cognitive, socioemotional, and physical skills. Lastly, this chapter will inspire ideas for future directions to advance the field of dance and movement therapy.*

DOI: 10.4018/978-1-6684-7856-1.ch009

## INTRODUCTION

Dance is considered one of the most fundamental art forms since it embodies expression directly from the individual. It has been used throughout history by an extensive number of cultures for entertainment, enjoyment, expression, celebration, tradition, and sacred practice. In the 1940s, dance was introduced into the field of psychology as a form of psychotherapy. It became a quickly growing field in the creative arts therapies, combining psychotherapy and embodiment. The American Dance Therapy Association (ADTA) was soon founded in 1966 to establish a set of high-quality standards among certified dance and movement therapists. The ADTA defines dance therapy as, "the psychotherapeutic use of movement as a process that furthers the emotional, cognitive, social, and physical integration of the individual" (Pratt, 2004, p. 831). There are two ways to become a registered dance and movement therapist in the United States. The first is to complete an approved ADTA graduate program, each with their own requirements and processes. The alternative way to achieve certification is from an already obtained master's degree in a related field of psychology, with additional dance and movement therapy training from a qualified teacher. Certified therapists work with clients to develop goals and improve movement quality, vocabulary, self-esteem, communication, and more. Today, dance and movement therapy is used in a variety of settings such as specialty schools, hospitals, and at home visits. Sessions are also often held at private practices, rehabilitation centers, and mental health clinics worldwide. The goal of dance therapy is different for each individual based on his or her current needs. However, most individuals who participate in dance therapy receive a multitude of both physical and mental health benefits, and an overall improved quality of life.

Anyone can participate in dance and movement therapy exercises as long as they are willing to engage with the therapist. Age of clients can range from infancy to older adults, with outcomes tailored to individual needs. For infants, motor exercises and facial expression practices are common to promote healthy developmental growth. Adolescents may partake in dance therapy for an increase in communication skills, self-esteem, or body image. Elders may choose to participate in dance therapy for an improved range of motion, as well as cognitive and emotional health benefits. A study conducted by Balgaonkar (2010), suggests that, "Dance helps increase the temporal and prefrontal activity to improve memory, multitasking, planning, and attention skills… [which] helps the older brain to form new interconnections and work faster" (p. 67). This is certainly beneficial for an aging brain to reinforce or create new connections, which may reduce the symptoms of Alzheimer's disease. Although dance therapy can be beneficial to individuals of all ages, genders, races, and cultures, the benefit to children is substantial. The present chapter will focus solely on children for several reasons. Dance and movement therapy is highly effective for children because of the countless creative aspects, play-like scenarios, and the plasticity, or malleability of the children's developing brains. Treatment for developmental disorders beginning in childhood also produce more successful outcomes compared to beginning treatment later in adulthood. Additionally, dance and other physical activities increase the release of endorphins, enhancing one's state of well-being and contributing to the enjoyment of the activity (Teixeira-Machado, 2017, p. 427). This is especially favorable when working with children to prevent boredom or refusal of engagement. Furthermore, the present chapter will introduce best approaches and treatments for children, as well as specific developmental disorders dance therapy has been shown to be valuable towards.

## Children Around the World

Dance and movement therapy has not only taken off in the United States, but in many other countries as well, including Israel, Germany, Korea, Sierra Leone, and Haiti. Other countries such as Greece do not offer as many creative arts therapy resources, but would benefit greatly from them. Each country has its own set of standards and certifications for dance therapists. While international programs are not approved by the ADTA, "the Dance/Movement Therapy Certification Board recommends applying via the Alternate Route if attending an international program" (American Dance Therapy Association, 2020). This alternative route requires a master's degree and additional training by an ADTA registered dance and movement therapist. From an international panel at the American Dance Therapy Association's Annual Conference, Capello (2008) reports on other countries' statuses on treatment plans and techniques for underprivileged or high risk children exercised by licensed dance therapists in each country. The international panel was conducted in the interest of, "acknowledging that early intervention is critical to the diagnosis and prevention of further pathology in adulthood" (Capello, 2008, p. 24). While some countries have brilliant dance therapy programs in place, affording children with a variety of psychological needs the opportunity to seek benefits and relief, others are lacking in these programs. For instance, many children with disabilities and other disadvantages are not receiving the care they need. The ADTA's objective from the panel is to learn from other countries' programs and approaches while integrating a number of cultures to enhance programs in the United States and to continue further research for developing children.

### Israel

Ever since its declaration of independence in 1948, Israel has been involved in a series of wars and conflicts that directly affects the Israeli citizens. The Hadassah

Hebrew Medical School conducted a study following 41 terrorist attacks near the nation's capital, Jerusalem. The study examined post-traumatic stress disorder (PTSD) symptoms in 163 children and adolescents brought to the emergency room of Hadassah Hospital. "Of the sample, 23.3% had to be admitted (three of whom died); the remaining 76.7% were discharged. Examination revealed that 42.9% of the children had the PTSD symptoms of re-experiencing, avoidance, or hyperarousal" (Tyano, 2003, p. 8). Dance and movement therapists in Israel have been working with similar children who were diagnosed with PTSD, acquired war related injuries, had experienced sexual assault, and homeless youth. They also work with children in areas that may not have experienced these conflicts, but are at a high risk to encounter them. The therapists offer emotional communication with children through the use of improvisation and one-on-one work, while also coordinating with parents throughout sessions to continue this work at home by addressing signals for physical and emotional needs.

## Germany

Professionals in Germany are currently using dance therapy in healthcare institutions, schools, and in private practices. Research and treatment have been conducted on children with eating disorders, learning disorders, psychiatric illnesses, autism, attention deficit/hyperactivity disorder (ADHD), sensory deficits, and physical disabilities. The professionals often use assessments such as the Laban Movement Analysis, a method for describing and interpreting human movement created by Rudolf Laban. Laban was a Hungarian/German choreographer and dance theorist of the early 20th century who quickly rose to fame as a pioneer of modern dance. Laban's analysis was often used in conjunction with the Chace approach, which involves articulating movement with symbolism, empathy, and rhythm. These methods have been deemed critical in Germany to working with children in terms of sensory integration and psychomotor practice.

## Korea

Children in Korea often lack many physical, social, and creative skills as playtime is greatly reduced compared to other countries in order to prioritize cognitive development and academic success. This concentration on academia may cause a lack of awareness on how to regulate relationships and emotions. According to Capello (2008), of 8,000 Korean school children, "67% experience tremendous stress in regard to academic performance and 57% show problems in peer relationships" (p. 29). Because of this, many children in Korea have shown symptoms of attention deficit disorders and behavioral issues. Dance therapy has been working for several years in schools as an impeccable communication channel to express feelings and discover emotional needs, while obtaining some additional physical exercise. Therapists work with children who have less opportunities to freely move their body, whether that be because of a strong focus on academic success, or other physical inabilities. Results of group dance therapy in Korea has shown significant improvements in children naturally relating to their peers by using a newly learned sense of self, body language, and social cues. Dance and movement therapy overall improved physical and mental development of children in the country.

## Sierra Leone

Professionals at the Center for Victims of Torture (CVT) in Sierra Leone often work with children who have suffered from child labor, abuse, and those who have been former child soldiers and orphans. The country has the highest mortality rate for children under five years of age. Similarly to Israel, many children suffer from symptoms of PTSD, anxiety, and depression because of traumatic life events or living conditions. Dance and movement therapy programs in trauma recovery centers have promoted a safe environment for these children along with the building of trust, confidence, relaxation, and grounding. David Alan Harris is an American dance and movement therapist who has worked in Sierra Leone teaching the basics of the psychotherapy to CVT professionals. Certain approaches aided him and other dance therapists in integrating past trauma into movement for coping and expression of emotions. Popular Sirena Leonean music was used with each session, blending tradition and new American techniques. “A safe environment was thus established in which this highly traumatized youth started to rebuild trust and regain their dignity” (Capello, 2008, p. 33). Despite most of the children not receiving any psychological evaluations or treatment beforehand, each participant was highly engaged and was reported to have an improved way of life, and reduced symptoms of anxiety, depression, and PTSD.

## Haiti

As one of the most underdeveloped countries in the world, Haiti often struggles with funding education and mental healthcare systems. Most government funding goes toward emergency food, shelter, and physical healthcare clinics. Despite Haiti’s economic, social, and political troubles, dance remains a significant pursuit and outlet for the people of Haiti. Traditional Haitian dance emphasizes the body as a medium for healing and prayer. The use of rhythm and drumming are accentuated in dance therapy sessions to unify and re-center communities, maintain traditions, and to embrace culture. Dance is also a powerful way of embracing their history and bravery, reminding them of their successful revolution in 1804 that freed thousands of slaves from European power. Procedures have been implemented by the American Dance Therapy Association in low income areas near Cap Haïtien to incorporate dance therapy into already existing education, counseling, and community building programs. Children of trafficking, torture, and violence are targeted to join these programs to reduce depression, anxiety, and symptoms of PTSD. "A unique aspect of these programs is their openness to working not only with children who are victims of violence, but also with their perpetrators, since violence is experienced as a means of survival" (Capello, 2008, p. 34). While victims and perpetrators do not work together in sessions, they both receive the numerous benefits of dance therapy and learn how to appropriately participate in daily life.

### Greece

While dance is a major part of Greek culture and history, therapeutic and psychosocial uses of dance therapy are not widely utilized. While there are some dance therapy programs found in inpatient hospitals and private practices, there is a scarcity of trained professionals working in public healthcare or education systems (Capello, 2008, p. 29). Despite the abundance of research that suggests only benefits to its use, the problem lies in Greece's special education system itself. Children with disabilities who would benefit from dance therapy are often underserved and secluded, while those who are able to receive these accommodations often lack transportation and resources to obtain it. Because dance is so strongly embedded in Greek culture, dance and movement therapy has the potential to become a standard practice in healthcare and education systems. There is a huge need for more government funded special education programs, psychological evaluations, and graduate programs to offer a path to becoming a dance therapist. However, these challenges offer opportunity for growth within the entire dance therapy community. More opportunities include working with current dance therapists to provide training and developing new approaches for early intervention.

## Approaches

The effectiveness of dance therapy on the child participant will be greatly impacted by how a therapist approaches the session and techniques. Dance therapy approaches are always based on psychological theories and prior studies conducted. Certified dance movement therapist Bräuninger (2014) introduces four dance therapy approaches that were shown to be relevant and beneficial to her study on the correlation between dance therapy and cognitive functioning. The findings suggested an improved relationship between client and therapist, a reduce in stress, and an improvement in the overall quality of life for the client. The four approaches used and discussed are the Chace approach, the Psychodynamic Oriented approach, the Authentic Movement approach, and integrated dance therapy.

The Chace approach established by Marian Chace, a dance therapy pioneer, involves participating in body symbolism, kinesthetic empathy, and group rhythm. The main goal of utilizing the Chace approach in a session is to improve clients' expression, communication, and emotional responses, typically in a group setting. Many of the activities or movements done involve two or more people, and communication can be entirely non-verbal. The Chacian Circle is an example of an intervention often used in the Chace approach which places group members and the therapist in one harmonic circle, equally distributing each person's presence. It is used to enhance the relationships of all group members and to create an equal ground, establishing a safe space to reflect and learn. Mirroring is also used throughout dance and movement therapy, but initially derived from the Chace approach. With the use of the mirroring technique, "the emotional repertoire of clients' movements is empathically mirrored to establish empathic connections and to promote empathic reflection" (Bräuninger, 2014, p. 446). Both the Chacian Circle and mirroring have shown to produce positive outcomes to clients' emotional and communicative skills.

The Psychodynamic Oriented approach to dance therapy combines several theories originated by famous psychodynamic psychologists including Sigmund Freud, Anna Freud, and Carl Jung. Topics such as the unconscious versus conscious, conflicts of past experiences, and underlying meanings are often explored. The Psychodynamic Oriented approach in dance therapy focuses on improvisation to initiate mind-body activity. The movement is unprompted and self-directed from the client, supposedly stemming from the unconscious or imagination. This allows the client to free his or her mind of any current obsessive thoughts, and allow the body to move as it needs to. The process of free association is encouraged, one movement spontaneously prompting the next and the next. Different styles of music can be added to assist in the kindling of this movement, or as a calming background noise. At the end of the session, a thorough reflection of this movement along with like experiences and relations to the group are shared.

The Authentic Movement approach is similar to the Psychodynamic Oriented approach in that individual, spontaneous movement is explored. However, rather than coming from the unconscious mind, movement is thought to be coming from the conscious individual which is then interpreted in an effort to explore his or her unconscious. According to Bräuninger (2014), it is "a form of dance meditation derived from movement in depth" (p. 446). Authentic movement is considered to be a self-directing form of movement, allowing for any meanings or thoughts to be shared. To thoroughly analyze movement together, fellow group members or instructors are encouraged to observe in an objective and supportive way. One of the major goals of this approach is to promote emotional communication and self-exploration. While this goal has been a common theme between most approaches, not all clients can achieve their goals the same way. These different approaches allow for unique avenues for clients to fulfill the beneficial socioemotional outcomes of dance and movement therapy.

Lastly, integrative dance therapy combines many of the interventions previously stated and emphasizes the practical use of each approach for appropriate usage with each individual. Improvisation, the concept of the free mind and body, and composition are all valuable techniques in integrative dance therapy. Although all four approaches have similarities in techniques, outcomes, and goals, one of the most significant correspondences is the presence of nonverbal communication through movement and transference. These processes have been shown to be beneficial to individuals, in particular children, with neurological and developmental disorders.

## Techniques

Techniques used by dance and movement therapists are tools for yielding certain desirable results from a client. They are strategies used to reach a certain objective or accomplishment, which differ from the methodological approaches previously discussed. Similar to different approaches, techniques intertwine and will often be used in combination with one another. Mirroring, synchrony, focusing, imaginative techniques, and enhanced robotics are just five techniques that are especially beneficial for children. These techniques can be used in a variety of approaches to produce certain results a client may need. Each touch on improving either emotional or behavioral issues, motor skills, relationships, engagement, or multiple areas, depending on the child's needs.

### Mirroring

Mirroring is a technique used by many dance and movement therapists to enhance the relationship with their clients, to improve socioemotional skills, and is suggested to enhance empathy. When therapists and clients engage in mirroring together, they may echo exact body movements, or make similar or coordinated movements. A therapist or client may also mirror by echoing the emotionality of a specific movement rather than exact motions. The result is an enhanced relationship and understanding of one another through non-verbal communication. Mirroring also increases the likelihood of a client making greater progress in dance and movement therapy sessions because of the trust built with the therapist through the technique (Koch et al., 2015, pp. 2-3). In the case of a child who is non-verbal and has autism from McGarry and Russo's (2011) research, mirroring the movements of this child allowed for a demonstration of acceptance and connection. Eventually, this child who never engaged in connections with others before, was able to express himself emotionally through dance movements.

The mirroring technique used in dance and movement therapy relies on the mirror neuron system of the brain. According to McGarry and Russo (2011), the mirror neuron system operates as, "sensory input is relayed to the premotor cortex and parietal cortex via the superior temporal sulcus" (p. 179). This input generates greater activation in the limbic system during observation and participation in emotional actions. In the same study, participants observed and mirrored facial expressions while brain activity was measured through a fMRI scan. The scan revealed parts of the brain involved in the mirror neuron system activating when engaging in the activity, as well as parts of the brain involved in eliciting emotional responses such as the amygdala. This evidence supports the idea that participants involved in mirroring not only understand the emotions they are witnessing and enacting, but they have the potential to feel them as well. In accordance with these findings, Winters (2008), conducted a study viewing body posture in comparison to mirror neurons. She found that participants were feeling the same emotional responses body postures were structured to evoke. This was accurate whether participants were observing a posture or embodying the same posture, which supports prior mirror neuron research. In connection to dance therapy, these shared feelings and emotions can be extremely beneficial, especially children with autism and who are non-verbal. They not only build relationships and trust to make for a more engaging environment, but help the child express feelings in a new way.

## Synchrony

Synchrony is a rhythmic technique used in dance and movement therapy to gain similar outcomes to mirroring. However, it has yet to be shown to be capable of activating the mirror neuron system. Since it is also a non-verbal technique, synchrony has been shown to be useful in settings with children with autism, children struggling with communicating emotions, and children with empathy deficits (Bräuninger, 2014, p. 447). Synchrony uses rhythm, timing, and effort to share experiences and emotions between therapist and client, as well as client and client in group settings. It is taught by sharing movement qualities of two or more individuals in the same or different body parts. For example, slow and flowy movements of the arms performed by a therapist might be carried out by the client as slow and flowy movements of the head and neck. This synchrony of movement quality reflecting emotions felt by one individual is experienced by another in their own unique ways. One may also choose to quicken the pace of a movement but remain in a similar rhythm to elaborate on a phrase or explore movement, emotions, and feelings within oneself.

## Focusing

The technique of focusing is used in dance and movement therapy when an individual may need more specific attention in one area of their needs. Focusing may be a beneficial technique to children with PTSD, trauma, or severe behavioral disorders to aid them in navigating through intense emotions. Focusing is more appropriate for one-on-one, therapist-client sessions, rather than in group settings. This allows the therapist to gain better control of the outcome and adapt sessions to the specific need of the individual, which is the main objective of the technique. A therapist might concentrate an entire session on an overall theme, feelings, or connotations prompted by the client, and is often determined prior to the session beginning. While engaging in focusing with a dance therapist, no specific type of body movement is required or limited. Focusing permits the actions of pausing, reflecting on experiences, and perceiving those experiences through a new lens. One disadvantage to the technique of focusing in dance and movement therapy is the risk of not attending to an individual's extensive needs. As an integrative therapy, multiple needs are typically addressed in each session, including improved overall well-being. However, focusing on one particular theme or emotion may limit a session and not allow a client to progress in other areas.

## Imaginative Techniques

Active imagination and mental imagination are two types of imaginative techniques used by dance and movement therapists, particularly with children. These techniques require more reflection by the client on sensations they feel, as well as movements they choose to make. Imaginative techniques are often used in the psychodynamic-oriented approach, reflecting one's inner and unconscious desires. According to Bräuninger (2014), active imagination refers to the physical expression of imagined or thought stimuli. It allows for individuals to use their internal sensations, emotions, images, scenarios, etc. and externally embody them. Mental imagination, also known as visualization, refers to the same concept of using internal sensations, but also imagining the embodiment of them. Rather than physically moving, the individual will imagine the movements they would want their body to make. This technique is ideal for individuals who are immobile or who have restricted movement capabilities. For example, a child with cerebral palsy may wish to express an intense feeling of anger through large movements such as jumping or stomping the floor. This child may not be able to fully embody these movements, but they can mentally imagine performing them, yielding similar results. This technique cannot be used alone in dance therapy as there is no physical movement involved, however, it is optimal for those who may need breaks from movement, while still receiving benefits from the therapy.

## NAO Robotics

Although dance therapy can be a more enjoyable form of therapy for children compared to other approaches, psychologists in Japan are working toward a new way to increase enjoyment, and to keep children engaged for a longer period of time, thus increasing the number of learning opportunities. A study was conducted by Suzuki et al. (2017), examining the performance of NAO, a robot designed as a teaching assistant in dance therapy. The purpose of this robot was not to replace the dance therapist but rather to engage and sustain the attention of children with autism. Three categories were assessed in this study since they were deemed to be the main deficits in children with autism: motor impairment, imitation behavior, and joint attention. Children were taught a sequence of movements in the form of a dance (head, shoulders, knees, clap), by both the robot and the therapist. They were tested on social responsiveness, response time, and correct body movements. The researchers hypothesized that NAO could perform similar tasks as a dance therapist to engage children and to have them carry out specific tasks with no significant differences between the robot and therapist. Results supported their hypothesis with no significant differences in social responsiveness nor response time, signifying that NAO works in a similar manner to the therapist and effectively keeps the children engaged. Although fluctuations were found in results of correct body movements, this did not affect the final consensus. Overall, the researchers concluded that robots such as NAO are effective for children with autism in teaching dance therapy, as well as making the session engaging; opening more opportunities for learning about their own mind and bodies.

## Developmental Disorders

According to the Centers for Disease Control and Prevention (2022b), "About 1 in 6 (17%) children aged 3–17 years were diagnosed with a developmental disability, as reported by parents, during a study period of 2009-2017." These disabilities included autism, ADHD, cerebral palsy, blindness, and others. Many treatment/therapy options available for these children are offered through the public education system in the United States. These options are often directed toward one single issue at a time, which sometimes causes other issues to be neglected. Since dance therapy is a holistic approach, intertwining the mind and body, sessions target children as a whole rather than only targeting one issue they may be having. Because of this, benefits are much greater to those participating and may extend past treatment for the disorder and into everyday life.

## Autism

Autism Spectrum Disorder is a developmental disability that affects the way one interacts, communicates, emotes, and learns. Since Autism is a spectrum, some individuals may need little support while others may need significant help with everyday tasks. According to the Center for Disease Control (CDC, 2022b), "About 1 in 44 children has been identified with an autism spectrum disorder." It is also four times more likely to be diagnosed in young boys than in girls. Dance therapy has been found to be extremely successful for improving social/communicative skills, motor awareness, and repetitive behavior patterns of children with autism. The three major functions dance therapy may target to improve the affected social skills are emotion, cognition, and bodily awareness.

A study conducted by Koch et al. (2015), analyzing the effects of dance therapy on autism, hypothesized that dance therapy would increase the overall well-being of participants as well as improve body awareness and self-distinction. The 31 participants in the treatment group underwent seven one-hour weekly sessions, which included a warm up routine, an interactive movement, a group circle, and lastly a verbal processing part. Results found that the treatment group improved in areas of psychological well-being, body awareness, self-other awareness, and social skills. Improvement of empathy was not significant. The results of the treatment group were compared to no significant differences in any areas from the control group. According to Koch et al. (2015), the data suggests that the increase of skills likely created the basic primary embodied skills from scratch (pp. 2-8). Overall, the therapy sessions were extremely successful for improving the well-being of the participants with autism, as well as building the social skills needed to propel them further in life and in their relationships.

## Cerebral Palsy

Cerebral Palsy is a group of developmental disorders that affects one's ability to perform motor tasks and maintain balance due to abnormal brain development in the cerebral motor cortex. As the most common motor disability affecting children, "About 1 in 345 children in the United States have been identified with CP" (CDC, 2022a). Similar to autism, cerebral palsy affects individuals in different ways. In a more severe case, individuals might need a wheelchair or medical equipment to aid them in walking. In more mild cases, individuals may have trouble with coordination and balance, but can walk unassisted. Dance and movement therapy can be beneficial even for children who cannot walk, or dance in the typical way individuals dance. Movements can be as small as facial or finger movements, but carry much expression and coordination.

In a clinical trial conducted by Teixeira-Machado (2017), 12 children and young adults with cerebral palsy participated in one-hour sessions of dance therapy, twice a week, for three months. The study was proposed because of concerns about the consequences of cerebral palsy in adulthood, affecting both physical and psychosocial components in everyday life. Areas focused on were global range of motion with coordination and rhythm, motor coordination of opposite directions and diagonals, body image or space-temporal orientation, and skill/agility with sequential movements. Participants took pre and post self-questionnaires including physical questions such as standing for 30-minute periods, getting dressed, washing one's whole body. There were also questions about social and cognitive functions such as learning a new task, maintaining friendships, and being emotionally affected by cerebral palsy. The questionnaires were in addition to observational data collected by psychologists during the dance therapy sessions and movement analysis. Results demonstrated that dance therapy improved development and restoration of motor functionality. The psychologists concluded that this means dance therapy can and should be recommended as a "biopsychosocial" treatment option to effectively improve symptoms of cerebral palsy (p. 429).

## Down Syndrome

Down syndrome is the most common genetic chromosomal disorder that impacts intellectual ability, receptive/expressive language, cognitive and neuro-motor functioning in the United States. According to the CDC (2020), "Each year about 6,000 babies are born with Down syndrome, which is about 1 in every 700 babies born." The prevalence rate of Down syndrome from 1979 to 2003 has increased by 30 percent. Likewise, the prevalence of the disorder increases with a mother's age, meaning an older mother would be more likely to have a child with down syndrome than a younger mother. Many individuals with down syndrome also experience other health conditions, in addition to the developmental deficits of the disorder including, heart defects, hearing loss, and eye diseases. Dance therapy can be substantially helpful for children with down syndrome since it is a holistic approach which aims to improve many different aspects of concern.

In an experiment conducted by DeFarias and Teixeira-Machado (2016), 12 participants with Down syndrome were assessed to test the efficacy of dance therapy on cognitive, social, and motor functioning in children with down syndrome. Dance therapy sessions were one hour long, twice a week, for 12 months. The dance was accompanied by playful music in an attempt to increase socialization among participants. The Functional Independence Measure (FIM) was used to measure independence on a scale from 18 to 126, with 18 being the lowest and 126 being the highest measure of independence. The Mini Mental State Examination (MMSE) was also used to examine cognitive ability. After treatment, the experimental group of participants showed significant improvement on the FIM with scores beginning at 65.5 and reaching 97.37 at the end of the sessions. This indicated an expansion of independence, psychosocial adjustments, and mobility. Data drawn from the MMSE testing cognitive impairment showed a slight increase in functioning, but it was not significant. Findings exhibited overall reduced limitations, and improvements in educational, emotional, and social performance. According to DeFarias and Teixeira-Machado (2016), "Although DS is characterized by substantial limitations in intellectual functioning, dance promoted adaptive behavior due to... mnemonic memory and its relatedness to affective learning" (p. 22). Dance therapy promotes autonomy and builds the capacity of these systems through simulating various skills used in real life scenarios. Thus, it prepares individuals to handle such skills in the ever-changing society we live in.

## Non-Verbal Children

As aforementioned, developmental disorders often affect more than one system in children, i.e., cognitive functioning, motor skills, cardiovascular systems, auditory systems. In addition to this, children can be non-verbal for several reasons. In autism, a lack of social and communication skills can result in a child who is non-verbal. In Down syndrome, receptive and expressive language can be impaired. In other cases, children may experience social or selective mutism caused by anxiety or poor relationships with family. Because dance and movement therapy is a multifaceted field, advantages are unrestricted and can range from generally improved physical fitness to improvements in non-verbal to verbal communications. Through entirely non-verbal exchange, dance and movement can be an avenue for expressive communication and shared emotions.

In a study conducted on infant communication intended on capturing dialogues between a mother and her infant, psychologists found that these dialogues can be seen through the infant's movements and direction of focus (Samaritter & Payne, 2013, p. 4). Imitation of gaze direction and facial expressions were found to be the root of this interaction. Infants are able to imitate facial expressions of adults from birth, which allow them, pre-linguistically, to recognize and copy emotion pre-linguistically. Parallel to the study on infancy, kinesthetic partnering in dance therapy with children and adult therapists is known to achieve mutual responsiveness. In partnering movements, both participants "feel, through direct perception, the kinetic qualities of their own movement patterns and those of their partner" (Samaritter &

Payne, 2013, p. 8). These actions may be through the use of gaze following, imitation, mirroring one another, or touch. This kinesthetic partnering and shared sense of emotion allows for an empathic attunement during the session exclusively through non-verbal interactions. It has been suggested that the mirror neuron system plays a principal role in the process of this exchange of sentiment.

## Case Study

Children with Autism Spectrum Disorder are some of the more common clients in dance and movement therapy. The goals and outcomes of this type of therapy are equivalent to many of the physical, socioemotional, and communicative needs for children with autism. The case study conducted by Teixeira-Machado (2015) demonstrates dance therapy's effects on a single 15-year-old male with autism. The study anticipated to examine effects of motor performance, common gestures, quality of life, and several mental skills. It was proposed that dance and movement therapy will be able to modify and correct the repetitive and stereotyped movement patterns, while also improving communication and socialization.

The 15-year-old participated in 30-minute dance and movement therapy classes twice a week for one year. This amounted to a total of 120 sessions, with the majority being individual and the last few being group sessions. Sessions were set at Academia Sergipana de Ballet, in Brazil. This was a typical dance studio with mirrors and a sound system. Approaches used in the sessions remains unknown, but techniques included mirroring and synchrony with a choreographic style of Brazilian ballroom. Choreography was changed every few weeks to complement the teenager's improvement. The Childhood Autism Rating Scale (CARS) was used to evaluate improvement throughout sessions. CARS is a 15-item scale that identifies and distinguishes autistic behaviors and developmental delays. A score of 15 to 30 is considered non-autistic, 30 to 36 is considered mild to moderate, and 36 to 60 is severe autism.

Results found a significant improvement in the severity of autism after the completed one year of dance and movement therapy sessions. "In the first evaluation, the teenager was found to have a 41.5-point score, and he was classified as been severely autistic… After a six-month intervention, the teenager's score was 37.5 points, and after twelve months of intervention, 32.5 points" (Teixeira-Machado, 2015). After 12 months, autism severity in the teenager dropped from a classification of severe to mild/moderate. As for specific skills, both static and dynamic movements, balance, replacement of repetitive movements, and social interaction were all seen to improve. The teenager's process in the sessions and learning of new skills overall improved his quality of life.

Even after sessions had finished, it was reported that the CARS score remained on the lower end indicating a mild severity of autistic behaviors. Repetitive movements and social interactions also remained at a similar level as to when sessions ended, signifying they did not worsen nor improve. It was found that, "Dancing, as a physical activity, fosters the reduction of atypical behaviors, as it physiologically modulates stereotyped actions through the release of specific neurotransmitters" (Teixeira-Machado, 2015). These results emphasize the seriousness of dance therapy intervention for correcting sensory-motor function in children with autism, thus allowing them to utilize their full physical, socioemotional, and cognitive capacities. Because dance and movement therapy touches on various areas of functioning sessions are seen to improve the overall quality of life of the participant. It is important to note that this study was only conducted on one individual and a larger sample of participants would be needed to generalize the effectiveness of dance therapy onto all people with Autism Spectrum Disorder.

## CONCLUSION

Since dance and movement therapy is still a relatively new field of study compared to the established psychological theories supporting it, there are an insufficient number of repeated experiments conducted to confirm the various findings discussed. One example of these types of limitations involves the mirror neuron system and empathy enhancement. Many psychologists, including McGarry and Russo (2011) and Winters (2008), have proposed the idea of using the mirror neuron system in the brain, which has been shown to elicit emotional responses in people when mirroring movements of others, to attempt to also elicit the feeling of empathy in children with autism. Since children with autism often lack the social skills needed to experience complex emotional constructs like empathy, there is not enough research to confirm these hypotheses yet. To progress forward, additional clinical studies would need to be performed directly testing empathy, whereas many current studies test more than one emotional response. Also to enhance the quality of this research, fMRI scans of the brain may be necessary to distinguish the mirror neuron system further.

Psychologists have already begun observing and measuring the benefits of the use of dance therapy in new contexts, such as in individuals with brain injuries, learning disorders, and eating disorders. However, research still remains extremely limited in these areas. Symptoms and effects of these newly studied disorders have the potential to carry over to other more-extensively studied disorders. For example, intellectual disabilities of a person with Down syndrome might experience similar cognitive limitations to a person with a learning disorder. In this context, researchers are able to predict certain benefits one with a learning disorder might achieve from dance therapy based on prior research conducted on cognition, but further studies are still required. In terms of areas more largely investigated, there is an extensive amount of data on the benefits of dance and movement therapy on children with cancer and other terminal illnesses, however this research is out of the scope in the current discussion. Furthermore, there has been considerable research conducted on elderly individuals with Alzheimer's disease that suggests dance therapy is capable of slowing the degeneration of neurons, but more time and funding are required to expand on the proposition.

For future directions of dance and movement therapy, it is crucial to the growth of the field that widespread acceptance of creative arts therapies is established as a treatment option for mental health issues. Such as in Greece where these holistic approaches are not easily accessible because of the lack of overall acceptance and government funding, the field of dance therapy has not yet had a chance to develop. An overwhelming amount of research has only reported benefits from the use of dance and movement therapy in schools, hospitals, rehabilitation centers, and more. With advantages to cognitive, social, emotional, and physical attributes of participants in dance therapy sessions, an overall improved quality of life is easily attainable.

## REFERENCES

American Dance Therapy Association. (2020). *Become a dance movement therapist: Frequently asked questions.* https://www.adta.org/become-a-dance-movement-therapist

Balgaonkar, A. V. (2010). Effect of dance/motor therapy on the cognitive development of children. *The International Journal of the Arts in Society*, *3*(11), 54–72.

Bräuninger, I. (2014). Specific dance movement therapy interventions—Which are successful? An intervention and correlation study. *The Arts in Psychotherapy*, *41*(5), 445–457. doi:10.1016/j.aip.2014.08.002

Capello, P. P. (2008). Dance/movement therapy with children throughout the world. *American Journal of Dance Therapy*, *30*(1), 24–36. doi:10.100710465-008-9045-z

Centers for Disease Control and Prevention. (2020, October 23). *Data & statistics on down syndrome.* CDC. https://www.cdc.gov/ncbddd/birthdefects/downsyndrome/data.html

Centers for Disease Control and Prevention. (2022a, May 2). *Data & statistics for cerebral palsy.* CDC. https://www.cdc.gov/ncbddd/cp/data.html

Centers for Disease Control and Prevention. (2022b, March 2). *Data & statistics on autism spectrum disorder.* CDC. https://www.cdc.gov/ncbddd/autism/data.html

De Farias, L. H. S., & Teixeira-Machado, L. (2016). Behind the dance: Educational, emotional and social contexts in Down syndrome. *International Journal of Humanities Social Sciences and Education, 3*(1), 20–23.

Koch, S. C., Mehl, L., Sobanski, E., Sieber, M., & Fuchs, T. (2015). Fixing the mirrors: A feasibility study of the effects of dance movement therapy on young adults with autism spectrum disorder. *Autism, 19*(3), 338–350. doi:10.1177/1362361314522353 PMID:24566716

McGarry, L. M., & Russo, F. A. (2011). Mirroring in dance/movement therapy: Potential mechanisms behind empathy enhancement. *The Arts in Psychotherapy, 38*(3), 178–184. doi:10.1016/j.aip.2011.04.005

Pratt, R. R. (2004). Art, dance, and music therapy. *Physical Medicine and Rehabilitation Clinics of North America, 15*(4), 827–841. doi:10.1016/j.pmr.2004.03.004 PMID:15458755

Samaritter, R., & Payne, H. (2013). Kinaesthetic intersubjectivity: A dance informed contribution to self-other relatedness and shared experience in non-verbal psychotherapy with an example from autism. *The Arts in Psychotherapy, 40*(1), 143–150. doi:10.1016/j.aip.2012.12.004

Suzuki, R., Lee, J., & Rudovic, O. (2017, March). Nao-dance therapy for children with ASD. *Proceedings of the Companion of the 2017 ACM/IEEE International Conference on Human-Robot Interaction*, 295-296. 10.1145/3029798.3038354

Teixeira-Machado, L. (2015). Dance therapy in autism: A case report. *Fisioterapia e Pesquisa, 22*, 205–211.

Teixeira-Machado, L., Azevedo-Santos, I., & DeSantana, J. M. (2017). Dance improves functionality and psychosocial adjustment in cerebral palsy: A randomized controlled clinical trial. *American Journal of Physical Medicine & Rehabilitation, 96*(6), 424–429. doi:10.1097/PHM.0000000000000646 PMID:27820729

Tyano, S. (2003). Post-traumatic stress disorder in Israeli children. *International Psychiatry : Bulletin of the Board of International Affairs of the Royal College of Psychiatrists, 1*(2), 7–8. doi:10.1192/S1749367600006421 PMID:31507661

Winters, A. F. (2008). Emotion, embodiment, and mirror neurons in dance/movement therapy: A connection across disciplines. *American Journal of Dance Therapy, 30*(2), 84–105. doi:10.100710465-008-9054-y

## KEY TERMS AND DEFINITIONS

**Affective Learning:** Learning that is related to the learner's feelings, experiences, and behavior.

**American Dance Therapy Association:** Organization created to establish and maintain standards and licensure among professional dance therapists in the United States.

**Attention Deficit/Hyperactivity Disorder:** Developmental disorder characterized by difficulty maintaining attention, impulsiveness, and hyperactivity.

**Biopsychosocial:** Interconnection between biological, psychological, and social factors.

**Endorphins:** Hormones that relieve pain and create a general feeling of well-being.

**fMRI: (Functional Magnetic Resonance Imaging):** Type of brain scan measuring the brain waves by detecting changes in blood flow.

**Kinesthetic Intersubjectivity:** Mutual attunement and understanding of interactions.

**Laban Movement Analysis:** Method of analyzing and interpreting human movement.

**Limbic System:** System of the brain responsible for emotional and behavioral responses.

**Mirror Neuron System:** System of the brain engaged when witnessing and embodying other's movements to produce emotional responses.

**Mnemonic Memory:** Techniques used to aid in memory retention or retrieval.

**Parietal Cortex:** Part of the brain responsible for sensations of touch, temperature, and pain.

**Post-Traumatic Stress Disorder:** Mental health disorder caused by a traumatic event with symptoms of flashbacks, nightmares, self-destructive behavior, anxiety, and depression.

**Premotor Cortex:** Part of the brain responsible for motor plans and voluntary movement.

**Superior Temporal Sulcus:** Part of the brain responsible for a variety of social activities including language perception and replicating the mental processes of others.

**Transference:** Process of directing one's feelings onto another person.

# Chapter 10
# Dance Movement Therapy Treatment for Eating Disorders and Disordered Eating

**Heather Kroesche**
*Marymount Manhattan College, USA*

## ABSTRACT

*Eating disorders impact a large number of individuals worldwide. Due to a rise in media standards on weight and appearance, prevalence rates of eating disorders are at an incline. Diagnoses include anorexia nervosa, bulimia nervosa, binge eating disorder, and emotional eating. Research in dance movement therapy as treatment for eating disorders suggest that dance movements' creative and physical attributes can positively affect individuals' recoveries from eating disorders as increased body-image satisfaction, self-awareness, and body awareness occurs. Dance movement therapy offers a range of intervention styles that can be tailored through individual therapy or be used to build community in group therapy. Additionally, different intervention designs tackle a myriad of components that plague eating disordered individuals such as attachment style, emotional distress response, and the mind-body connection. Dance movement therapy's treatment has a prominent focus on the therapist/patient relationship, development of physical practice and confidence, and personal reflection.*

DOI: 10.4018/978-1-6684-7856-1.ch010

## INTRODUCTION

Eating disorders (ED) and disordered eating are a unique group of psychological disorders. While EDs are characterized as mental health disorders, the physicality of the body is concurrently a concern for those who suffer. EDs are more common in Western and Asian countries, and up to 30 million people in the U.S. are affected (Bucharová, Malá, Kantor, & Svobodová, 2020). Characteristics of EDs can involve undereating or overeating, but EDs are truly defined by the individual's attitude toward food, when the relationship to food is the top priority of the individual.

The pathology of EDs proves to be a complex system of factors involving psychological stress, distorted body-image, low self-esteem, media influences, material and environmental surroundings, and attachment styles. Krueger and Schofield (1986) discuss how individuals with eating disorders tend to have impaired self-regulation and rely on external cues like counting calories or measuring exact amounts of food. Internal bodily sensations and messages are lost as the individual ignores or suppresses the body's message of hunger. This innately creates a divide between mind and body. A characteristic that has been found to be coexistent with EDs is alexithymia, a personality trait described as the inability to identify one's feelings and body sensations which often exists with depression, anxiety, and social phobias (Bucharová et al., 2020).

These symptoms, characteristics, and risks indicate how the disease is multifaceted and affects a large number of individuals; it necessitates a multimodal approach that addresses behavioral, biological, psychological, and social factors. Traditional treatments prescribed for EDs like cognitive behavior therapy or talk therapy have low long-term success rates. Some believe this is due to the nature of the disorder running deeper than health behaviors and that it affects the psyche, but also the physical body.

Research in Dance Movement Therapy (DMT) challenges the depth and range of the therapeutic experience, since embodied practices have the ability to decrease objectification and ignorance toward the body and increase the mind-body connection to experience self. Embodiment integrates internal and external experiences, as well as relational, environmental, cultural, and existential parts of oneself (Perey & Cook-Cottone, 2020). Approaches from DMT to treat EDs vary in specific techniques and foci, which allows for a nuanced experience for the participants experiencing it. On the whole, DMT interventions promote an increase in self-awareness, building a subjective relationship to one's body, and strengthening the mind-body connection.

## Eating Disorders

Externally, disordered eating can look like many things and similarly, the internal turbulence of an individual with an ED is no different. Krantz (1999) suggested that psychodynamic, cultural, and gender conflicts are all components of disordered eating, causing a dissatisfaction with body-image. Body-image is developed through internal cognitions like kinesthetic sensations, somatic experiences, and aspects that encompass the psychological self. There is a reported increase in the prevalence of EDs worldwide, which is in part due to changes in diagnostic criteria and to a surge in social media, with a focus on the body aesthetic as well as gender roles (Bucharová et al., 2020).

Historically, social factors have always influenced the perception of EDs in general as well as treatment as interventions influenced by feminist and post-feminist theories were developed as a way to understand issues that women encounter in our society, socially and culturally. The transgender community is a highly at-risk population as approximately one in five transgender individuals suffer from an eating disorder, while 1.8 percent of cisgender women and 0.2 percent of cisgender males suffer in the U.S. (Griffiths & Yager, 2019). Media holds idealistic images of masculinity and femininity. Transgender individuals are more likely to suffer from body dysmorphia surrounding extreme thinness as a feminine trait and "reverse anorexia" or the intense psychological desire to be muscular as a masculine characteristic. As gender is interpreted through the perception or acceptance of others, the transgender community is susceptible to disordered eating as a means of fulfilling normative gender expectations.

A core risk factor of EDs is body-image disturbance, or distorted body-image. Body-image is developed from birth and is influenced internally through sensations and proprioception, and externally through perceptions of the body from the individual or others. Measuring body-image requires a combination of emotions, attitudes, self-esteem and identity (Savidaki, Demirtoka & Rodríguez-Jiménez, 2020). The non-verbal nature of DMT can promote unconscious insights of a client's beliefs, behaviors, and perceptions, suggesting that the creative therapies are a beneficial intervention strategy since they require active participation, self-expression, and imagination. Emotional detachment, apathy, and/or alexithymia in tandem with poor self-efficacy and self-esteem are key components of the disease. These characteristics may be related to weak levels of secure attachment, which can be caused by a lack of tactile interaction from a caregiver which offers infants psychological and physical soothing, or maltreatment as a child. ED treatment that focuses on improving attachment security had a positive effect on interpersonal relationships. DMT practices build self-esteem, improve empathic behaviors emotionally and physically, and increase levels of secure attachment.

## Anorexia Nervosa

Anorexia Nervosa (AN) is a type of eating disorder that is most prevalent in adolescent girls. It involves an intense fear of weight gain and a continuous refusal of food. Women and girls may lose their menstrual cycle due to low body weight and due to a lack of nutrients. Perry and Cook-Cattone (2020), explained that this disorder creates a distorted perception of the body which allows individuals with AN to pursue unattainable body standards and ultra-thinness.

On a social level, Eli and Lavis (2021) examined the disorder through a philosophical lens, describing ultra-thinness in literature and media as having the greatest effect on individuals with anorexia. Media consistently objectifies (almost exclusively female) bodies where the subjectivity of *woman* doesn't exist. Therefore, this influence perpetuates the aesthetic of ultra-thinness while simultaneously supporting the voicelessness of this character. It can be argued that a body that has lost its agency socially and has restricted self-awareness physically will likely psychologically suffer, as well. Researching and examining these connections is crucial when analyzing treatment plans for patients with AN.

## Bulimia Nervosa

Bulimia Nervosa (BN) is defined by a recurring cycle of binging or uncontrolled overeating, and purging which may include self-induced vomiting, use of laxatives, strict dieting, and over-exercising to prevent weight gain (Trably, Gorwood, & Di Lodovico, 2022). This system places self-evaluation solely on physical appearance, resulting in low body-image and self-esteem, and is distinctive because of destructive thoughts about food, body, weight and impulsive eating behaviors.

Similar to AN, bulimia suppresses bodily sensations and feelings of hunger and satisfactions, inhibiting the relationship between the physical body and an internal sense of self. Fewer than half of sufferers with AN and BN recover completely and have relatively low longevity of recovery and there is high risk of relapse. Additionally, AN and BN present the highest mortality rate of any mental health disorder (Krantz, 1999).

## Binge Eating Disorder

Binge Eating Disorder (BED) is similar to BN due to the presence of binging episodes as a response to emotional distress or stressful life events, however, it lacks the compensatory behavior of purging seen in bulimia. The presence of psychological distress that causes compulsive binging is distinctive to BED. This cycle can be induced through extreme dieting followed by failure to follow through or a lack of weight loss contributing to or causing distress and leading to a binging episode.

One sample study found that almost 20 percent of obese individuals suffer from BED. Those most at risk for BED tend to be those who are women, white, young, and overweight (Meekums, 2005). Another sample offered that four out of five patients with BED suffered trauma and/or maltreatment in adolescence and early childhood. While BED-specific research is in its infancy, interventions including cognitive behavioral therapy, interpersonal therapy, and mindfulness therapy that focus on a distress response have been shown to reduce binging.

### Emotional Eating

Emotional eating is overeating as a reaction to emotional states. Obese individuals may suffer from lower self-acceptance and self-esteem and struggle with everyday interpersonal discrimination. Emotional eating is similar to, but is not technically diagnosed BED and instead is dependent on self-report and linkage between overeating in relation to the absence of hunger, low self-esteem, psychological discomfort, and negative body-image (Meekums, Vaverniece, Majore-Dusele, & Rasnacs, 2012). Obese individuals are likely to suffer from social avoidance, where stigmatization of obesity discourages participation in exercise or physical activity, as well as in other social settings.

The World Health Organization reported in 2011 that obesity rates have doubled between 1980 and 2010. This could be due to increased media stigmatization of obesity and emphasis on thinness. Obese individuals are a vulnerable population for overeating as social stigmatization, or failed dieting or exercise interventions decrease body-image and self-esteem, perpetuating the cycle of coping with emotion through food.

## Dance/Movement Therapy

Causes and effects of EDs can range from genetic, biological, behavioral, psychological, and social factors. Anxiety and depression are common in patients with EDs, and individuals may display perfectionistic, neurotic, and obsessive tendencies (Bucharová et al., 2020). Some argue that the DMT could be more detrimental than healing for ED patients. Sufferers of AN or BN are particularly vulnerable to over-exercising as a symptom of their ED. Due to a paucity of research in this area, it is unknown whether the inclusion of an embodied and physical treatment would trigger individuals who over-exercise. While physical activity is known to release endorphins, for these individuals who have little to no internal reference of self, exercise and food behaviors intend to please or get recognition from others. DMT intrinsically combats this since it utilizes techniques of muscle relaxation, breathing exercises, and guided imagery to create a sense of self and an awareness of the body.

Dance movement therapy addresses these issues in treatment by nurturing a strong non-hierarchical relationship between the therapist and patient. One technique that is used in DMT is *Mirroring,* where the therapist is involved in the movement practice and the client follows along. This is not only a beneficial starting point for those beginning DMT, it also deconstructs the hierarchy between therapist and client that is often present during verbal psychotherapy, as well as other therapies. This creates a positive environment where vulnerability can be present.

The fact that media connects thinness to attractiveness, success, and sexual acceptance highlights how sexual trauma can be related to the development of an ED (Krantz, 1999). The physical nature of DMT can uniquely address developmental regressions as well as trauma- related sexual and physical abuse since it provides an outlet for individuals to be vulnerable and to address traumatic events of their past. Improvisation may be used as a tool to practice expression of emotional content and an associated memory. Therefore, DMT is distinctly equipped to treat all components of EDs.

DMT integrates the emotional, physical, social and spiritual aspects of self. Through physicality, DMT increases self-awareness, kinesthetic empathy and kinesthetic awareness and additionally requires reflections from participants. Whether it is verbal, written, drawn, or recorded through visual art, individuals can reflect on the emotions that they uncover first through movement and then can interpret on paper.

## Individual Therapy

Individual therapy is mostly used for clients working through specific and personal trauma-based emotions and events. Characteristics such as feeling invisible or inadequate can be addressed by creating a vulnerable space for an individual to embody particular action words or through characterizations of people in their lives, or as themselves whether it be past or present. A beneficial tool used in individual therapy is improvisation, which not only builds one's own agency, but can also become a coping skill since free associations can be processed through movement, can defend against emotional or physical repression, and can address apathy and tension.

Mobility and strength in the body is also a component of DMT, and within an individual therapy setting, the therapist is able to demonstrate and prescribe certain exercises to the client. This is not only for the body, but for energetic pathways to be opened to release emotional tension. For example, depression, which can often be comorbid with ED, can be physicalized through a sunken chest, lethargic movement, and hunched shoulders (Krantz, 1999) and can be addressed specifically and strategically within an individual therapeutic session, where strengthening and mobilizing techniques and exercises can be prescribed for the individual. Additionally, specific practices may be repeated particularly by reenacting situations that cause distress or anxiety. This provides alternative tools for the client when faced with these situations in their day-to-day life.

## Group Therapy

Group therapy programs normally consist of a developed structure or syllabus designed to guide the group through the intervention together to gain self-awareness but also to build group cohesion and trust. Savidaki et al. (2020) examined a 12-week-long group therapy intervention of 90 minute sessions. Each session included check-in, warm-up, guided imagery, movement exploration, and written personal reflection. Remembering that DMT heavily focuses on the lack of hierarchy between the patient and therapist to create a collaborative and creative environment that builds confidence in the individuals receiving treatment, the first four sessions of the intervention focused on building a positive and safe environment where trust with the therapist was developed, and also between participants within the group. Additionally, there was value placed on trusting oneself and creating a subjective relationship with one's physicality.

Sessions five to ten facilitated group cohesion as an empathy building experience, where participants explored movement in pairs and increased self- and body-awareness. The last two sessions focused on preparing closure of the intervention and drew attention to examining inter and intrapersonal connections. Self-reports from participants reported improved body satisfaction and a decrease in anxiety. Additionally, improved self-awareness and a mention of internal and external connectedness were common. DMT sessions promoted mind-body connections through practicing identification of feelings, setting boundaries, and experiencing internal thoughts or memories through an external reality.

Another example of a group therapy program is described by Meekums et al. (2012). This intervention consisted of ten sessions and focused on emotional eating for female individuals who were obese. The sessions introduced the group to different components of dance and movement. First, they practiced rhythm and responding to music, the next session focused on movement quality and how time, space, and flow may be interpreted psychologically. The subsequent group of sessions developed vulnerability and intimacy. Participants focused on concepts such as moving from different body parts, actions of giving or receiving, safety and comfort. These then developed into more intense and direct interpretations of embodying emotions, like body-image and self-acceptance. The last two weeks of ten weekly sessions was the closure stage, where participants represented, "Me: present and future" and lastly, "Parting."

Treatment of obese individuals with emotional eating suggests a relationship between eating habits, self-esteem, body-image distress, and well-being. After a ten-session group intervention program, the control group had no change in psychological symptoms, whereas the DMT group showed decreased symptoms of anxiety and depression, and increased body-image satisfaction and self-esteem (Meekums et al., 2012). These findings are valuable to develop in the dialogue of how DMT can be helpful in deconstructing underlying emotional issues of overeating. By offering a treatment that was not solely based on behavior change, DMT still includes a bodily component and is more sustainable than traditional weight loss interventions and increases self-esteem and self-awareness in tandem with behavior change.

Both designs of group therapy interventions created a safe environment, offering participants time to develop their comfort in movement and slowly relate it to their emotions, and lastly to reflect on the experience and decipher how exact exercises influenced their feelings.

## Embodiment and Materiality

Eli and Lavis (2021) defines anorexic embodiment through "being-in-the-world with anorexia," When discussing embodiment and the embodied experience for those living with an ED, materiality of mundane objects as well as environments are crucial to examine as a component of how these relationships relate to an individual's illness and recovery.

Field studies were conducted throughout the years 2005–2011 in anorexia recovery clinics in the UK and Israel. Eli and Lavis (2021) specifically surveyed the material items of everyday life and their effects on thoughts, perceptions and how they influence self and identity in individuals with anorexia. The importance of these materials or objects are examined in a recovery setting, since these comforts 'became extensions of self,' and 'question compliance and resistance, illness and health, belonging and difference.'

One case study investigates the objectivity of a simple chair within the recovery clinic. Patients are observed and monitored while they eat, as well as after meal times and are required to sit for a period of time after meals. They are unable to walk around or move about, and while individuals in recovery comply with these rules, minute signs of resistance within even a simple object as the chair becomes evident. One individual in the clinic would move around on the chair by stretching and yawning. While this behavior seems harmless, the movement is a way to obey the rules, while pushing the boundaries. This embodied act can be interpreted as superficial, but it is representative of internal conflict faced by someone in recovery for an ED, where a negotiation between illness and identity is explored, questioned, and practiced.

This research extends beyond a sole focus on the body and creates a holistic network of objects and materials that individuals interact with. It highlights an area of EDs that is not considered in traditional literature. It questions the implications that the environment has on individuals, and the complexity of the illness. This analysis contributes to DMT as treatment for EDs since it addresses physicality and behavioral practice as a mode of recovery.

## Symbolism as Treatment

Franks and Fraenkel (1991) explain that individuals with disordered eating utilize food and body weight or size to attain control in their lives since these factors turn into symbols of control and success. Since the media idealizes thinness as attractiveness and success, symbolism as treatment for eating disorders can be effective. This seminar specifically examines how fairy tales through DMT can benefit individuals with EDs by offering physical practice through a mode grounded in symbolism outside of food and body.

Fairy tale and DMT seminars were 8–12-week interventions that included individuals with AN, BN, and/or obesity. This approach was pedagogical and therapeutic. The focus of fairy tales explores a metaphorical approach to DMT, as symbiotic relationships create a way of indirectly addressing difficult emotional barriers through embodiment. Fairy tales offer non-threatening narratives that can be contextualized within culture, yet open the door for creative interpretation, and can be correlated with playfulness and imagination.

Through dramatization, embodying clear personality traits or characters, individuals can physicalize new versions of their physical selves and mediate their own thoughts and feelings by finding relevant components of the symbols or characters they are embodying. This develops not only improvisation skills, but also allows expression of dissatisfaction, perfectionism, interpersonal distress, and other emotions that affect disordered eaters, providing a new way of experiencing subjectivity outside of behaviors related to food.

Parallel to most DMT practices, this seminar also included a written component from the participants. As they were assigned specific stories to read, they were asked to write about characters that stood out as well as the relationships that the stories produced. The writings also included the expectations of what participants thought would be present and then what actually was present. Writing practice as well as embodying symbolic characters demonstrated a positive effect on individuals' ability to relate to their subjectivity and cope with unconscious emotions contributing to their disordered eating through metaphor in fairy tales. Case studies from participants in the seminar showed how the intervention allowed clients to tangibly physicalize intangible archetypes. Unconscious realizations took place and allowed a new understanding of real-life relationships and experiences were introduced through fairy tale embodiment.

### Yoga/Mindfulness as Treatment

Similar to DMT treatment, yoga has been an exploratory treatment for EDs. It is a valuable study in embodiment that follows similar goals to DMT, where individuals develop the mind-body connection through physicality and connection to self through somatic awareness, and subjectivity (Perey & Cook-Cottone, 2020). The embodied practice of yoga is a valuable treatment technique since it focuses on breath work, muscle relaxation, mindfulness, self-regulation, self-compassion, and body awareness. While research on this niche area is slim, yoga shows a promising future in the treatment of eating disorders since it can address varying aspects of low body-image, emotional distress, and self-esteem.

## CONCLUSION

Considering the pathology of eating disorders, it is evident how many factors in various spheres of life, including social, environmental, external and internal areas, influence the development of disorders, behaviors, and risks. Eating disorders like anorexia, bulimia, binge eating and emotional eating affect millions of people each day. These disorders are destructive to the mind and body connection of an individual, since disordered behaviors ignore bodily sensations of discomfort or hunger. Low body-image or body-image dissatisfaction consist of low self-esteem and an image of oneself that is negative and distorted from reality. This can cause anxiety and depression as well as a lack of self-awareness signaled through emotional detachment. Recovery programs for EDs traditionally offer talk therapy as well as cognitive behavioral therapy among others. EDs, specifically anorexia, have low long-term recovery rates and hold the title of having the highest mortality rate out of all psychiatric disorders.

To question the physical effects that EDs have on individuals, embodied research is critical. As a whole, DMT lacks quantitative data due to small sample sizes in the research that has been conducted. An additional implication of DMT research related to EDs, is the specific nature of field studies that have been done, with each intervention being customized to one individual or of a small recovery group, general research on the benefits of DMT have not been published. Large scale data of how dance movement interventions improve different classifications of eating disorders such as binge eating disorder or bulimia, would begin to cover the gaps of research within the field.

So far, the research conducted on analyzing dance movement therapy in conjunction with eating disorder recovery shows how the values of dance movement such as its lack of hierarchy between patient and therapist and its emphasis on emotional confidence and self-awareness prove to benefit many factors of EDs (Savidaki et al., 2020). Many cases found improvements in body satisfaction, body-image and emotional states.

## REFERENCES

Bucharová, M., Malá, A., Kantor, J., & Svobodová, Z. (2020). Arts therapies interventions and their outcomes in the treatment of Eating disorders: Scoping review protocol. *Behavioral Sciences (Basel, Switzerland)*, *10*(12), 188. doi:10.3390/bs10120188 PMID:33316926

Eli, K., & Lavis, A. (2021). Material environments and the shaping of anorexic embodiment: Towards a materialist account of eating disorders. *Culture, Medicine and Psychiatry*, *46*(2), 344–363. doi:10.100711013-021-09715-8 PMID:33826076

Franks, B., & Fraenkel, D. (1991). Fairy tales and dance/movement therapy: Catalysts of change for eating-disordered individuals. *The Arts in Psychotherapy*, *18*(4), 311–319. doi:10.1016/0197-4556(91)90070-Q

Good Therapy. (2018, May 15). *Dance /Movement therapy (DMT)*. Dance/Movement Therapy. https://www.goodtherapy.org/learn-about-therapy/types/dance-movement-therapy

Griffiths, S., & Yager, Z. (2019). Gender, embodiment, and eating disorders. *The Journal of Adolescent Health*, *64*(4), 425–426. doi:10.1016/j.jadohealth.2019.01.016 PMID:30904090

Krantz, A. M. (1999). Growing into Her Body: Dance/Movement therapy for women with eating disorders. *American Journal of Dance Therapy*, *21*(2), 81–103. doi:10.1023/A:1022104603189

Krueger, D. W., & Schofield, E. (1986). Dance/movement therapy of eating disordered patients: A model. *The Arts in Psychotherapy*, *13*(4), 323–331. doi:10.1016/0197-4556(86)90033-X

Meekums, B. (2005). Responding to the embodiment of distress in individuals defined as obese: Implications for research. *Counselling & Psychotherapy Research, 5*(3), 246–255. doi:10.1080/17441690500317119

Meekums, B., Vaverniece, I., Majore-Dusele, I., & Rasnacs, O. (2012). Dance movement therapy for obese women with emotional eating: A controlled pilot study. *The Arts in Psychotherapy, 39*(2), 126–133. doi:10.1016/j.aip.2012.02.004

Milton, A., Hambleton, A., Roberts, A., Davenport, T., Flego, A., Burns, J., & Hickie, I. (2021). Body-image distress and its associations from an international sample of men and women across the adult life span: Web-based survey study. *JMIR Formative Research, 5*(11), e25329. Advance online publication. doi:10.2196/25329 PMID:34734831

Perey, I., & Cook-Cottone, C. (2020). Eating disorders, embodiment, and yoga: A conceptual overview. *Eating Disorders, 28*(4), 315–329. doi:10.1080/10640266.2020.1771167 PMID:32964817

Savidaki, M., Demirtoka, S., & Rodríguez-Jiménez, R.-M. (2020). Re-inhabiting one's body: A pilot study on the effects of dance movement therapy on body-image and alexithymia in eating disorders. *Journal of Eating Disorders, 8*(1), 22. Advance online publication. doi:10.118640337-020-00296-2 PMID:32426135

Trably, F., Gorwood, P., & Di Lodovico, L. (2022). Art therapy in eating disorders. A systematic review of literature. *European Psychiatry, 65*(S1), S151. Advance online publication. doi:10.1192/j.eurpsy.2022.405

Wolff, K. (2018, March 18). *Materiality*. Society for Cultural Anthropology. https://culanth.org/fieldsights/materiality#:~:text=Materiality

## KEY TERMS AND DEFINITIONS

**Anorexia Nervosa:** An eating disorder, occurring most frequently in adolescent girls, that involves persistent refusal of food, fear of weight gain, and obsession with thinness that is insatiable causing disturbed perception of body-image.

**Binge Eating:** Consuming abnormally large quantities of food in a short time period with feelings of loss of control. Recurrent binge eating is associated with numerous adverse characteristics, such as increased risk of obesity as well as depression.

**Binge Eating Disorder:** A disorder marked by recurring episodes of uncontrolled consumption of food, caused by emotional distress.

**Body-Image Distress:** Occurs when there is a discrepancy between how an individual views their body (actual body-image) and how they want it to be (ideal body-image). Dissatisfaction, over evaluation, and preoccupation are considered as contributing factors to body-image distress.

**Bulimia Nervosa:** An eating disorder involving recurrent cycle of binge eating followed by inappropriate compensatory behaviors, or purging that may include self-induced vomiting, misuse of laxatives, fasting, excessive exercise.

**Embodiment:** The thesis that the human mind is largely determined by the structures of the human body through somatic and kinesthetic experiences and its interactions with the physical environment. This concept emerged from work in late 20th century linguistics, philosophy, and cognitive psychology.

**Improvisation:** Creative movement exploration that is sometimes prompted and is open-ended. In Dance Movement Therapy it can be used as a tool for expression of emotions, release of tension, and increase of body-awareness.

**Materiality:** The anthropological definition explains materiality as a two-way relationship between material items as a social projection of culture, but also a determinant of culture influencing socialization.

**Mind-Body Connection:** A psychological and philosophical concept that describes how biological, behavioral, and physical components of an individual influences and is influenced by psychological and mental components. Together the physical and mental factors create a holistic experience of self and surroundings.

**Purge:** The activity of expelling food that has just been ingested, usually by vomiting, over-exercising, extreme dieting, or the use of laxatives. Its purpose is to eliminate or reduce real or imagined weight gain.

# Chapter 11
# The Positive Effects of Music Therapy on Stress

**Hunter Lloyd**
*Marymount Manhattan College, USA*

## ABSTRACT

*Music therapy has significant positive effects on stress and stress management. Many individuals suffer from daily and chronic stress. Stress is a risk factor for several ailments and serious diseases. This includes both mental, emotional, and physical stress. Music-based interventions play a significant role in decreasing stress levels. Music is effective in decreasing a variety of different stressors on both the mental and physical levels. Music can support individuals in dealing with uncomfortable stress in a noninvasive and accessible way. This chapter will describe what stress is and why it is so common. Also, it will include the background of music therapy and numerous ways music therapy can help reduce stress. We are only beginning to learn how healing music can be to our nation's current stress epidemic.*

## INTRODUCTION

This chapter discusses the relationship between music and stress. Music therapy is a new and innovative practice in the medical field for reducing stress levels. Music is well-known vastly throughout the world and in all cultures. In modern day America, chronic stress is increasing both in our minds and body. Music can support individuals in contending with uncomfortable stress in a noninvasive and accessible way. This chapter will describe what stress is and why it is so common. In addition, it will present the background of music therapy and numerous ways music therapy can help reduce stress. Brene Brown, a famous researcher and author,

DOI: 10.4018/978-1-6684-7856-1.ch011

states in her book *The Gifts of Imperfection,* "Whether it's a hymn at church, the national anthem, a college fight song, a song on the radio, or the carefully scored soundtrack to a movie, music reaches out and offers us connection- something we really can't live without" (Brown, 2010, p. 119). We are only beginning to learn how healing music can be to our nation's current stress epidemic.

## The Stress Epidemic

Chronic stress is a national epidemic. Chronic stress includes both mental and physical stress. Connolly et al. (2019) explains that the national epidemic of stress is due to a challenging combination of our socioeconomic, mental, environmental, physiological and spiritual lifestyles. On average, our culture is over-productive and neglects rest. Resisting rest and ignoring our bodily cues to slow down lead to burnout. Our society too often stigmatizes rest which encourages us to become overloaded with stress. This creates tension in our bodies and brains, which restricts us from moving freely and with ease. Stress negatively impacts almost every aspect of our health, including our vitality, mood, and longevity. Witte (2020) concludes that stress is a risk factor for several diseases including cancer and cardiovascular diseases. It is also a risk factor for mental health disorders, including anxiety, depression, and eating disorders. Although chronic stress is prevalent today, there are several, diverse forms of stress. These can include physical pain, anxiety, depression, autoimmune diseases, lifestyle changes, and many other factors. Connolly (2019) describes additional factors that can impact modern day stress levels, these include financial instability, social isolation, permeable boundaries, and a poor work-life balance. Prolonged stress not only affects the body, but it can also affect our mind and soul.

All ages, ethnicities, and classes can be affected by stress. Acute stress was helpful years ago when we were running away from potential danger (Shmerling, 2020). Today, most individuals are no longer running away from dangerous animals, but our stress levels are still chronically high (Shmerling, 2020). This chronic stress no longer serves us and is actually harmful. Stress is scary because it is not always visible (Shmerling, 2020). It can easily become a slippery slope and a gateway to many serious illnesses.

According to Delta (2015), stress can manifest in the brain and body in several different ways. It can stem from a lack of quality sleep, loneliness, and burnout. It can also accumulate in tense work or in the family environment. Additionally, life changes can be anxiety-provoking and stress-inducing. This can include new relationships, career changes, location changes, and grievances. Life is always changing and evolving. The only aspect of life that is constant is, paradoxically, change.

There are two main types of stress, physiological and psychological (Witte, 2020). Both types of stress are common and can adversely impact our health. Unfortunately, anxiety and depression levels in the world are on the rise. Anxiety and depression can both contribute to stress and stress can lead to symptoms of anxiety and depression. The most problematic form of stress is the chronic stress most individuals experience daily (Delta, 2015). Chronic stress can manifest physiologically and psychologically (Witte, 2020). This is harmful to the human body because it removes us from our natural state of homeostasis. Our body always wants to be in homeostasis or in a state of balance. When it is out of this state, the body is alerted to stress (Delta, 2015). This leaves our hormones imbalanced and our cortisol levels, the body's stress hormone, dangerously elevated (Delta, 2015).

Culturally, Americans are so stressed that they do not even recognize that they are stressed. They are constantly wired, but tired (Delta, 2015). This phenomenon relates to the feeling of being wired at night when the body should be sleeping. However, during the day, they are depleted and exhausted. It is a vicious cycle when the body's natural sleep rhythms are off (Delta, 2015). Many individuals suffer from insomnia and a dysregulated circadian rhythm. Having a normal and consistent sleep-wake cycle is important for stress and hormonal health. Lack of quality sleep is one main reason why the nation is experiencing chronic stress.

Furthermore, society does not only have mental and emotional stressors, but also external stress factors that negatively impact us. According to Kandarakis et al. (2009), endocrine- disrupting chemicals (EDCs) are in our environment. This includes the toxins we breathe in and the hormones we ingest from specific foods. These are known as endocrine disruptors. Endocrine disruptors surround us every day and pollute our world. These disruptors interfere and negatively affect our hormones and bodily functions. These toxins add more stress to our already stressed- out systems. The increase in environmental toxins today may significantly impact our overall stress levels.

## Women and Stress

In the modern world, women are expected to assume more roles than decades ago. Women are expected to do and be so much nowadays, including pursuing jobs and diverse societal roles. Women are expected to be wives, mothers, daughters, entrepreneurs, and friends. It is revolutionary that women can do and pursue much more than they have in the past, but it is also costly. Women's health may suffer. As aforementioned, the United States is a country that encourages over- productivity and criticizes rest. This is harmful, especially to women, who are in a state of chronic stress and near burn-out. This is especially true for women in their reproductive years, since it is easy for hormones to become unbalanced. Kandarakis (2009) posits that the environment's endocrine-disrupting chemicals (EDCs) and the stresses women experience may explain why reproductive conditions such as endometriosis and Polycystic Ovary Syndrome (PCOS) are on the rise. Women would greatly benefit from stress reduction and stress management. Additionally, Connolly's (2019) research indicates that 28% of women admit that their appearance causes them stress. These findings are disheartening, but provide more areas of data where women experience routine stress.

Additionally, pregnancy and birth are very stressful on the women mentally and physically. Having a newborn baby and contending with life postpartum are stress-inducing. Stewart et al. (2018) conclude that women in their mid-life have a vast number of stressors and life changes occurring. These changes occur within their careers, family lives, caregiving, and even due to discrimination. Their stress levels have adverse effects on their health, especially their cardiovascular health. This study focuses on the relationship between stress and the heart health of women. Unfortunately, mid-life is not the only stressor on women. On average, women are juggling various facets of their lives and the stress can affect all of them. Stewart (2018) defines midlife as the years between 40 to 65. This is a stressful time for women because their bodies are transitioning from perimenopause to menopause. This life transition happens for all women at a certain point in their lives which is why having stress-relieving modalities, like music therapy, is important. Hormonal changes are stress-inducing on the body. Having alternative ways to counterbalance the stress is vital (Stewart, 2018).

## Music as Medicine

Today, millions of individuals are utilizing pharmaceuticals to help manage their stress levels. Unfortunately, many of these medications have adverse effects and can take a negative toll on our bodies. Often when individuals are contending with stress, they tend to be susceptible to bad habits, including alcohol, non- prescription drugs, and other addictions. There are non- pharmaceutical modalities that can provide great benefits to our health and wellbeing. Music therapy is one of these interventions with known potential. Music as medicine is widely used for stress management. Witte (2020) states that music has been used for years to provide relaxation. Calming our nervous system with feelings of rest and relaxation are crucial components for fighting stress. Music is a very potent form of medicine. It even has the power to move us emotionally which is a key component to music being effective in reducing stress. Healing with a holistic view of an individual is important when discussing treatments for stress.

## What Is Music Therapy?

Witte (2020) explains that music therapy is the use of music to accomplish goals to meet our mental, emotional, and psychological needs. Though all music can be therapeutic, music therapy in a clinical setting should be conducted with a trained music therapist (Witte, 2020). Specifically, the individual should be licensed with the proper training in psychology and medicine (Witte, 2020). For this chapter's purpose we are including all forms of music- based interventions, not only clinical music therapy with a licensed practitioner.

Although clinical music therapy is highly effective, other music-based interventions also show great benefit for stress reduction. Music is universal and is listened to throughout the world (Simon, 2015). All cultures listen to and produce music (Simon, 2015). Music's accessibility makes it a wonderful field for achieving therapeutic needs (Fallon, 2020). It is easily accessible regardless of one's socioeconomic status (SES). Individuals can listen to it on the radio, television, smart phones, and in nature. Music allows the body to slow down and rest (Witte, 2020). It allows the mind to relax, open, and connect (Simon, 2015). It allows the nervous system to enter a parasympathetic mode. This presence and stillness can allow space for stress reduction (Simon, 2015).

## Physiological Stress

Witte (2020) explains that just listening to music is strongly correlated with stress reduction. This occurs by lowering our physiological arousal by decreasing our stress hormone, cortisol, and lowering our heart rate. Cortisol levels are our body's stress hormones. It is normal for our cortisol hormones to be elevated in the morning and to decrease as the day goes on. It is harmful when our cortisol levels are chronically elevated. For some individuals, these levels are chronically high. Music can help lower our body's arousal, and can therefore alleviate stress. Fallon (2020) discovered that stress interrupts our body's hypothalamic-pituitary-adrenal axis (HPA) and the sympathetic nervous system (SNS). Having both of these systems disrupted leads to increased cortisol in the body. Music can be therapeutically used to counterbalance this disruption. Furthermore, Novotney (2013) discovered how music improves our immune system function in addition to reducing stress. Moreover, Novotney (2013) describes how listening to music can increase our body's antibody of immunoglobulin A. Listening to music can also increase our body's production of our natural killer cells. These particular cells help the body prevent viruses and infections from attacking us. Music reduces inflammatory cytokines in the body. Reducing inflammation in the body may impact our overall well-being. Having a healthy body with a strong immune system helps in aiding stress (Novotney, 2013).

According to Simon (2015), musical tempos that are slow are beneficial to the body's cardiovascular system. Slow music tempos can lower both our heart rate and blood pressure. Slow music can also assist in vasodilation which can help reduce the body's stress. The more consistently music therapy sessions are held, the more consistent the results are. This means that if music is utilized daily, then the benefits of reduced stress are more likely to be sustained over time. Rhythmic music has a plethora of benefits including calmness, relaxation, and feelings of safety.

At this time, autoimmune diseases and chronic illness are currently on the rise. According to Shmerling (2020), stress may be causing autoimmune diseases. Research has found a strong correlation between individuals who had a stress-related disorder and later developed an autoimmune disease. The results showed that individuals who were diagnosed with a stress disorder were more likely to develop an autoimmune disease compared to those who were not diagnosed with one. Shmerling (2020) describes stress as a feeling of tension relating to the physiological, mental, or emotional body. What causes stress for one individual may not cause stress for another (Shmerling, 2020). It is how our particular body perceives and responds to stress. Research suggests there is a significant difference between experiencing stress and having a stress disorder (Shmerling, 2020). Individuals experiencing stress-related disorders may have severe stress, such as post- traumatic stress disorder (PTSD) (Shmerling, 2020). Chronic illnesses are becoming more common today and this is partially due to stress (Shmerling, 2020). Music therapy can be utilized to reduce the severity of stress and to ease tension.

## Stress as Pain

According to Bernatzky et al. (2011), surgery and pain are known to be two of the most physiological stressful occurrences in an individual's life. Surgery and pain can also comprise mental and emotional stressors. This study used self-report on stress and pain for post-surgical patients who used music therapy. Findings suggest that not only did music-based interventions reduce self-reported pain levels, but they also reduced the need for pharmaceutical interventions. This shows that musical interventions can provide less invasive and therapeutic remedies for pain. Bernatzky (2011) concludes that music therapy can also be conducted in combination with other forms of intervention to increase their effectiveness. Music therapy is a relatively newer and effective modality for treating stress and pain. In addition to musical interventions treating pain, they also treat anxiety, sleep, and life quality. Since music therapy is a non- pharmacological and non-invasive form of therapy, it may be used with children. Bernatzky (2011) reports that pharmaceuticals are not widely studied in children, therefore, music interventions would be a safer option. These findings suggest promising effects of music as medicine.

Bradt and colleagues (2016) suggest that a diagnosis of cancer can influence a variety of stressful emotions. Not only is living with cancer physically stressful on the body, but it also is mentally and emotionally taxing. Chemotherapy is a treatment many individuals with cancer receive. Though the treatment may help eliminate the cancer, it takes a toll on the body's strength and immune system. Pharmaceutical interventions can place additional stress on the body, so it is important to discover other treatment modalities and interventions. Music therapy can include listening to music, composing music, playing an instrument, and combining music interventions with other forms of therapy. The findings in this study explain that music therapy is significant in reducing stressful emotions in patients with a cancer diagnosis. More research should be conducted to see if music therapy can reduce stress in patients with other diagnoses and illnesses. The results show that music significantly reduces anxiety in individuals diagnosed with cancer. There is also a strong reduction in depression and fatigue found in the study. Additionally, music-based interventions for cancer patients can reduce the use of anesthetics and analgesics.

Novotney (2013) described a study observing the relationship between music and stress. The study tested if music could aid in soothing patients in the pediatric emergency room. The study included 42 children. The patients were between the ages of 3 and 11. The researchers from the University of Alberta discovered a significance in patients reporting less pain when listening to music while receiving an IV insertion. The patients listening to music during the IV insertion also reported less distress and tension compared to the patients who did not listen to music. Additionally, the health-care workers reported that the IVs were easier to insert on the patients listening to music compared to the patients who did not listen to music. The findings suggest that music significantly reduced stress in pediatric patients, ages 3 to 11.

Novotney (2013) also discovered music can significantly help adult patients, as well. In Singapore, researchers found that patients reported relief from chronic pain when they participated in live music therapy sessions. These patients were engaged in different forms of music-based interventions including singing, playing instruments, and song writing. These modalities helped the patients work through introspection and acceptance, specifically with their health conditions. Music therapy helped give the patients the space and permission for them to accept and feel peace with their chronic pain. By allowing this, music helped reduce their chronic pain levels.

## Cortisol Levels and Music

Hasanah et al. (2020) tested to see if music could reduce cortisol levels. The study included children who were receiving an IV insertion. As stated above in the previous study, an IV insertion for children can cause pain and can increase stress levels. The children who received the IV-line insertion had leukemia, adding still more stress to their bodies. The experiment employed a pre and post-test design to examine cortisol levels via saliva. Music therapy was used by placing headphones on 30 children with leukemia. The researchers used an enzyme-linked immunosorbent assay (ELISA) test to analyze the salivary cortisol levels. The findings suggest that music has an impact on reducing cortisol levels. Music therapy is accessible, easy, and effective compared to other interventions. In the brain, the sound of music alerts the hypothalamus to stimulate the pituitary gland. Then, the pituitary gland releases endorphins into the body. Endorphins are known as the body's natural analgesic, or pain reliever. This study found that music reduces cortisol levels of children receiving an IV insertion. By lowering the body's cortisol levels, children's stress levels decrease. Music helped reduce stress and agitation in the patient (Hasanah et al., 2020).

Fallon et al. (2020) discuss the significance that stress has on the body. Stress disrupts the body's hypothalamic-pituitary-adrenal axis (HPA) along with our nervous system regulation and hormones. Stress specifically raises our body's cortisol by having it become chronically high. Studies suggest that music can help lower these levels. Listening to music is also known to be pleasurable. Pleasure is great for our bodies, especially when it can reduce our body's stress levels. Chronic cortisol levels can increase the body's inflammatory response. Music can lower the body's cortisol levels by decreasing stress. Music and pleasure greatly reduce stress which makes music a great and effective form of therapy. Music, unlike most therapies, is easily accessible. Accessibility is important when discussing therapies and treatments because the most effective therapy is the one that can be easily acquired and utilized.

## The Brain and Music

The brain responds to music in very unique ways. Witte (2020) posits that music activates certain brain areas like the mesolimbic reward system and the amygdala. Both of these processes are involved in emotional activities. Music has a significant impact on the human brain. Music positively affects specific brain systems. This may be due to the certain sounds music emits. Sound healing is well-known throughout the world. The tempo of music can have an impact on relaxation or arousal of the individual. Witte (2020) states that meditative music or music with a slower tempo and rhythm can reduce heart rate. When it does, it allows for an individual to become more relaxed.

Music has neurological effects on the brain, as well. Our brains are wired to distinguish between music and other noises. Simon (2015) concludes that our brain's auditory nerve can send electrical pulses of music to the brain's temporal lobe. In the temporal lobe, there is an area that can perceive the pitch in music. Then, our brain's cerebellum can signal and process the pitch, while the frontal lobe perceives the emotional sectors of sound. Certain musical sounds can stimulate our brain's reward center. This is a similar to stimulation that our brain receives from substances like alcohol, drugs, or chocolate. According to Fallen (2020), the pleasure our brains receive from music is due to a high dopamine release in our brain's striatal reward system. This stimulation and release of pleasure can cause feelings of euphoria by increasing the body's Oxytocin. Oxytocin can be referred to as the body's trust hormone, and promotes feelings of happiness and togetherness.

Novotney (2013) explains that music is a combination of sounds and vibrations. Researchers, including Lee Bartel, Ph.D., a professor of music at the University of Toronto are examining whether musical vibrations can help ease disease symptoms, specifically in depression, Parkinson's disease, and fibromyalgia. This therapy utilizes sounds of low frequency to apply the vibrations to the body. The name of this intervention is called vibroacoustic therapy. Novotney (2013) describes the intervention with patients lying down relaxed on a bed embedded with speakers. The speakers use specific vibrations that are auditory and tactile. The findings of the research show improvement of symptoms, especially in patients with Parkinson's Disease. This research suggests that music offers benefits for easing symptoms in diseases. Relieving a variety of symptoms, it helps the body relax and counterbalance the chronic stress of living with a disease.

According to Novotney (2013), Lee Bartel is also studying the effects of music therapy on patients with Alzheimer's disease. He is using vibroacoustic therapy to see if it can improve communication, especially among certain brain regions. Just after four weeks of treatment, one patient is showing better memory recall. She is able to remember more, including the names of her grandchildren. Improving your memory and communication can aid in relieving stress. Vibroacoustic therapy has significant benefits for relieving symptoms of this very stressful disease.

## Maternal and Infant Stress

Newborns experience stress coming into a new environment. Mothers who have just given birth also experience significant stress after suffering a major physical and emotional life change. Furthermore, preterm infants have the added stress of coming into the world before they are fully developed. Kraft et al., (2021) examine stress on a mother and her preterm infant. In the Neonatal Intensive Care Unit (NICU), infants who are preterm can experience immense amounts of stress, along with their mothers. This study employed music therapy as a modality to alleviate stress levels in both the baby and mother. Some of the results music therapy had on the preterm infant included improving vital signs, neurodevelopment, and movement. Some of the benefits music therapy had on the mother were lowering overall stress levels and increasing mother-child bonding. Anxiety and stress levels are lowered in both child and mother when music therapy is administered.

## Psychological Stress

Simply listening to music can help lift our mood and help us get more in tune with our emotions. It also cues our nervous system to tell us to slow down and to be present. Slower music can help our minds relax and can thereby help alleviate stress. Witte (2020) states that music can help reduce anxious thoughts and restlessness while promoting a happier well-being. Having a peaceful and joyous wellbeing helps our bodies and brains stay grounded. We feel more secure, and become less susceptible to everyday life stressors. When our nervous systems are calm and steady, we are less reactive to life's challenges. This helps humans avoid additional chronic and perceived stress.

Witte (2020) discovered that listening to music lowers stress levels by allowing our minds to temporarily forget about tension-inducing thoughts. Music provides individuals with the mental and emotional space of becoming present and mindful. Mindfulness is important for controlling stress and anxiety. Music is a strong emotional outlet that encourages people to become connected to the present moment. Music, especially slow and meditative forms, gives us the permission to access a mindful state of being. Being mindful creates an internal environment of introspection and restoration. Both of these states allow the body to release emotional and physical tension. According to Fallon (2020), music can alter our moods by increasing relaxation and decreasing anxiety. By increasing rest and reducing tension, our bodies can come closer to homeostasis.

Additionally, as aforementioned, Witte (2020) explains that music can help the body release specific neurotransmitters, such as oxytocin and endorphins. By releasing these neurotransmitters, our body's feel connection, safety, and trust. When we feel safe, our body's stress system naturally relaxes. Experiencing feelings of togetherness and community are vital for our health. As stated earlier, stress is a gateway to many serious medical conditions. Stress is debilitating. Having ways to modulate and regulate stress is important for both our current states and longevity.

Fallen (2020) explains that music can help express a plethora of emotions depending on how the listener perceives it. Different types of music can create different feelings. For instance, slow music may be calming and upbeat music can be energizing. Also, music may be interpreted differently by different individuals. We are all individuals, who perceive stimuli differently. Music that helps one person, may not help another. Additionally, individuals may experience different emotions listening to the same music. Meditative music may help person A become more relaxed, and may help person B become happier. This is why in some studies participants are encouraged to select the music of their choice. Additionally, this is another advantage of music itself being so accessible. Most people have the ability to listen to music of their own choice and can select certain types that allow them to experience the feelings they crave.

Morinville et al. (2013) concluded that music can provide feelings of happiness and global happiness. Joy and happiness are known to reduce feelings of anxiousness and stress. Happiness promotes wellbeing, and can counteract negative feelings. The presence of negative feelings is important to recognize and acknowledge when dealing with stress. Morinville (2013) focused their research on adolescence. Morinville (2013) states that music is both pleasurable and energizing for adolescents. Music may increase pleasure in creative activities that adolescents take part in. Moreover, the researcher suggested that music could provide a happy state of mind. Pleasure is an experience most humans crave. Even neurotransmitters like dopamine crave the feeling of pleasure. Morinville's (2013) study on adolescence assessed whether or not music could add artistic and creative qualities to their lives. This study examined the benefits of music on global well-being and subjective well-being. This study used a self- determination model that compared music listening to subjective well-being. The benefits suggest that listening to music is positively correlated with higher levels of well-being in adolescence. People, specifically adolescents, are happier when listening to music they choose. If music can provide this, it will then aid in releasing our happy, feel good neurotransmitters. Music can be used medicinally for this reason. Stress hinders our quality of life, which is why counteracting it is vital to our wellbeing.

## Emotional Stress

It is common to experience mental and emotional stress. Many individuals journal, meditate, or partake in daily exercise to help combat these unwanted stressors. In research by Bernatzky (2011), patients reported a reduction in pain receptors when listening to music. This study tested if music can reduce self-reported pain levels. Additionally, research suggested that music specifically selected by the patient has more consistent positive benefits for reducing self-reported pain levels. The study discussed how music has an extensive history of alleviating pain in the medical world. It has been utilized in many cultures in the past to regulate painful emotions and physical pain. We do not yet fully recognize how many facets of stress music can help. Research shows that music helps regulate emotions through its neurophysiological effects. Specifically, musical interventions can counterbalance negative feelings associated with stress. Music also helped alleviate the common feeling of helplessness for patients in the hospital.

Music can be utilized to soothe the emotional body and teach us to self-soothe. Bernatzky (2011) concluded that music stimulates the socioemotional systems of the body. By stimulating our socioemotional bodily systems, our moods lift and we experience health benefits. Music is used universally, which is why it can easily be dismissed as a potent medical treatment. According to Bernatzky (2011), music therapy has a great effect on our emotional body because it releases oxytocin and endogenous opiates. Having the ability to self-soothe with music is a wonderful therapeutic and readily accessible tool for healing stress and other emotional ailments.

## DISCUSSION

Music is used universally in gyms, restaurants, and films. Most art forms, like music, are seen as healing. The creative arts are becoming more widely used and studied. The creative art therapies are more accessible than other modalities, such as pharmaceuticals. Because of music's impact on our brain and nervous system, it is known to be an effective treatment. Music can reduce stress in clinical and therapeutic settings, and also in recreational settings. Unlike other medical interventions, music is easily accessible. It is usually free to listen to and to stream online.

Music-based interventions can be designed and performed in several different ways. This includes listening to pre-recorded music, listening to live music, playing an instrument, composing music, improvising, and coupling music with other forms of therapy. All of these forms of music-based interventions are effective in reducing stress and other ailments. More research on music as medicine will result in the medical community accepting and advocating for this innovative form of therapy. Creative art therapies are effective because they touch us deeply in our bodies, brains, emotions, and spirits. Music therapy also poses little to no risk for the individual receiving it, unlike other medical interventions.

It would be helpful to see further research on music-based interventions on individuals with chronic stress. Since chronic stress is very prevalent today, this research would be beneficial to the vast majority of the public. Connolly (2019) states that people today are suffering from panic attacks and anxiety. We also tend to neglect how much of an impact stress has on our physical bodies and brain. Symptoms, such as fatigue and brain fog, are often overlooked in relation to stress.

## CONCLUSION

Stress adversely impacts the majority of individuals. Having healthy, non-invasive, and accessible ways to reduce our stress levels is key to a healthier society. Chronic stress can affect all ages and demographics of society, especially women. Music is a form of therapy that can be utilized to alleviate various stressors. Music therapy has significant benefits for pain, emotional stress, chronic stress, birth stress, and physical stress. Both acute and chronic stress can decrease with music-based interventions.

Future research can more comprehensively examine the efficacy of music therapy for reducing emotional stress. Anxiety, depression, addiction, and eating disorders are areas that may be effectively addressed with studies on music therapy. Pairing music therapy with talk therapy may be particularly beneficial for patients with various mental health disorders. Additionally, further research can include more pre and post-test designs. These will be helpful to see the immediate effectiveness of music on stress. Longitudinal studies will be helpful to observe the long-term effects of music for stress reduction. More research will aid in making musical interventions more popular and more accessible. Music therapy should serve as a common go-to for treating stress, especially in medical settings. Additionally, research can examine the effect of music-based interventions on symptom management. Managing symptoms of illnesses can be a significant source of stress and distress in the body. Utilizing music therapy to further address this stress can be a key area for future research.

As aforementioned, music can be an important part of the healing process. Besides reducing stress, music is known to help improve sleep and to increase energy levels. Music therapy is relatively new compared to other non-pharmaceutical therapies and treatments. More research on music therapy could be beneficial to the public in a variety of ways. This may also encourage more individuals to become certified as music therapists and to make music more accessible in various clinical settings. Unlike pharmaceuticals, using music-based interventions over the long-term could be helpful therapeutically, without leading to side-effects or additional health concerns.

## REFERENCES

Aalbers, S., Fusar-Poli, L., Freeman, R. E., Spreen, M., Ket, J. C., Vink, A. C., Maratos, A., Crawford, M., Chen, X. J., & Gold, C. (2017). Music therapy for depression. *Cochrane Database of Systematic Reviews*, *11*(11), CD004517. Advance online publication. doi:10.1002/14651858.CD004517.pub3 PMID:29144545

Bernatzky, G., Presch, M., Anderson, M., & Panksepp, J. (2011). Emotional foundations of music as a non-pharmacological pain management tool in modern medicine. *Neuroscience and Biobehavioral Reviews*, *35*(9), 1989–1999. doi:10.1016/j.neubiorev.2011.06.005 PMID:21704068

Bradt, J., Dileo, C., Magill, L., & Teague, A. (2016). Music interventions for improving psychological and physical outcomes in cancer patients. *Cochrane Database of Systematic Reviews*, (8), CD006911. Advance online publication. doi:10.1002/14651858.CD006911.pub3 PMID:27524661

Brown, B. (2010). *Gifts of imperfection, the*. Hazelden Information & Educational Services.

Connolly, M., & Slade, M. (2019). The united states of stress 2019. *Everyday Health,* https://www.everydayhealth.com/wellness/united-states-of-stress/

Delta. (2015). *Stressed and Exhausted? Tired and Wired?* FxMed Centers. https://fxmedcenters.com/2015/07/27/stressed-and-exhausted-tired-and-wired/

Fallon, V. T., Rubenstein, S., Warfield, R., Ennerfelt, H., Hearn, B., & Leaver, E. (2020). Stress reduction from a musical intervention. *Psychomusicology: Music, Mind, and Brain, 30*(1), 20–27. doi:10.1037/pmu0000246

Hasanah, I., Mulatsih, S., Haryanti, F., & Haikal, Z. Effect of music therapy on cortisol as a stress biomarker in children undergoing IV-line insertion. *Journal of Taibah University Medical Sciences, 15*(3), 238-243. https://www.sciencedirect.com/science/article/pii/S1658361220300421

Kandarakis, E., Bourguignon, J., Giudice, L., Hauser, R., Prins, G., Soto, A., Zoeller, R. T., & Gore, A. (2009). Endocrine-disrupting chemicals: an endocrine society scientific statement. *National Library of Medicine, 30*(4), 293-342, https://www.ncbi.nlm.nih.gov/pmc/articles/PMC2726844/

Kraft, K. E., Jaschke, A. C., Ravensbergen, A. G., Feenstra-Weelink, A., van Goor, M., de Kroon, M., Reijneveld, S. A., Bos, A. F., & van Dokkum, N. H. (2021). Maternal anxiety, infant stress, and the role of live-performed music therapy during NICU stay in the Netherlands. *International Journal of Environmental Research and Public Health, 18*(13), 7077. doi:10.3390/ijerph18137077 PMID:34281014

Morinville, A., Miranda, D., & Gaudreau, P. (2013). Music listening motivation is associated with global happiness in Canadian late adolescents. *Psychology of Aesthetics, Creativity, and the Arts, 7*(4), 384–390. doi:10.1037/a0034495

Novotney, A. (2013). Music as medicine. *American Psychological Association, 44*(10), 46. https://www.apa.org/monitor/2013/11/music

Shmerling, R. H. (2020). *Autoimmune diseases and stress: is there a link?* Harvard Health Publishing. https://www.health.harvard.edu/blog/autoimmune-disease-and-stress-is-there-a-link-2018071114230

Simon, B. H. (2015). Music as medicine. *The American Journal of Medicine, 128*(2), 208–210. doi:10.1016/j.amjmed.2014.10.023 PMID:25448175

Stewart, A., Kathawalla, U., Wolfe, A., & Everson-Rose, S. (2018). Women's heart health at mid-life: what is the role of psychosocial stress. *National Library of Medicine, 4*(11). https://www.ncbi.nlm.nih.gov/pmc/articles/PMC6297972/

Witte, M. D., Pinho, A., Stams, G. J., Moonen, X., Bos, A. E. R., & van Hooren, S. (2020). Music therapy for stress reduction: A systematic review and meta-analysis. *Health Psychology Review, 16*(1), 134–159. https://www.tandfonline.com/doi/full/10.1080/17437199.2020.1846580

## KEY TERMS AND DEFINITIONS

**Autoimmune Disease:** A disease in which the body's immune system attacks healthy cells.

**Cerebellum:** The part of the brain at the back of the skull in vertebrates. Its function is to coordinate and regulate muscular activity.

**Circadian Rhythm:** The natural cycle of physical, mental, and behavior changes that the body goes through in a 24-hour cycle.

**Cortisol:** The body's main stress hormone.

**Endorphins:** Any of a group of hormones secreted within the brain and nervous system and having a number of physiological functions. They are peptides which activate the body's opiate receptors, causing an analgesic effect.

**Homeostasis:** Homeostasis is the state of steady internal, physical, and chemical conditions maintained by living systems. This is the condition of optimal functioning for the organism and includes many variables, such as body temperature and fluid balance.

**Hypothalamic:** Pituitary-adrenal axis (HPA). The HPA axis is a term used to represent the interaction between the hypothalamus, pituitary gland, and adrenal glands; it plays an important role in the stress response.

**Oxytocin:** Oxytocin triggers feelings of love and protection, which naturally occurs when parents and children look into one another's eyes or when they embrace. Other relationship-enhancing effects also include empathy, trust, and the processing of bonding cues.

# Chapter 12
# The Creative Arts and Its Impact on Foster Children Within Their Critical Developmental Years

**Kayleen Cabrera**
*Marymount Manhattan College, USA*

**Nava R. Silton**
*Marymount Manhattan College, USA*

## ABSTRACT

*A child being put into the foster care system comes with various trials. This begins with the foster child's original household dynamic either consisting of neglect or ill-treatment. Other cases being a parent who may not have the capacity to raise the child. To contextualize the creative arts and how they may benefit foster children, this review uses research collected from previous literature to examine prevalence rates, a child's needs, at-risk youth, how the brain reacts to the creation of art, music therapy, and its effects on foster youth, including after-school programs and support that is provided to children that implement the use of creative arts. Significant findings were compiled about the arts activating parts of the brain, consistently stimulating the same three neurotransmitters (oxytocin, serotonin, and dopamine). Furthermore, the implementation of the arts in foster children's lives can reverse social and developmental delays they may have encountered as a result of trauma.*

DOI: 10.4018/978-1-6684-7856-1.ch012

## INTRODUCTION

The foster care system has had a notorious reputation of infrastructures being overcrowded; the ratio of children to attend to versus the number of workers available strikingly differ. This leads to the exhaustion of workers and overlooked children (Clausen et al., 2012). This can contribute to the desensitization of individuals leaving a child's life without proper notice. Further abandonment issues encountered by foster youth can lead to instability of future relationships (Clausen et al., 2012). Foster children are a very high-risk population, many encountering abuse, mistreatment, rape, mental illness, lack of medical care, etc. Foster youth are placed into situations where they must grow up quicker than others due to a large sense of independence at an age range where children are not typically able to defend themselves in society. Having a lack of individuals to look up to in their lives, inner-city foster youth have often looked up to music artists as role models due to the consistency music can have in one's life, contrary to what this demographic may be used to (Camilleri, 2007, chapter 8, p. 94). There is a large inconsistency in quantitative data collection in the foster care system due to data not being reported or offered to the public, with the statistics being disclosed within seven to sixteen-year increments (Roehrkasse, 2021). This begs the question of whether this population will continue to receive the services they need and if policies will be set into place to assist this demographic.

### Breakdown of the Foster Care System

In the year 2018, around 437,000 children were in foster care with 263,000 of those children entering the system that year. Twenty-four percent of children came from ill-treated and negligent homes while 16% had been victims of physical abuse (Child welfare outcomes 2018, 2021). A list of outcomes was used to measure the effectiveness and overall assistance that was offered to children in foster care nationally in 2018, statistically, this list consisted of:

- **Outcome 1:** Reduce recurrence of child abuse and/or neglect.
    - Regarding state performance, the percentage of child victims experiencing a recurrence of child maltreatment within a 6-month period was 5.5 percent. Nationally, child maltreatment declined between 2014 and 2018 (Child Welfare outcomes 2018, 2021).
- **Outcome 2:** Reduce the incidence of child abuse and/or neglect in foster care.
    - Regarding national median performance, the maltreatment of children in foster care was 0.26 percent and a range from 0.00 percent to 1.8

    - percent…The maltreatment of children in foster care was 0.26 percent in both 2014 and 2018 (Child welfare outcomes 2018, 2021).

- **Outcome 3:** Increase permanency for children in foster care.
    - States were mostly successful in achieving permanency (I.e., discharged to reunification, adoption, or legal guardianship) for all children leaving foster care with a median performance of 90.3 percent…less success in achieving permanency for children who had a diagnosed disability and children who entered care when they were older than 12 (Child welfare outcomes 2018, 2021).
- **Outcome 4:** Reduce time in foster care due to reunification without increasing reentry.
    - In 43 states (84 percent), at least half of reunifications occurred within 12 months from the time of entry into foster care…National performance over time has declined consistently over the past five years, showing an overall decrease of 7.8 percent since 2014…Of all children who entered foster care during 2018, a median of 7.1 percent had re-entered care within 12 months (Child welfare outcomes 2018, 2021).
- **Outcome 5:** Reduced time in foster care to adoption.
    - States continued to struggle with achieving timely adoptions in 2018, with a median of 2.7 percent of children discharged to a final adoption within 12 months of the latest removal (Child welfare outcomes 2018, 2021).
- **Outcome 6:** Increase placement stability.
    - In 2018, the majority of children in foster care for fewer than 12 months achieved placement stability (i.e., having had two or fewer placement settings in a single foster care episode), with a median performance of 83.5 percent…States were less successful in achieving placement stability the longer a child spent in foster care (Child welfare outcomes 2018, 2021).
- **Outcome 7:** Reduce placement of young children in group homes or institutions.
    - For half the states (50 percent), 3.1 percent or less of children entering foster care below the age of 12 were placed in group homes or institutions in 2018 (Child welfare outcomes 2018, 2021).

The demographics of children waiting to be adopted in 2017 were also recorded, with males (52%), females (48%), White (44%), Hispanic Origin (22%), and Black or African American (22%). Males were adopted less frequently than their female counterparts. White children were the largest demographic in foster care, children of

Hispanic origin (any race) were the second largest demographic, and Black/African American children were the third largest demographic in foster care.

Approximately 700,000 children in the U.S. are separated from their families due to issues such as neglect (62%), parent substance abuse (36%), parents' inability to cope with parenting (14%), or physical abuse (13%) (U.S. Department of Health & Human Services, 2020 as cited by Font & Gershoff, 2020). In various cases, children placed into the foster care system may suffer from a continuation of neglect, sent from home to home, and could go into late adolescence without being adopted into a legal family. In contrast, some foster children could find a healthy permanent home either through kinship (a blood relative) or through a non-kinship placement (unrelated adoptive parent). Some may even be able to be reunify with their original families (Font & Gershoff, 2020). Children accepted to live with a foster parent through kinship reduces behavioral issues, decreasing chances of mental health disorders such as Depression, Anxiety, etc. Being placed with a foster parent through kinship also reduces the chance that the child will be placed back into the foster care system (Jacobsen et al., 2020). With physical and mental health needs, children need a caregiver or a parent figure to protect them from harm and to ensure stability. Children in foster care are eligible for Medicaid to help them receive the health services they need. The downside of this coverage is that many providers do not accept patients who rely on Medicaid, which can result in neglect for mental and physical health concerns (Font & Gershoff. 2020).

Long-term maltreatment and abuse can take a toll on both the cardiovascular system and immune system (Bakema et al., 2020; Do Prado et al., 2017 as cited by Font & Gershoff, 2020), with psychological issues, including, difficulty learning, brain damage, and low self-esteem. These complications can influence substance abuse (Child Welfare Information Gateway, 2017). The effects of child abuse can consist of disruptive, disorganized, and unstable characteristics (Clausen et al., 2012). The foster care system differs in rules and regulations within the U.S. on a state-by-state basis. A state has the right to remove a child from a household that has been reported as unsafe or if the child is in a life-threatening or dangerous situation (Font & Gershoff, 2020). Federal policy establishes rules to ensure that prospective foster parents undergo a criminal and child maltreatment background check. However, if a child is unsuccessful in receiving a permanent home, states can offer to fund children who have aged out of the system (Font & Gershoff, 2020).

## At-Risk Youth

There is an issue of overpopulation and lack of resources in large cities such as New York, Washington D.C., Chicago, and Los Angeles. There can be a range of violence, poverty, exclusion, and trauma with poor health service coverage

(Camilleri, 2007, pp. 15-16). Living in these environments can have effects on the development, mental, and physical well-being of inner-city youth. Approximately 30% of residents in these cities are youth under the age of 19 as noted by Camilleri (2007, p.16). There have been concerns about foster care and the correlation to racial disparities between Native American and Black children within the system. Some even connect these two populations in a historical context to the separation of children and families during the time of the Indian Removal Act of 1830 and slavery with the exclusion of children from underprivileged races from protective services (Font & Gershoff, 2020).

Foster children are at risk for developing problems in social and emotional functioning. Possibly due to prior neglect and the abuse they may have encountered from a caregiver(s) which may relate to the challenge for some children of remaining in permanent homes (Jacobsen et al., 2020). Inner-city youth within foster care are more susceptible to continued abandonment issues, community violence, and financial instability (Camilleri, 2007, p. 93). These children are especially disadvantaged if they were never taken into a permanent home, were switched from one foster parent to another, did not have a family that could help pay for the continuance of their education and/or did not have a parent figure who was there to listen and guide them. Foster children in these situations may become more violent and may perform poorly in school. Certain groups of children fall victim to negligence and abuse more than others within the United States, girls at a rate of 9.6 per 1,000 others and boys 8.7 out of 1,000. Native American children fall within 5.2 per 1,000 and African American children at a rate of14.0 out of 1,000 (Child welfare outcomes 2018, 2021, p. 81).

## A Child's Needs

Undoubtedly, children within foster care do not always have their needs met, whether it be on an emotional, psychological, or physiological level. The Center for Disease Control and Prevention (CDC, 2021) presents milestones and basic expectations for the early stages of development, such as the healthy development of a growing child and effective parenting styles. The components that assist in healthy development are allowing a child to have the space to sing, dance, play, communicate, with the upkeep of their education, emotional support, and health needs (CDC, 2021). Parenting styles may look different for everybody. The factors that should be consistent in raising a healthy child are empathy and compassion, setting routines and household rules, promoting safety and wellness, using appropriate discipline without being harsh, and having a consistent parenting style.

Foster children tend to have a history of trauma and ill-treatment, resulting in placement difficulties. This includes feelings of loneliness and abandonment (Steenbakkers et al., 2018). If proper care and attention are given to these children who have been misplaced, it can provide further opportunities for bright, healthy futures with stable family placement (Steenbakkers et al, 2018). Maslow's Hierarchy of Needs (Maslow, 1943) identifies the necessities for a human, which help them develop and grow. At the very base of his pyramid are physiological needs (food, water, etc.). As you move up the pyramid, you see that a human has safety needs (resources, health, and wellness), then needs for love and belonging (relationships, friendships), then esteem needs (feeling accomplished, confidence, self-esteem), and finally needs for self-actualization (problem-solving, morality) (Mcleod, 2018). A child separating from his/her biological parents can cause a rift in the child's development and attachment style. Children may feel alienated from their biological family and may be forced to build a relationship with a new adoptive family (Steenbakkers et al., 2018).

Due to the foster child's need for a secure attachment, a foster caretaker must show the foster child that he/she is in a secure household with a trustworthy caregiver. There are four attachment styles that can describe a potential attachment of an individual who has experienced different child-rearing styles (Bowlby, 1969). These styles of attachment present themselves as secure attachment (a caregiver who provides security to a child and the child does not have a fear of abandonment), ambivalent attachment (children both pull toward and push away the caregiver), avoidant attachment (caregiver only provides necessities but no emotional support, which leads the child to avoid their feelings and thoughts to prevent conflict), and disorganized attachment (caregiver constantly fails to provide for the child, causing a child to have trust issues, fear of abandonment, avoiding closeness with others, etc.) (Huang, 2020; Bowlby, 1969).

Offering children an opportunity to develop relationships with other children, family members and professionals can help provide them with a sense of permanency. In addition, it can help children develop social interaction and communication skills. Steenbakkers et al.'s (2018) systematic review of literature on foster children's needs suggests that a foster parent who can fulfill a child's need to belong, may parallel assistance in the management of a foster child's behavior and emotions. This can be observed though actively listening to the child's past experiences, assisting them in establishing regular contact with biological relatives such as siblings, nurturing and even assisting with grooming and hair care such as braiding an African American child's hair, etc. (Steenbakkers et al., 2018). Fulfilling these needs can lead to a safe, loving, and welcoming environment where positive social cues are in place. Steenbakkers et al. (2018) further discuss physiological and self-actualization needs. The physiological needs consist of an understanding and sensitive parenting style, being attentive to what may trigger the child and how their traumas have affected them. When these characteristics are present in an adoptive parent, it can reduce signs of depression in a child (Stoner et al., 2015 as cited by Steenbakkers et al.,

2018). Self-actualization needs include support in schooling and encouragement in continuing education, with providing a consistent school experience (not constantly transferring a child from school to school) (Hudson 2013; Mendis et al. 2015; Quest et al. 2012).

Due to early inadequate parenting and neglect, the needs expressed in Maslow's hierarchy of needs tend to not be addressed. This leads to a child encountering a lack of emotional, financial, and social support following their adolescent years. With a hard time accepting emotions, a foster child's ego may be easily overcome by sexual and violent energy starting from the early adolescent years. This may drive an adolescent to act out their feelings in self-destructive ways due to their lack of restraint and self-expression (Berkovitz 1995 as cited by Camilleri, 2007, p. 94). Foster children in their teenage years may have a harder time trusting others and building relationships; frequently experiencing significant bouts of anger, anxiety, and sadness. At times, they may wonder whether they are to blame for their own predicament and this fear coupled with an unstable living environment can elevate their feelings of abandonment and hopelessness (Berkovitz 1995; Herman 1992 as cited by Camilleri, 2007, p. 94). Being placed into a secure and nurturing home can reverse the damage of abandonment, alongside difficulties in schooling, and depression among other things, since the needs of a foster child are unique and tend to differ on a case-by-case basis (Steenbakkers et al, 2018).

When a foster child is placed into a new home, the child may encounter internalizing and externalizing problems which could cause stress to the legal guardians. Internalizing problems include: anxiety, depression, disordered eating, etc. External problems may manifest as behavioral issues, hostility, or antisocial behavior. Foster children often encounter damaged attachment styles through neglect and abuse from their original caregivers. On the other hand, the child may have had a healthy relationship with their biological parent, but the parent could no longer take care of them, which still leads to a broken family with a threatened attachment (Goemans et al., 2018). Goemans et al. (2018) investigate the connection between foster children's internalizing and externalizing behaviors to the stress of adoptive parents. The training offered before becoming a foster parent provides the tools of how to handle the stressors of taking care of foster youth. In Goemans et al. (2018) study, it was found that those who had been trained would not take out their stress or anger on the child. The parents exercised self-control and did not add another burden of trauma onto their foster child. While foster parents' stress may not have a direct correlation to foster children's internal and external problems, a biological parent's stress can show adverse effects on child development (Baker et al., 2003 as cited by Goemans, 2018).

Moreover, Jacobsen et al. (2020) discuss how externalizing behaviors can cause disruptions in placement with foster children encountering behavioral problems by the age of eight. A study on Norwegian foster children and their socioemotional functioning was tested by Jacobsen et al., (2020) to see how emotional difficulties discovered during toddlerhood can correspond with behavioral patterns in 8-year-old foster youth. Moreover, Jacobsen et al. (2020) suggest that the earlier behavioral problems are identified, the better chance a child may have of receiving support and assistance. Children often require caregivers to guide them on how to be emotionally stable. Early detection and resolution of emotional instability offers a higher acceptance rate for placement permanency (Jacobsen et al., 2020). The study had shown results of foster children indeed having unstable emotions including behavioral issues, compared to the results of the average 8-year-old population. Training and guidance for foster parents to help manage their mental health was also suggested as a tactic to reduce behavioral problems within this demographic (Jacobsen et al. 2020).

## The Modes of Creative Art Therapies

The creative arts are useful in a multitude of ways to provide an avenue for individuals to communicate in ways they may have not attempted before. Through creative arts (CA) therapies, patients can analyze their emotions and experiences outside of verbalization, utilizing artistic cues as a form of self-expression. Creative arts also offer children the opportunity to be heard, stand out, and be loud in a world where they're consistently shut out (Bannister, 2003, p. 48). Creative practices have been recognized throughout history for their healing properties; bringing people together through music, rituals, dance, storytelling, art, etc. (Bannister, 2003, p. 41). There are multiple modalities within the creative arts sector, including dance therapy, drama therapy, music therapy, art therapy, play therapy, etc. With a diverse range of settings, creative art therapists can work in education, hospitals, mental health facilities, private practice, prisons, and can even hold a variety of specializations and certifications (Shafir et al., 2020).

### Dance and Movement Therapy (DMT)

Dance Movement Therapy (DMT) has been shown to assist patients in learning about self-preservation and stability, which has been attributed to innovative learning techniques provided by the creative arts. Certain movements in dance therapy were designed to pull emotions out of participants, embodying the feelings, thoughts, and experiences that patients may have a hard time verbally expressing. DMT has assisted in the improvement of mental health by reducing anxiety and depression. Thus, providing a better quality of life with an increase in social and cognitive functioning (Shafir et al., 2020).

## Drama Therapy

Another mode of Creative Arts Therapies, drama therapy also known as psychodrama has been used across many demographics, in helping translate what one may want to express to another through openness in therapy sessions (Shafir et al., 2020). Drama therapy can assume the role of spontaneously acting out one's emotions and experiences, including the use of mirroring (one imitating another), soliloquy (thoughts or sayings addressed to self), and doubling (mediator speaking between two conflicting parties to assist in understanding one another). Identity is normally developed with the help of a mother or primary caregiver starting from ages two to three. If the relationship with the caregiver/mother is severed or halted by traumatic experiences, the identity of the child becomes threatened (Bannister, 2003, p. 44). Psychodrama has introduced healing and regrowth for children who have encountered these experiences; helping them slowly repair their sense of self and identity (Bannister, 2003, p.4 4). Individuals who have used drama therapy as their therapy of choice have seen its effects in providing relief from stress and loneliness, emphasizing empathy, relatability, and support for others (Shafir et al., 2020). Drama therapy has the benefit of improving self-actualization like dance movement therapy, enhancing a sense of self and life, and assisting in coping with sorrow and grief.

## Music Therapy

The third Creative Arts Therapy modality, music therapy, has been found to aid groups with neurological disabilities through songwriting programs. These programs assist in the development of a sense of self and identity (Shafir et al. 2020). Through practices of music therapy, participants display resilience and a break away from previous trauma, developing healthy coping strategies, and developing a new perspective on the world. Music therapy has also been shown to enhance one's purpose in life, boosting confidence with feeling more socially accepted (Shafir et al., 2020).

## Art Therapy

The fourth mode of Creative Arts Therapies, art therapy, has been helpful in the development of parent-child relationships and interpersonal skills using self-expression. Art therapy has helped individuals in their personal and professional growth cope with stressors and perceptions of self. Art therapy has also been able to contribute to the analysis of where an individual's headspace may be. For instance, activities such as drawing a "person picking an apple from a tree" given to children with and without special needs can help showcase a child's views of their parental figures and the way they're treated at home (Shafir et al., 2020). The creative arts are needed to locate new and innovative ways for therapists and clients to build relationships and connect with a client beyond the verbal level.

## Play Therapy

Play therapy has also been effective for foster youth and children alike and has been considered to be less of an abstract form of therapy. Play therapy has helped young children stabilize their emotions, with the ability to practice role-playing, develop innovative problem-solving skills, and the chance to express their interests (Landreth, 2002 as cited by Clausen et al., 2012). Clausen et al. (2012) delved into the topic of play therapy and its effect on foster children, examining the way older foster youth express themselves on a verbal level compared to younger foster youth who are more expressive and less verbal. An example of children demonstrating their fear of abandonment can surface through play therapy, an older foster child may say "I want to talk about why I worry so much about people leaving me" while a younger foster child may use hide-and-seek, to convey a similar message (Clausen et al., 2012). Play therapy can heal a child from trauma, providing children with a nurturing form of therapy, self-expression, and self-awareness. Long-term therapy is effective for foster youth primarily due to this population's feelings of rejection or little to no one having truly taken the time to get to know them due to transient individuals in their lives, whether it be social workers, being transferred from home to home, and their biological family being unable to take care of them (Clausen et al., 2012). Through the incorporation of long-term therapy, foster youth have the opportunity to address repressed or unconscious emotions, alongside past trauma that they had encountered and never felt comfortable discussing. This form of trauma has the possibility of impacting their self-image and views of the world (Clausen et al., 2012). Within the study, Clausen et al. (2012) had a sample of predominantly male participants, in the 70th percentile, a culmination of 30% of various races, 35% Black/African American, and 30% white between the ages of 5-10 years at the beginning of the study. An individual therapist was assigned to each foster child for approximately three years. Significance was found in the improvement of participant relationships, with a decrease in anxiety, violence, depression, and dissociation alongside improvement in sleep and educational experiences. These outcomes showed that long-term therapy assists in learning to develop functional and stable relationships, which greatly benefits foster youth. These findings suggest that the development of a secure and impactful relationship can reduce the chances of a child experiencing a challenging future (Clausen et al., 2012).

## Music Therapy and Its Effects on Adolescents in Foster Care

Music therapy had been utilized by Camilleri (2007, pp. 92-103) while working with a group of adolescent foster children from Brooklyn at Turtle Bay Music School, located in New York City in the years 1991-2004. During the adolescent years, identity and self-image are continuously questioned, and changes are evident in cognitive, physiological, social, and psychological development (Camilleri, 2007, p. 93). These changes in the self are amplified in a foster child when he/she is thrust into early independence, having adverse effects on their development. Music is an influential and effective way to assist teens in their stages of development because rhythm and sound can be seen as a constant in most people's lives; a song has the potential to connect to one's memories. Music is also able to fill the void of an inconsistent caregiver, being able to reveal the way a child feels about him or herself and the world (Camilleri, 2007, p. 94). The goal for these specific children was to provide a mechanism to learn how to work cohesively in a group, boost self-esteem, confidence, and self-expression. Due to the skepticism that African American and Latino communities have about therapy, the music therapy sessions were offered under the guise of being purely music lessons.

There were challenges to encouraging teens to participate since adolescents do not always want to follow rules or listen to an individual who they cannot identify with, race-wise. This age group tends to have a fear of rejection by peers, opening up or allowing oneself to be vulnerable regarding private matters can be challenging. Some would especially find it difficult since many did not ever have a safe person to confide in about personal matters (Austin & Dvorkin, 1993; Milman & Goldman, 1987 as cited by Camilleri, 2007, p. 96). The kids were instructed to create their own rules, and what these rules would look like to prevent power struggles between one another. Their rules were often stricter than the facilitator's own rules, Camilleri (2007, p. 98), since they disallowed cursing, spitting, or being rude to one another. It was inferred that their rules reflected the make-up of mistreated and neglected children (Blos, 1962 as cited by Camilleri, 2007, p. 98). Four months later, Camilleri (2007, p. 97) observed the children weaving multiple parts of their personalities together; not fearing how the group would think of them, accepting parts of themselves that they had repressed. The girls within the group would bring in CDs containing songs that resonated with their plight. All but one girl in the therapy group, had encountered sexual abuse where it was then suggested that a group poem was to be created. Every participant wrote one to two lines about their feelings towards sexual assault. This helped in opening the group up to reducing any feelings of alienation and the lack of trust in people and their surroundings; these emotions resonated most within this demographic (Camilleri, 2007, p. 99). Through Turtle Bay's music therapy program, many youth groups were able to leave celebrating the positive impact the program had on their development; providing a sense of community and trust during a coming-of-age time frame for them (Camilleri, 2007, p. 103).

## The Creative Arts and Its Effects on the Brain

At times, complex issues require complex solutions. Creative thinking through the arts can help demographics such as children by opening them up to diverse forms of critical thinking, aiding them in contextualizing thoughts, ideas, and communication. With fallacies being spread by the media about the brain, Dow and Kozlowski (2020) delve into the misconceptions of the right and left hemispheres taking hold of specific functions of an individual. For instance, the right brain being in control of both creative and artistic functions and the left brain dominating mathematical and scientific capabilities. When the right and left brain interchangeably control the functions of an individual, the brain can work together as one. When an individual is executing a creative work, picturing a situation, or solving a problem, brain function/movement has been found through procedures such as Functional Magnetic Resonance Imaging (fMRI) and Positron Emission Tomography (PET scan). These procedures can identify blood flow to areas of the brain when performing these tasks, demonstrating how pervasive creative assignments can be to the brain. Other tests such as Electroencephalograms (EEG) use a method that measures the electrical impulses of brain wave patterns using tiny, innocuous electrodes fastened to the scalp using gel and tape, have also found brain activity throughout creative tasks.

Brain studies bring new findings, three parts of the brain are activated when participating in a creative activity. These three networks include: *The Salience Network, the Imagination Network,* and the *Central Executive Network* (Beaty et al., 2015; Koontz, 2019 as cited in Dow & Kozlowski, 2020). Dow and Kozlowski (2020) go into the three networks, the *Imagination Network* stimulates the occipital lobe, parietal lobe, and prefrontal cortex. These parts of the brain have a function in the way children connect to individuals and can feel empathy for others, coupled with the ability to produce ideas and daydream. The *Central Executive Network* ties into the parietal lobe like the Imagination Network and the frontal lobe, assisting in finding solutions to problems and helping kids in being able to focus and make decisions concerning difficult tasks. Authors Dow and Kozlowski (2020) then recall the final network, the *Salience Network*, combining the Imagination and Central Executive Networks, helping filter out information that may not be needed to fulfill a task, and using the frontal and temporal lobes to execute this. All three networks need to work together to ensure the solution to a situation or a creative thought process (Dow & Kozlowski, 2020). Additionally, neurotransmitters normally deemed happy hormones such as oxytocin, serotonin, and dopamine are present when participating in the creative arts through group activities, imaginative thinking, and the generation of thoughts and ideas. It has been found that Dance and Movement Therapy (DMT) can depict a client's emotions by mirror neurons being activated during the process of moving (Shafir et al., 2020). Dow and Kozlowski (2020) note that the neurotransmitter, cortisol which normally relates to the fight or flight response and increased stress levels can create stagnation in the creative process, stunting concentration and causing irritability. Dow and Kozlowski (2020) conclude by affirming the belief that through creative and interactive teaching using group assignments, where a potential award is given, can assist in helping children learn from mistakes and find creative solutions in the process.

## Creative Arts, After-School, and Support for Youth

The National Conference of State Legislatures (NCSL, 2022) shared that schooling takes a large portion of a child's early and adolescent years, and the incorporation of extra-curricular activities such as community-based support and after-school programs can further assist in a child's development. NCSL (2022) noted that programs offered to kids assist them in forging relationships outside of schooling, mentorship, academic assistance, and more. It has been reported that notable, quality after-school programs have been shown to improve students' academic performance, a wish to attend school often, and an ability to connect to their peers socially and emotionally. It has also been found that through consistent attendance at after-school programs, children from low-income communities have been able to receive opportunities and resources, which can bridge the gap between underprivileged communities and college/career readiness, with a decrease in school attrition rates (NCSL, 2022). The positive effects of after-school do correlate with student success through regular attendance, properly trained professionals leading teams, and quality support through well-thought-out programming. There has been a lack of funding for after-school programs since 2014 and thereafter due to inflation and federal funding not matching the rise in costs. This leaves after-school programs to bear the brunt of the loss, with programs needing to hold fundraisers, asking for funding from the state, the communities they reside in, and families (NCSL, 2022).

School programs such as the Boys and Girls Club of America have made a name for themselves due to their innovative and engaging programs offered such as health and wellness, arts, sports and recreation, character and leadership development, education assistance, etc., offered to kids ages 6-18. In the art program offered, children are given a voice to express themselves through their work whether it be through music-making, painting, drama/theater, photography, etc. Data was presented where 76% of low-income children between the ages of 12 to 18 were able to receive A's and B's in their classes through the help of the Boys and Girls Club and their encouragement of continued education; compared to their peers nationally falling in the 67th percentile (Boys and Girls Club of America, n.d.). The Boys and Girls Club (2017, p. 3) has also been trying to further develop its creative arts department, bringing attention to the effectiveness of the arts and self-expression, participant retention rates, and significance in social-emotional development. The Boys and Girls Club of America (2017, p. 3) acknowledges that the arts have had a tremendous impact on the youths' sense of self, improving critical thinking and communication skills, in addition to learning important fundamentals of being a leader and a team player. The implementation of showcasing student artwork (with their permission) through exhibitions, libraries, and Chambers of Commerce events helps a child develop a sense of pride and advocacy for being recognized in their capabilities. The Boys and Girls Club of America (2017, p. 20) have been seeking out creative arts organizations to partner with, in assisting youth with their growth and success, which is a way to expand and find innovative ways to improve the quality of the arts programs they offer.

Similarly, the creative arts program, The Performing Arts Troupe has aided foster youth in Bridgeport, Connecticut since 1999 with the help of Casey Family Services. They're meeting foster youth where they are in their developmental stages to assist in their mental and emotional growth. This program provides a support system by allowing youth to partake in CA therapies through the incorporation of expressing themselves as a unit, employing through group therapy sessions (Greene et al., 2009). Many sessions would be provided for urban youth as well at The Performing Arts Troupe, since these demographics need support because feelings of despair and helplessness are not uncommon for individuals in these communities. Feelings of despair and helplessness can potentially lead to the destruction of low-income communities, with a lack of care for what may happen next in an individual's life due to the circumstances at-hand (Greene et al., 2009). The self-expression and healing from trauma through the vulnerable populations they work with, coupled with programs that promote resilience, assist in the character development of participants. These milestones were expressed as a youth participant learning to have emotional stability, a positive self-outlook, self-advocacy, the ability to build foundational relationships with others, and to learn to work and assist others for their betterment and personal fulfillment (Greene et al., 2009).

On the contrary, Holochwost et al. (2021) discusses the gaps within creative arts programs, a lack of solid evidence of activities provided being truly effective. It is expressed that research needs to go further than surface level such as research findings consistently speaking on the Creative Arts (CA's) helping children learn to be empathic towards others. Holochwost et al. (2021) expresses that research behind studies like this needs to have a more scientific basis through a socioemotional lens with reducing such broad findings. A large multitude of Creative Arts programs are fully or partially funded by donors, other organizations, or on the federal level, and the impact the Creative Arts has on youth is of interest to policymakers, practitioners, etc. Inquiries arise as to what exact aspects of the arts causes change and stimulation in youth and socio-emotional development (Holochwost et al., 2021). Holochwost et al. (2021) further questions what is required of an individual to be artistically inclined and whether these requirements are different for each form of Creative Arts (dance, drama, music, art), and how creating art has a different impact compared to witnessing art. It is expressed that the best way to demonstrate the effectiveness of a program on children's socioemotional development is through contextualizing the experiences of the individuals with the mission of an arts program and receive personal accounts of the effects thereafter. It is important to unite these groups to devise a research question of value that can aid in the study of participant development and how the programs benefit society. Holochwost et al. (2021) suggests that the study of the correlation between the arts and child development would provide a rich understanding of something that needs to be further researched.

## CONCLUSION

The research compiled in this chapter discussed how foster youth are in critical need of additional resources and assistance. Foster children are a demographic that is most vulnerable to encountering hardships such as abandonment, difficulties in schooling, sexual assault, violence, etc. Series of events like this do cause adverse effects such as a lack of trust in others, an absence of expression, resulting in living through survival tactics instead of living the life of a child. The readings mentioned within the paper offer insight into how creative arts therapies have a positive effect on foster children and similar groups. A decrease in the number of children within the foster care system from 2014 to 2018 was discussed, but there is a paucity of data provided on how these numbers look now (2023). There are many gaps within the quantitative data regarding the foster care system, the last relevant source of quantitative data dates to 2018 but no sooner than that. There are a number of necessities that come with raising a child and there is a tendency for foster children to not receive the adequate care they need, resulting in many of these children facing a future of hardship. It was noted that further research needs to be conducted to actualize the needs of foster care children rather than only addressing the issues they face alongside the developmental makeup of a foster child's sense of identity and autonomy (Steenbakkers et al., 2018).

Roehrkasse (2021) also discusses further research that needs to be conducted concerning the factors of foster care implementation, and reasoning, whether it be violence, female imprisonment, welfare, and other varying components that differ across ethno-racial backgrounds. According to the different attachment styles, it is predicted that foster children would have a mix of disorganized and ambivalent attachment. These children have encountered multiple unstable relationships that have come in and out of their lives but also have the desire to be understood, yearning for a stable connection with somebody. Further research can be conducted to assist in finding validity in this prediction. The author of this paper was surprised by the large number of Caucasian children in foster care. Looking into the readings it was stated that roughly, 60-70% of the U.S. population is white, while this demographic of children accounts for 44% of the average foster care population (Child welfare outcomes 2018, 2021). Clinicians in the Creative arts therapies are also attempting to implement the facilitation of art therapy through virtual reality in the future (Shafir et al., 2020). As foster children continue to encounter traumatic events, there is hope that further policies will be put into place soon to protect this population and offer them the care that they need to grow into healthy, capable adults.

## REFERENCES

Austin, D. (2007). Lifesongs: Music therapy with adolescents in foster care. In V.A. Camilleri (Ed.), Healing the inner city child: Creative arts therapies with at-risk youth (pp. 92-103). Jessica Kingsley Publishers.

Austin, D., & Dvorkin, J. M. (1993). Resistance in individual therapy. *The Arts in Psychotherapy*, *20*(5), 423–429. doi:10.1016/0197-4556(93)90049-8

Bakema, M. J., van Zuiden, M., Collard, D., Zantvoord, J. B., de Rooij, S. R., Elsenburg, L. K., & Lok, A. (2020). Associations between child maltreatment, autonomic regulation, and adverse cardiovascular outcome in an urban population: The HELIUS study. *Frontiers in Psychiatry*, *11*, 69. doi:10.3389/fpsyt.2020.00069 PMID:32256391

Baker, B. L., McIntyre, L., Blacher, J., Crnic, K., Edelbrock, C., & Low, C. (2003). Pre-school children with and without developmental delay: Behaviour problems and parenting stress over time. *Journal of Intellectual Disability Research*, *47*(4–5), 217–230. doi:10.1046/j.1365-2788.2003.00484.x PMID:12787154

Bannister, A. (2003). *Creative therapies with traumatized children*. Jessica Kingsley Publishers.

Beaty, R. E., Benedek, M., Barry Kaufman, S., & Silvia, P. J. (2015). Default and executive network coupling supports creative idea production. *Scientific Reports*, *5*(1), 10964. doi:10.1038rep10964 PMID:26084037

Berkovitz, I. H. (1995). *Adolescents grow in groups: Experiences in adolescent group psychotherapy*. Jason Aronson Inc.

Blos, P. (1962). *On adolescence: A psychoanalytic interpretation*. The Free Press.

Bowlby, J. (1969). Attachment and Loss: Volume I. Attachment. Hogarth Press.

Boys and Girls Club of America. (2017). *Partnering with community arts organizations: A pathway to a high-quality club experience*. https://www.bgca.org/-/media/Documents/Programs/3154-17_FormingArtsPartnerships_FINAL_REV.pdf

Boys and Girls Club of America. (n.d.). https://www.bgca.org/programs/the-arts

Camilleri, V. A. (2007). The inner city. In V. A. Camilleri (Ed.), *Healing the inner city child: Creative arts therapies with at-risk youth* (pp. 15–20). Jessica Kingsley Publishers.

Center for Disease Control and Prevention. (2021). *Child developmental basics*. https://www.cdc.gov/ncbddd/childdevelopment/facts.html

Child Welfare. (2017). *Long-term consequences of child abuse and neglect*. https://www.childwelfare.gov/pubpdfs/long_term_consequences.pdf

Child Welfare Outcomes 2018: Report to Congress. (2021, May 14). https://www.acf.hhs.gov/cb/report/cwo-2018

Clausen, J., Ruff, S., Wiederhold, W., & Heineman, T. (2012). For As Long As It Takes: Relationship-Based Play Therapy for Children in Foster Care. *Psychoanalytic Social Work, 19*(1), 43–53. doi:10.1080/15228878.2012.666481

Do Prado, C. H., Grassi-Oliveira, R., Daruy-Filho, L., Wieck, A., & Bauer, M. E. (2017). Evidence for immune activation and resistance to glucocorticoids following childhood maltreatment in adolescents without psychopathology. *Neuropsychopharmacology, 42*(11), 2272–2282. doi:10.1038/npp.2017.137 PMID:28664925

Dow, G. T., & Kozlowski, K. (2020, May 1). *The creative brain*. ASCD. https://www.ascd.org/el/articles/the-creative-brain

Font, S. A., & Gershoff, E. T. (2020). Foster care: How we can, and should, do more for maltreated children. *Social Policy Report, 33*(3), 1–40. doi:10.1002op2.10 PMID:33833492

Goemans, A., Geel, M. V., & Vedder, P. (2018). Foster children's behavioral development and foster parent stress: Testing a transactional model. *Journal of Child and Family Studies*, *27*(3), 990–1001. doi:10.100710826-017-0941-z PMID:29568216

Greene, A. H., Goldenberg, L., & Freundlich, M. (2009). The use of expressive therapies and social support with youth in foster care: The performing arts troupe. *Journal of Youth Development*, *4*(1), 1. doi:10.5195/jyd.2009.275

Herman, J. L. (1992). *Trauma and Recovery*. Basic Books.

Holochwost, S. J., Goldstein, T. R., & Wolf, D. P. (2021). Delineating the benefits of arts education for children's socioemotional development. *Frontiers in Psychology*, *12*, 624712. doi:10.3389/fpsyg.2021.624712 PMID:34054643

Huang, S. (2020, Nov 3). *Attachment styles*. Simply Psychology. www.simplypsychology.org/attachment-styles.html

Hudson, A. L. (2013). Career mentoring needs of youths in foster care: Voices for change. *Journal of Child and Adolescent Psychiatric Nursing*, *26*(2), 131–137. doi:10.1111/jcap.12032 PMID:23607825

Jacobsen, H., Bergsund, H. B., Wentzel, T., Smith, L. L., & Moe, V. (2020). Foster children are at risk for developing problems in social-emotional functioning: A follow-up study at 8 years of age. *Children and Youth Services Review*, *108*, 104603. doi:10.1016/j.childyouth.2019.104603

Koontz, A. (2019, March). The circuitry of creativity: How our brains innovate thinking. *Cal Tech Letters*.

Landreth, G. L. (2002). *Play therapy: The art of the relationship* (2nd ed.). Brunner-Routledge.

Maslow, A. H. (1943). A theory of human motivation. *Psychological Review*, *50*(4), 370–396. doi:10.1037/h0054346

McLeod, S. A. (2018, May 21). *Maslow's hierarchy of needs*. Simply Psychology. https://www.simplypsychology.org/maslow.html

Mendis, K., Gardner, F., & Lehmann, J. (2015). The education of children in out-of-home care. *Australian Social Work*, *68*(4), 483–496. doi:10.1080/0312407X.2014.963134

Milman, D., & Goldman, G. (1987). *Techniques of Working with Resistance*. Jason Aronson.

Quest, A. D., Fullerton, A., Geenen, S., & Powers, L. (2012). Voices of youth in foster care and special education regarding their educational experiences and transition to adulthood. *Children and Youth Services Review, 34*(9), 1604–1615. doi:10.1016/j.childyouth.2012.04.018

Shafir, T., Orkibi, H., Baker, F. A., Gussak, D., & Kaimal, G. (2020). Editorial: The state of the art in creative arts therapies. *Frontiers in Psychology, 11*, 68. doi:10.3389/fpsyg.2020.00068 PMID:32116898

Steenbakkers, A., Van Der Steen, S., & Grietens, H. (2018). The needs of foster children and how to satisfy them: A systematic review of the literature. *Clinical Child and Family Psychology Review, 21*(1), 1–12. doi:10.100710567-017-0246-1 PMID:29075894

Stoner, A. M., Leon, S. C., & Fuller, A. K. (2015). Predictors of reduction in symptoms of depression for children and adolescents in foster care. *Journal of Child and Family Studies, 24*(3), 784–797. doi:10.100710826-013-9889-9

U.S. Department of Health and Human Services. (2019). *The AFCARS Report: Preliminary FY1 2018 Estimates as of August 22, 2019* (No. 26). https://www.acf.hhs.gov/sites/default/files/documents/cb/afcarsreport26.pdf

Wallace, A. (2021, March 2). *Supporting student success through afterschool program.* NCSL. https://www.ncsl.org/research/education/expanding-learning-opportunities-through-afterschool-programs.aspx

## KEY TERMS AND DEFINITIONS

**At-Risk:** An individual who may encounter life-threatening or negative events in the future because of previous circumstances (Camilleri, 2008, p. 17).

**CA:** Creative Arts.

**DMT:** Dance and Movement Therapy.

**Dopamine:** A neurotransmitter that helps in the feeling of reward and pleasure.

**Frontal Lobe:** Located in the front part of the brain, the frontal lobe has to do with cognitive functions such as emotions, memories, solving problems, etc.

**Occipital Lobe:** Located in the back of the head, the occipital lobe has to do with perception, assisting in the way one views the world such as color, movement, etc.

**Oxytocin:** A neurotransmitter that oversees attachment, bonding with others, and decreasing stress.

**Parietal Lobe:** A major lobe of the brain that has to do with sensory information such as touch, taste, etc.

**Prefrontal Cortex:** Assisting in the creation of one's personality, deciphering and understanding behaviors of self and others.

**Serotonin:** A neurotransmitter that can assist in stabilizing mood.

**Social-Emotional Functioning/Development:** The ability for an individual to be able to communicate and build relationships with others in their lives such as a parent, friends, and significant others.

# Compilation of References

Aalbers, S., Fusar-Poli, L., Freeman, R. E., Spreen, M., Ket, J. C., Vink, A. C., Maratos, A., Crawford, M., Chen, X. J., & Gold, C. (2017). Music therapy for depression. *Cochrane Database of Systematic Reviews, 11*(11), CD004517. Advance online publication. doi:10.1002/14651858. CD004517.pub3 PMID:29144545

AATA National Office. (2021, February 10). *About our members: AATA at a glance 2021.* American Art Therapy Association. https://arttherapy.org/news-member-infographic/

Acosta, M. A. (2021). *Exploring the acceptability of an improv-based workshop series for college student stress and anxiety.* [Doctoral dissertation, University of Hartford]. ProQuest Dissertations Publishing.

Aday, R. H., Dye, M. H., & Kaiser, A. K. (2014). Examining the traumatic effects of sexual victimization on the health of incarcerated women. *Women & Criminal Justice, 24*(4), 341–361. doi:10.1080/08974454.2014.909758

Agosin, M. (1996). *Tapestries of hope, threads of love: The arpillera movement in Chile, 1974–1994* (C. Kostopulos-Cooperman, Trans.). University of New Mexico Press.

Agosin, M. (2014). *Stitching resistance: Women, creativity, and fiber arts.* Solis Press.

Aguilar, B. (2017). The Efficacy of Art Therapy in Pediatric Oncology Patients: An Integrative Literature Review. *Journal of Pediatric Nursing, 36*, 173–178. https://doi.org/ doi:10.1016/j.pedn.2017.06.015

AlDabbagh, M. (2014). Positive Art Impact On healing therapy "Review Study". Brewster, L. *The Impact of Prison Arts Programs on Inmate Attitudes and Behavior: A Quantitative Evaluation.*

Alden, A. (2000, June 30). Sewing comfort out of grief. *Midwifery Today, 43*(54).

Alders, A. (2011). Perceived self-efficacy and its role in education-related cognitive performance in Latino American elderly. *Journal of Latinos and Education, 10*(4), 299–319. doi:10.1080/15348431.2011.605680

Allan & Crandall. (1986). The Rosebush: a visualization strategy. *Elementary School Guidance & Counseling, 21*(1), 44–51. https://www.jstor.org/stable/42871035

Alzheimer's Association. (2020). 2020 Alzheimer's Disease Facts and Figures. *Alzheimer's & Dementia, 16*(3), 391–460. doi:10.1002/alz.12068

Alzheimer's Association. (2022). *Alzheimer's disease facts and figures.* Alzheimer's Disease and Dementia. https://www.alz.org/alzheimers-dementia/facts-figures

American Art Therapy Association. (2017). *About Art Therapy.* American Art Therapy Association. https://arttherapy.org/about-art-therapy/

American Dance Therapy Association. (2020). *Become a dance movement therapist: Frequently asked questions.* https://www.adta.org/become-a-dance-movement-therapist

American Psychiatric Association. (2013). *Diagnostic and statistical manual of mental disorders* (5th ed.). doi:10.1176/appi.books.9780890425596

Amiri, S. (2022). Prevalence of suicide in immigrants/refugees: A systematic review and meta-analysis. *Archives of Suicide Research, 26*(2), 370–405. doi:10.1080/13811118.2020.1802379 PMID:32780682

APA. (2017). *Diagnostic and statistical manual of mental disorders: Dsm-5.* CBS Publishers & Distributors, Pvt. Ltd

Appleton, V. (2002). Avenues of hope: Art therapy and the resolution of trauma. *Art Therapy: Journal of the American Therapy Association, 5*, 6–13.

Applied Improvisation Network. (2022). *About.* AIN. https://www.appliedimprovisationnetwork.org/

Arain, M., Haque, M., Johal, L., Mathur, P., Nel, W., Rais, A., ... Sharma, S. (2013). Maturation of the adolescent brain. *Neuropsychiatric Disease and Treatment, 9*, 449. PMID:23579318

Arkin, S. (2007). Language-enriched exercise plus socialization slows cognitive decline in alzheimer's disease. *American Journal of Alzheimer's Disease and Other Dementias, 22*(1), 62–77. doi:10.1177/1533317506295377 PMID:17534004

Art Therapy Credentials Board, Inc. (2017). *What is Art Therapy?* Art Therapy Credentials Board, Inc. https://www.atcb.org/what-is-art-therapy/

Austin, D. (2007). Lifesongs: Music therapy with adolescents in foster care. In V.A. Camilleri (Ed.), Healing the inner city child: Creative arts therapies with at-risk youth (pp. 92-103). Jessica Kingsley Publishers.

Austin, D., & Dvorkin, J. M. (1993). Resistance in individual therapy. *The Arts in Psychotherapy, 20*(5), 423–429. doi:10.1016/0197-4556(93)90049-8

Baird, A., Garrido, S., & Tamplin, J. (2019). Music and Dementia: From Cognition to Therapy. In *Google Books.* Oxford University Press. doi:10.1093/oso/9780190075934.001.0001

Bakema, M. J., van Zuiden, M., Collard, D., Zantvoord, J. B., de Rooij, S. R., Elsenburg, L. K., & Lok, A. (2020). Associations between child maltreatment, autonomic regulation, and adverse cardiovascular outcome in an urban population: The HELIUS study. *Frontiers in Psychiatry, 11*, 69. doi:10.3389/fpsyt.2020.00069 PMID:32256391

Baker, B. L., McIntyre, L., Blacher, J., Crnic, K., Edelbrock, C., & Low, C. (2003). Pre-school children with and without developmental delay: Behaviour problems and parenting stress over time. *Journal of Intellectual Disability Research*, *47*(4–5), 217–230. doi:10.1046/j.1365-2788.2003.00484.x PMID:12787154

Balgaonkar, A. V. (2010). Effect of dance/motor therapy on the cognitive development of children. *The International Journal of the Arts in Society*, *3*(11), 54–72.

Ball, M. (1977). Neuronal loss, neurofibrillary tangles and granulovacuolar degeneration in the hippocampus with ageing and dementia. *Acta Neuropathologica, 37*(2), 111–118. doi:10.1007/BF00692056

Ball, E. L., Owen-Booth, B., Gray, A., Shenkin, S. D., Hewitt, J., & McCleery, J. (2020). Aromatherapy for dementia. *Cochrane Database of Systematic Reviews, 8. The Cochrane Library, 2020*(8). doi:10.1002/14651858.CD003150.pub3 PMID:32813272

Ballon, B. C., Silver, I., & Fidler, D. (2007). Headspace theater: An innovative method for experiential learning of psychiatric symptomatology using modified role-playing and improvisational theater techniques. *Academic Psychiatry*, *31*(5), 380–387. doi:10.1176/appi.ap.31.5.380 PMID:17875623

Bandura, A. (1993). Perceived self-efficacy in cognitive development and functioning. *Educational Psychologist*, *28*(2), 117–148. doi:10.120715326985ep2802_3

Bannister, A. (2003). *Creative therapies with traumatized children.* Jessica Kingsley Publishers.

Barraza, E., Sanchez, C., & Solis, C. (2015). *An arts-based exploration of immigration and acculturation through the lenses of first, second, and third generation clinical art therapists.* [Theses, Loyola University].

Barua, A., Ghosh, M. K., Kar, N., & Basilio, M. A. (2010). Distribution of depressive disorders in the elderly. *Journal of Neurosciences in Rural Practice, 01*(02), 067–073. doi:10.4103/0976-3147.71719

Basting. (2006). Arts in Dementia Care: "This is not the end... it's the end of this chapter." *Generations, 30*(1), 16–20. https://www.ingentaconnect.com/content/asag/gen/2006/00000030/00000001/art00004

Baumeister, R. F., Bratslavsky, E., Finkenauer, C., & Vohs, K. D. (2001). Bad is stronger than good. *Review of General Psychology*, *5*(4), 323–370. doi:10.1037/1089-2680.5.4.323

Beaty, R. E., Benedek, M., Barry Kaufman, S., & Silvia, P. J. (2015). Default and executive network coupling supports creative idea production. *Scientific Reports*, *5*(1), 10964. doi:10.1038rep10964 PMID:26084037

Beck, A. T. (1963). Thinking and depression: I. Idiosyncratic content and cognitive distortions. *Archives of General Psychiatry*, *9*(4), 324–333. doi:10.1001/archpsyc.1963.01720160014002 PMID:14045261

Belknap, J. (2020). *The invisible woman: Gender, crime, and justice*. SAGE Publications.

Bender, K. A. (2023). Incarcerated Women's Perceptions of the Role Model Prison Officer as Procedurally Just. *International Journal of Offender Therapy and Comparative Criminology*, *0*(0), 0306624X2211442. Advance online publication. doi:10.1177/0306624X221144287 PMID:36601909

Bensimon, M., Amir, D., & Wolf, Y. (2012). A pendulum between trauma and life: Group music therapy with post-traumatized soldiers. *The Arts in Psychotherapy*, *39*(4), 223–233. doi:10.1016/j.aip.2012.03.005

Benson, E. (2003). Rehabilitate or Punishment? *American Psychological Association.* https://www.apa.org/monitor/julaug03/rehab

Berkovitz, I. H. (1995). *Adolescents grow in groups: Experiences in adolescent group psychotherapy*. Jason Aronson Inc.

Bermant, G. (2013). Working with(out) a net: Improvisational theater and enhanced well-being. *Frontiers in Psychology*, *4*, 1–6. doi:10.3389/fpsyg.2013.00929 PMID:24339820

Bernatzky, G., Presch, M., Anderson, M., & Panksepp, J. (2011). Emotional foundations of music as a non-pharmacological pain management tool in modern medicine. *Neuroscience and Biobehavioral Reviews*, *35*(9), 1989–1999. doi:10.1016/j.neubiorev.2011.06.005 PMID:21704068

Blomdahl, C., Gunnarsson, A. B., Guregård, S., & Björklund, A. (2013). A realist review of art therapy for clients with depression. *The Arts in Psychotherapy*, *40*(3), 322–330. doi:10.1016/j.aip.2013.05.009

Bloom, B., & Covington, S. (2008). Addressing the mental health needs of women offenders. In R. Gido, L. Dalley, & D. McDonald (Eds.), *The unmet mental health needs of women across the criminal justice system*. Prentice-Hall/Pearson.

Bloom, S. L. (1995). Creating sanctuary in the school. *Journal for a Just and Caring Education*, *1*(4), 403–433.

Blos, P. (1962). *On adolescence: A psychoanalytic interpretation*. The Free Press.

Boron, J. B., Turiano, N. A., Willis, S. L., & Schaie, K. W. (2007). Effects of cognitive training on change in accuracy in inductive reasoning ability. *The Journals of Gerontology. Series B, Psychological Sciences and Social Sciences*, *62*(3), P179–P186. doi:10.1093/geronb/62.3.P179 PMID:17507586

Bowlby, J. (1969). Attachment and Loss: Volume I. Attachment. Hogarth Press.

Boys and Girls Club of America. (2017). *Partnering with community arts organizations: A pathway to a high-quality club experience*. https://www.bgca.org/-/media/Documents/Programs/3154-17_FormingArtsPartnerships_FINAL_REV.pdf

Boys and Girls Club of America. (n.d.). https://www.bgca.org/programs/the-arts

Bradt, J., Dileo, C., Magill, L., & Teague, A. (2016). Music interventions for improving psychological and physical outcomes in cancer patients. *Cochrane Database of Systematic Reviews*, (8), CD006911. Advance online publication. doi:10.1002/14651858.CD006911.pub3 PMID:27524661

Bräuninger, I. (2014). Specific dance movement therapy interventions—Which are successful? An intervention and correlation study. *The Arts in Psychotherapy*, *41*(5), 445–457. doi:10.1016/j.aip.2014.08.002

Bremner, J. D., Vermetten, E., Schmahl, C., Vaccarino, V., Vythilingam, M., Afzal, N., Grillon, C., & Charney, D. S. (2005). Positron emission tomographic imaging of neural correlates of a fear acquisition and extinction paradigm in women with childhood sexual-abuse-related post-traumatic stress disorder. *Psychological Medicine*, *35*(6), 791–806. doi:10.1017/S0033291704003290 PMID:15997600

Brewster, L. (2014). The Impact of prison arts programs on inmate attitudes and behavior: A Quantitative evaluation. *Justice Policy Journal*, *11*(2). https://repository.usfca.edu/cgi/viewcontent.cgi?article=1008&context=pna

Brewster, L. (2014). The Impact of Prison Arts Programs on Inmate Attitudes and Behavior: A Quantitative Evaluation. *Justice Policy Journal*, *11*(2), 1–28.

Brittle, Z. (2015). Turn towards instead of away. *The Gottman Institute Blog*. https://www.gottman.com/blog/turn-toward-instead-of-away/

Bronson, J., & Berzofsky, M. (2011). *Indicators of mental health problems reported by prisoners and jail inmates*. U.S. Department of Justice. https://www.bjs.gov/content/pub/pdf/imhprpji1112.pdf

Brown, C. J., Chirino, A. F. C., Cortez, C. M., Gearhart, C., & Urizar, G. G. (2020). Conceptual Art for the Aging Brain: Piloting an Art-Based Cognitive Health Intervention. *Activities, Adaptation & Aging, 45*(1), 39–69. Taylor & Francis Online. doi:10.1080/01924788.2020.1719584

Brown, B. (2010). *Gifts of imperfection, the*. Hazelden Information & Educational Services.

Brown, L. S., & Wright, J. (2001). Attachment theory in adolescence and its relevance to developmental psychopathology. *Clinical Psychology & Psychotherapy*, *8*(1), 15–32. doi:10.1002/cpp.274

Buchalter (2011). Art Therapy and Creative Coping Techniques for Older Adults. In *Google Books*. Jessica Kingsley Publishers.

Buchalter, S. (2015). *Raising self-esteem in adults: An eclectic approach with art therapy, CBT. and DBT-based techniques*. Jessica Kingsley Publishers.

Bucharová, M., Malá, A., Kantor, J., & Svobodová, Z. (2020). Arts therapies interventions and their outcomes in the treatment of Eating disorders: Scoping review protocol. *Behavioral Sciences (Basel, Switzerland)*, *10*(12), 188. doi:10.3390/bs10120188 PMID:33316926

Bugos, J. A., Perlstein, W. M., McCrae, C. S., Brophy, T. S., & Bedenbaugh, P. H. (2007). Individualized Piano Instruction enhances executive functioning and working memory in older adults. *Aging & Mental Health, 11*(4), 464–471. Taylor & Francis Online. https://doi.org/doi:10.1080/13607860601086504

Buschert, V., Bokde, A. L. W., & Hampel, H. (2010). Cognitive intervention in Alzheimer disease. *Nature Reviews. Neurology*, *6*(9), 508–517. doi:10.1038/nrneurol.2010.113 PMID:20717104

Camilleri, V. A. (2007). The inner city. In V. A. Camilleri (Ed.), *Healing the inner city child: Creative arts therapies with at-risk youth* (pp. 15–20). Jessica Kingsley Publishers.

Campbell, M., Decker, K. P., Kruk, K., & Deaver, S. P. (2016). Art therapy and cognitive processing therapy for combat-related PTSD: A randomized controlled trial. *Art Therapy: Journal of the American Art Therapy Association*, *33*(4), 169–177. doi:10.1080/07421656.2016.1226643 PMID:29332989

Canul, G. D. (2017). Genealogical-PhotoTherapy as a tool for integrating my Mayan and Spanish origins. *MindConsiliums, 17*(3), 1-16. https://mindconsiliums.org/pub/2017/03/2017-03-Canul-G-D-genealogical-phototherapy-integrating-my-mayan-and-spanish-origins.pdf

Capello, P. P. (2008). Dance/movement therapy with children throughout the world. *American Journal of Dance Therapy*, *30*(1), 24–36. doi:10.100710465-008-9045-z

Carnwell, R. (2017). Essential differences between research and evidence-based practice. *Nurse Researcher*, *8*(2), 65–68.

Carocci, M. (2010). Textiles of healing: Native American AIDS quilts. *Textile (Oxford)*, *8*(1), 68–84. doi:10.2752/175183510X12580391269986

Case, C., & Dalley, T. (2014). *The Handbook of Art Therapy*. Routledge. doi:10.4324/9781315779799

Center for Disease Control and Prevention. (2021). *Child developmental basics*. https://www.cdc.gov/ncbddd/childdevelopment/facts.html

Center for Medicare & Medicaid Services. (2018). Survey and Enforcement Process for Skilled Nursing Facilities and Nursing Facilities. In *State Operations Manual*. Center for Medicare & Medicaid Services. https://www.cms.gov/Regulations-and-Guidance/Guidance/Manuals/Downloads/som107c07pdf.pdf

Centers for Disease Control and Prevention. (2020, October 23). *Data & statistics on down syndrome.* CDC. https://www.cdc.gov/ncbddd/birthdefects/downsyndrome/data.html

Centers for Disease Control and Prevention. (2022a, May 2). *Data & statistics for cerebral palsy.* CDC. https://www.cdc.gov/ncbddd/cp/data.html

Centers for Disease Control and Prevention. (2022b, March 2). *Data & statistics on autism spectrum disorder.* CDC. https://www.cdc.gov/ncbddd/autism/data.html

Chancellor, B., Duncan, A., & Chatterjee, A. (2014). Art Therapy for Alzheimer's Disease and Other Dementias. *Journal of Alzheimer's Disease, 39*(01), 1–11. doi:10.3233/JAD-131295 PMID:24121964

Chapman, L., Morabito, D., Ladakakos, C., Schreier, H., & Knudson, M. M. (2001). The effectiveness of art therapy interventions in reducing post traumatic stress disorder (PTSD) symptoms in pediatric trauma patients. *Art Therapy: Journal of the American Art Therapy Association, 18*(2), 100–104. doi:10.1080/07421656.2001.10129750

Charland, W. (2011). War rugs: Woven documents of conflict and hope. *Art Education, 64*(6), 25–32. doi:10.1080/00043125.2011.11519149

Child Welfare Outcomes 2018: Report to Congress. (2021, May 14). https://www.acf.hhs.gov/cb/report/cwo-2018

Child Welfare. (2017). *Long-term consequences of child abuse and neglect.* https://www.childwelfare.gov/pubpdfs/long_term_consequences.pdf

Chillag, A. (2018, August 20). How an improv class is relieving anxiety. *CNN Health.* https://www.cnn.com/2018/07/05/health/improv-for-anxiety-staying-well/index.html

Chilton, G., & Wilkinson, R. (2016, January 6). *Exploring strengths through masks: Art therapy from a positive psychology perspective.* Retrieved from https://arttherapy.org/exploring-strengths-masks-art-therapy-positive-psychology-perspective/

Chilton, G. (2013). Art therapy and flow: A Review of the literature and applications. *Art Therapy: Journal of the American Art Therapy Association, 30*(2), 64–70. doi:10.1080/07421656.2013.787211

Chin, M. H. (2020). Lessons from improv comedy to reduce health disparities. *JAMA Internal Medicine, 180*(1), 5–6. doi:10.1001/jamainternmed.2019.5930 PMID:31816039

Chin, M. H., Clarke, A. R., Nocon, R. S., Casey, A. A., Goddu, A. P., Keesecker, N. M., & Cook, S. C. (2012). A roadmap and best practices for organizations to reduce racial and ethnic disparities in health care. *Journal of General Internal Medicine, 27*(8), 992–1000. doi:10.100711606-012-2082-9 PMID:22798211

Choi, S. S. (2021). *Foreigner to Third Culture Kid: Exploring Intersectional Self-Identity through Phototherapy*. [Thesis, Pratt Institute]. ProQuest Dissertations & Theses Global. (2555973384). https://www.proquest.com/dissertations-theses/foreigner-third-culture-kid-exploring/docview/2555973384/se-2

Ciasca, E. C., Ferreira, R. C., Santana, C. L. A., Forlenza, O. V., dos Santos, G. D., Brum, P. S., & Nunes, P. V. (2018). Art therapy as an adjuvant treatment for depression in elderly women: A randomized controlled trial. *Revista Brasileira de Psiquiatria (Sao Paulo, Brazil)*, *40*(3), 256–263. doi:10.1590/1516-4446-2017-2250 PMID:29412335

Clapp, L. A., Taylor, E. P., Di Folco, S., & Mackinnon, V. L. (2018). Effectiveness of art therapy with pediatric populations affected by medical health conditions: A systematic review. *Arts & Health*, *11*(3), 183–201. doi:10.1080/17533015.2018.1443952 PMID:31038441

Clausen, J., Ruff, S., Wiederhold, W., & Heineman, T. (2012). For As Long As It Takes: Relationship-Based Play Therapy for Children in Foster Care. *Psychoanalytic Social Work*, *19*(1), 43–53. doi:10.1080/15228878.2012.666481

Cloitre, M., Stovall-McClough, K. C., Nooner, K., Zorbas, P., Cherry, S., Jackson, C. L., Gan, W., & Petkova, E. (2010). Treatment for PTSD related to childhood abuse: A randomized controlled trial. *The American Journal of Psychiatry*, *167*(8), 915–924. doi:10.1176/appi.ajp.2010.09081247 PMID:20595411

Cohen, G. (2009). New theories and research findings on the positive influence of music and art on health with ageing. *Arts & Health*, *1*(1), 48–62. doi:10.1080/17533010802528033

Cohen, J. S., & Miller, L. J. (2009). Interpersonal mindfulness training for well-being: A pilot study with psychology graduate students. *Teachers College Record*, *111*(12), 2760–2774. doi:10.1177/016146810911101202

Cohen, R. A. (2013). Common threads: A recovery programme for survivors of genderbased violence. *Intervention (Amstelveen, Netherlands)*, *11*(2), 157–168. doi:10.1097/01.WTF.0000431118.16849.0c

Cole, J. (2016). *I've got your back: Utilizing improv as a tool to enhance workplace relationships.* [Master's Thesis, University of Pennsylvania]. University of Pennsylvania Scholarly Commons.

Collier, A. F. (2011). The well-being of women who create with textiles: Implications for art therapy. *Art Therapy: Journal of the American Art Therapy Association*, *28*(3), 104–112. doi:10.1080/07421656.2011.597025

Connolly, M., & Slade, M. (2019). The united states of stress 2019. *Everyday Health*, https://www.everydayhealth.com/wellness/united-states-of-stress/

Cook, R. (1994). *An historical and psychological context for the phenomenon of art therapy* [Thesis, Edith Cohen University].

Costa, D. S. J., Mercieca-Bebber, R., Rutherford, C., Tait, M.-A., & King, M. T. (2021). How is quality of life defined and assessed in published research? *Quality of Life Research: An International Journal of Quality of Life Aspects of Treatment, Care and Rehabilitation, 30*(8), 2109–2121. doi:10.100711136-021-02826-0 PMID:33792834

Creswell, J. W. (2014). *Research design: Qualitative, quantitative and mixed methods approaches* (4th ed.). Sage.

Crocq, M., & Crocq, L. (2000). From shell shock and war neurosis to posttraumatic stress disorder: A history of psychotraumatology. *Dialogues in Clinical Neuroscience, 2*(1), 47–55. doi:10.31887/DCNS.2000.2.1/macrocq PMID:22033462

Csikszentmihalyi, M. (1990). *Flow: The psychology of optimal experience*. Harper Perennial Modern Classics.

Curl, K. (2008). Assessing stress reduction as a function of artistic creation and cognitive focus. *Art Therapy: Journal of the American Art Therapy Association, 25*(4), 164–169. doi:10.1080/07421656.2008.10129550

Czamanski-Cohen, J., & Weihs, K. L. (2016). The bodymind model: A platform for studying the mechanisms of change induced by art therapy. *The Arts in Psychotherapy, 51*, 63–71. doi:10.1016/j.aip.2016.08.006 PMID:27777492

Dalebroux, A., Goldstein, T. R., & Winner, E. (2008). Short-term mood repair through art-making: Positive emotion is more effective than venting. *Motivation and Emotion, 32*(4), 288–295. doi:10.100711031-008-9105-1

Davis, K. L. (1999). Alzheimer's disease: Seeking new ways to preserve brain function. Interview by Alice V. Luddington. *Geriatrics, 54*(2), 42–48. PMID:10024872

Davis, R. N., Massman, P. J., & Doody, R. S. (2001). (2001). Cognitive Intervention in Alzheimer Disease: A Randomized Placebo-Controlled Study. *Alzheimer Disease and Associated Disorders, 15*(1), 1–9. https://tinyurl.com/yfwa7h9t. doi:10.1097/00002093-200101000-00001 PMID:11236819

De Farias, L. H. S., & Teixeira-Machado, L. (2016). Behind the dance: Educational, emotional and social contexts in Down syndrome. *International Journal of Humanities Social Sciences and Education, 3*(1), 20–23.

de Guzman, A. B., Santos, J. I., Santos, M. L., Santos, M. T., Sarmiento, V. V., Sarnillo, E. J., & Sarsagat, J. M. (2010). Traditional Filipino arts in enhancing older people's self-esteem in a penal institution. *Educational Gerontology, 36*(12), 1065–1085. doi:10.1080/03601270903534713

de Vugt, M., & Dröes, R.-M. (2017). Social health in dementia. Towards a positive dementia discourse. *Aging & Mental Health, 21*(1), 1–3. doi:10.1080/13607863.2016.1262822 PMID:28098498

Deaver, S. (2002). What Constitutes Art Therapy Research? *Art Therapy, 19*(1), 23–27. doi:10.1080/07421656.2002.10129721

Degges-White, S., & Davis, N. L. (Eds.). (2017). Integrating the expressive arts into counseling practice: Theory-based interventions. Springer Publishing Company.

Delta. (2015). *Stressed and Exhausted? Tired and Wired?* FxMed Centers. https://fxmedcenters.com/2015/07/27/stressed-and-exhausted-tired-and-wired/

DeMichele, M. (2015). Improv and ink: Increasing individual writing fluency with collaborative improv. *International Journal of Education & the Arts*, *16*(10). http://www.ijea.org/v16n10/

DeMichele, M., & Kuenneke, S. (2021). Short-form, comedy improv affects the functional connectivity in the brain of adolescents with complex developmental trauma as measured by qEEG: A single group pilot study. *NeuroRegulation*, *8*(1), 2–13. doi:10.15540/nr.8.1.2

Dhikav, V., & Anand, K. S.Dhikav & Anand. (2012). Hippocampus in health and disease: An overview. *Annals of Indian Academy of Neurology*, *15*(4), 239. doi:10.4103/0972-2327.104323 PMID:23349586

Dillehay, R. (1990). Caregivers for Alzheimer's Patients: What We Are Learning from Research. *The International Journal of Aging and Human Development*, *30*(4), 263–285. https://doi.org/doi:10.2190/2P3J-A9AH-HHF4-00RG

Do Prado, C. H., Grassi-Oliveira, R., Daruy-Filho, L., Wieck, A., & Bauer, M. E. (2017). Evidence for immune activation and resistance to glucocorticoids following childhood maltreatment in adolescents without psychopathology. *Neuropsychopharmacology*, *42*(11), 2272–2282. doi:10.1038/npp.2017.137 PMID:28664925

Dohe, K., & Pappas, E. (2017). Lessons from the field: What improv teaches us about collaboration. *Library Leadership & Management*, *32*(1), 1–16.

Doric-Henry, L. (1997). Pottery as Art Therapy with Elderly Nursing Home Residents. *Art Therapy: Journal of the American Art Therapy Association*, *14*(3), 163–171. doi:10.1080/07421656.1987.10759277

Douglass, A., Walterfang, M., Velakoulis, D., & Abel, L. (2018). Behavioral Variant Frontotemporal Dementia Performance on a Range of Saccadic Tasks. *Journal of Alzheimer's Disease*, *65*(1), 231–242. doi:10.3233/JAD-170797 PMID:30040708

Dow, G. T., & Kozlowski, K. (2020, May 1). *The creative brain.* ASCD. https://www.ascd.org/el/articles/the-creative-brain

Drinko, C. (2021). *Play your way sane.* Simon & Schuster.

Dunlosky, J., Cavallini, E., Roth, H., McGuire, C. L., Vecchi, T., & Hertzog, C. (2007). Do self-monitoring interventions improve older adult learning? *The Journals of Gerontology: Series B*, *62*(Special_Issue_1), 70–76. doi:10.1093/geronb/62.special_issue_1.70

Eaton, L. G., Doherty, K. L., & Widrick, R. M. (2007). A review of research and methods used to establish art therapy as an effective treatment method for traumatized children. *The Arts in Psychotherapy*, *34*(3), 256–262. doi:10.1016/j.aip.2007.03.001

Edwards, D. (2004). *Art therapy*. Sage Publications.

Eekelaar, C., Camic, P. M., & Springham, N. (2012). Art galleries, episodic memory and verbal fluency in dementia: An exploratory study. *Psychology of Aesthetics, Creativity, and the Arts*, *6*(3), 262–272. APA PsycArticles. https://psycnet.apa.org/doi/10.1037/a0027499

*Effects of Art Therapy* 20. Petrillo, L. & Winner, E. (2005) Does Art Improve Mood? A Test of a Key Assumption Underlying Art Therapy. *Art Therapy, 22*(4), 205-212, doi:10.1080/07421656.2005.10129521

Egan, M. F., Kost, J., Voss, T., Mukai, Y., Aisen, P. S., Cummings, J. L., Tariot, P. N., Vellas, B., van Dyck, C. H., Boada, M., Zhang, Y., Li, W., Furtek, C., Mahoney, E., Harper Mozley, L., Mo, Y., Sur, C., & Michelson, D. (2019). Randomized Trial of Verubecestat for Prodromal Alzheimer's Disease. *The New England Journal of Medicine*, *380*(15), 1408–1420. doi:10.1056/NEJMoa1812840 PMID:30970186

Ehlers, A., & Clark, D. (2003). Early psychological interventions for adult survivors of trauma: A review. *Biological Psychiatry*, *53*(9), 817–826. doi:10.1016/S0006-3223(02)01812-7 PMID:12725974

Eli, K., & Lavis, A. (2021). Material environments and the shaping of anorexic embodiment: Towards a materialist account of eating disorders. *Culture, Medicine and Psychiatry*, *46*(2), 344–363. doi:10.100711013-021-09715-8 PMID:33826076

Emblad, S. Y. M., & Mukaetova-Ladinska, E. B.Emblad & Mukaetova-Ladinska. (2021). Creative Art Therapy as a Non-Pharmacological Intervention for Dementia: A Systematic Review. *Journal of Alzheimer's Disease Reports*, *5*(1), 353–364. doi:10.3233/ADR-201002 PMID:34189407

Erickson, B. (2008). *Art Therapy Treatment with Incarcerated Women.* [Doctoral Dissertation, University of Central Florida]. STARS.

Erickson, B. J. (2008). *Art therapy treatment with incarcerated women* [Unpublished doctoral dissertation, University of Central Florida].

Fallon, V. T., Rubenstein, S., Warfield, R., Ennerfelt, H., Hearn, B., & Leaver, E. (2020). Stress reduction from a musical intervention. *Psychomusicology: Music, Mind, and Brain*, *30*(1), 20–27. doi:10.1037/pmu0000246

Fan, D.-Y., & Wang, Y.-J. (2019). Early Intervention in Alzheimer's Disease: How Early is Early Enough? *Neuroscience Bulletin*, *36*(2), 195–197. doi:10.100712264-019-00429-x PMID:31494835

Federal Bureau of Prisons. (2023, February 25). *BOP Statistics: Average Inmate Age.* Federal Bureau of Prisons. https://www.bop.gov/about/statistics/statistics_inmate_age.jsp

Feen-Calligan, H., Mcintyre, B., & Sands-Goldstein, M. (2009). Art Therapy Applications of Dolls in Grief Recovery, Identity, and Community Service. *Art Therapy: Journal of the American Art Therapy Association*, *26*(4), 167–173. doi:10.1080/07421656.2009.10129613

Felitti, V. J., Anda, R. F., Nordenberg, D., Williamson, D. F., Spitz, A. M., Edwards, V., Koss, M. P., & Marks, J. S. (1998). Relationship of childhood abuse and household dysfunction to many of the leading causes of death in adults: The Adverse Childhood Experiences (ACE) Study. *American Journal of Preventive Medicine*, *14*(4), 245–258. doi:10.1016/S0749-3797(98)00017-8 PMID:9635069

Felsman, P., Gunawardena, S., & Seifert, C. M. (2020). Improv experience promotes divergent thinking, uncertainty tolerance, and affective well-being. *Thinking Skills and Creativity*, *35*, 100632. Advance online publication. doi:10.1016/j.tsc.2020.100632

Ferguson & Goosman. (1991). A foot in the door: Art therapy in the nursing home. *American Journal of Art Therapy*, *30*(1), 2–3. https://pubmed.ncbi.nlm.nih.gov/10114781/ PMID:10114781

Ferszt, G. G., Hayes, P. M., DeFedele, S., & Horn, L. (2004). Art therapy with incarcerated women who have experienced the death of a loved one. *Art Therapy: Journal of the American Art Therapy Association*, *21*(4), 191–199. doi:10.1080/07421656.2004.10129695

Fjell, A. M., McEvoy, L., Holland, D., Dale, A. M., & Walhovd, K. B. (2013). Brain Changes in Older Adults at Very Low Risk for Alzheimer's Disease. *The Journal of Neuroscience : The Official Journal of the Society for Neuroscience*, *33*(19), 8237–8242. doi:10.1523/JNEUROSCI.5506-12.2013 PMID:23658162

Fletcher, A. (2012). *Allegory: The theory of a symbolic mode*. Princeton University Press. doi:10.1515/9781400842049

Fonagy, P. (2012) Art Therapy and Personality Disorder. *International Journal of Art Therapy*, *17*(3), 90. doi:10.1080/17454832.2012.740866

Font, S. A., & Gershoff, E. T. (2020). Foster care: How we can, and should, do more for maltreated children. *Social Policy Report*, *33*(3), 1–40. doi:10.1002op2.10 PMID:33833492

Forsberg, L., & Douglas, T. (2020). What is Criminal Rehabilitation? *Criminal Law and Philosophy*, 1–24. doi:10.100711572-020-09547-4 PMID:35530429

Franks, B., & Fraenkel, D. (1991). Fairy tales and dance/movement therapy: Catalysts of change for eating-disordered individuals. *The Arts in Psychotherapy*, *18*(4), 311–319. doi:10.1016/0197-4556(91)90070-Q

Freedman, V. A., Cornman, J. C., & Kasper, J. D. (2021). *National Health and Aging Trends Study Trends Chart Book: Key Trends, Measures and Detailed Tables* (48th ed., Vol. 4). National Institute on Aging., https://micda.isr.umich.edu/research/nhats-trends-dashboards

Frewen, P., Thornley, E., Rabellino, D., & Lanius, R. (2017). Neuroimaging the traumatized self: fMRI reveals altered response in cortical midline structures and occipital cortex during visual and verbal self- and other-referential processing in women with PTSD. *European Journal of Psychotraumatology*, *8*(1), 1314164. doi:10.1080/20008198.2017.1314164 PMID:28649298

Frith, C., & Law, J.Frith & Law. (1995). Cognitive and Physiological Processes Underlying Drawing Skills. *Leonardo*, *28*(3), 203–205. https://muse.jhu.edu/pub/6/article/607018/summary. doi:10.2307/1576075

Frydman, J. S., & McLellan, L. U. C. Y. (2014). *Complex trauma and executive functioning: envisioning a cognitive-based, trauma-informed approach to drama therapy. In Trauma Informed Drama Therapy: Transforming Clinics, Classrooms, and Communities*. Thomas.

Gantt, L. M., & Anderson, F. (2009). The formal elements art therapy scale: A measurement system for global variables in art. *Art Therapy: Journal of the American Art Therapy Association*, *26*(3), 124–129. doi:10.1080/07421656.2009.10129372

Gao, L., Peranson, J., Nyhof-Young, J., Kapoor, E., & Rezmovitz, J. (2019). The role of "improv" in health professional learning: A scoping review. *Medical Teacher*, *41*(5), 561–568. doi:10.1080/0142159X.2018.1505033 PMID:30428747

Garai, J. (1984). New Horizons of Holistic Healing through Creative Expression. *Art Therapy: Journal of the American Art Therapy Association*, *1*(2), 76–82. doi:10.1080/07421656.1984.10758751

Gardner, H. (1974). *The shattered mind*. Vintage Books.

Garlock, L. R. (2016). Stories in the cloth: Art therapy and narrative textiles. *Art Therapy: Journal of the American Art Therapy Association*, *33*(2), 58–66. doi:10.1080/07421656.2016.1164004

Giano, Z., Wheeler, D. L., & Hubach, R. D. (2020). The frequencies and disparities of adverse childhood experiences in the U.S. *BMC Public Health*, *20*(1), 1327. doi:10.118612889-020-09411-z PMID:32907569

Glass, T. A., Leon, C. F. M. D., & Berkman, L. F. (2016). Social Engagement and Depressive Symptoms in Late Life: Longitudinal Findings. *Journal of Aging and Health*, *18*(4). Sage Journals. https://doi.org/ doi:10.1177/0898264306291017

Goemans, A., Geel, M. V., & Vedder, P. (2018). Foster children's behavioral development and foster parent stress: Testing a transactional model. *Journal of Child and Family Studies*, *27*(3), 990–1001. doi:10.100710826-017-0941-z PMID:29568216

Gold, K. J., & Marcus, S. M. (2008). Effect of maternal mental illness on pregnancy outcomes. *Expert Review of Obstetrics & Gynecology*, *3*(3), 391–401. doi:10.1586/17474108.3.3.391

Good Therapy. (2018, May 15). *Dance /Movement therapy (DMT)*. Dance/ Movement Therapy. https://www.goodtherapy.org/learn-about-therapy/types/dance-movement-therapy

Goodwin, R. D., Dierker, L. C., Wu, M., Galea, S., Hoven, C. W., & Weinberger, A. H. (2022). Trends in U.S. depression prevalence from 2015 to 2020: The widening treatment gap. *American Journal of Preventive Medicine*, *63*(5), 726–733. doi:10.1016/j.amepre.2022.05.014 PMID:36272761

Graves-Alcorn, S. L. (1994). *Expressions of healing: Embracing the process of grief.* Bookbaby.

Green, M. (2017, Mrs. 23). The History of Post-Traumatic Stress Disorder and How We Treat it. *Newsweek.*

Greene, A. H., Goldenberg, L., & Freundlich, M. (2009). The use of expressive therapies and social support with youth in foster care: The performing arts troupe. *Journal of Youth Development*, *4*(1), 1. doi:10.5195/jyd.2009.275

Griffiths, S., & Yager, Z. (2019). Gender, embodiment, and eating disorders. *The Journal of Adolescent Health*, *64*(4), 425–426. doi:10.1016/j.jadohealth.2019.01.016 PMID:30904090

Gross, J., & Haynes, H. (1998). Drawing facilitates children's verbal resorts of emotion laden events. *Journal of Experimental Psychology*, *4*, 163–179.

Guerra, C., Toro, E., Taylor, E. P., Lobos, P., & Pinto-Cortez, C. (2022). Design considerations for group interventions for adolescent victims of interpersonal violence in Chile. *Journal of Aggression, Maltreatment & Trauma*, *31*(10), 1318–1336. doi:10.1080/10926771.2022.2089864

Gussak, D. (2004). Art therapy with prison inmates: a pilot study. *Art Therapy with Prison Inmates: A Pilot Study, 31*(4), 245–259. https://pascal-francis.inist.fr/vibad/index.php?action=getRecordDetail&idt=16112574

Gussak, D. (2014). The Distinction Between Male and Female Inmates in Art Therapy. *Psychology Today*. https://www.psychologytoday.com/us/blog/art-trial/201401/the-distinctions-between-and-inmates-in-art-therapy

Gussak, D. (2016). Art Therapy in Prison Is Social Justice. *Psychology Today.* www.psychologytoday.com/gb/blog/art-trial/201602/art-therapy-in-prison-is-social-justice

Gussak, D. (2004). Art therapy with prison inmates: A pilot study. *The Arts in Psychotherapy*, *31*(4), 245–259. doi:10.1016/j.aip.2004.06.001

Gussak, D. (2006). Effects of art therapy with prison inmates: A follow-up study. *The Arts in Psychotherapy*, *33*(3), 188–198. doi:10.1016/j.aip.2005.11.003

Gussak, D. (2009). Comparing the effectiveness of art therapy on depression and locus of control of male and female inmates. *The Arts in Psychotherapy*, *36*(4), 202–207. doi:10.1016/j.aip.2009.02.004

Gussak, D. (2009). The effects of art therapy on male and female inmates: Advancing the research base. *The Arts in Psychotherapy*, *36*(1), 5–12. doi:10.1016/j.aip.2008.10.002

Gussak, D. E., & Rosal, M. L. (Eds.). (2016). *The Wiley Handbook of Art Therapy*. John Wiley & Sons, Inc.

Ha, B. C., & Robinson, G. (2011). Chronic care model implementation in the California state prison system. *Journal of Correctional Health Care, 17*(2), 173–182. doi:10.1177/1078345810396859 PMID:21525120

Haber, D. (2006). Life review: Implementation, theory, research, and therapy. *International Journal of Aging & Human Development, 63*(2), 153–171. doi:10.2190/DA9G-RHK5-N9JP-T6CC PMID:17137032

Habib, H. A., & Ali, U. (2015). Efficacy of Art Therapy in the Reduction of Impulsive Behaviors of Children with ADHD Co-Morbid Intellectual Disability. *Pakistan Journal of Psychology, 46*(2). http://pjpku.com/index.php/pjp/article/view/72

Haeyen, S., Chakhssi, F., & Van Hooren, S. (2020). Benefits of Art Therapy in People Diagnosed With Personality Disorders: A Quantitative Survey. *Frontiers in Psychology, 11*, 686. https://doi.org/https://doi.org/10.3389/fpsyg.2020.00686. doi:10.3389/fpsyg.2020.00686 PMID:32351431

Halpern, C., Close, D., & Johnson, K. (1994). *Truth in comedy: The manual of improvisation*. Meriwether Publishing.

Hanes, M. J. (2008). Signs of suicide: Using road drawings with inmates on suicide observation at a county jail. *Art Therapy: Journal of the American Art Therapy Association, 25*(2), 78–84. doi:10.1080/07421656.2008.10129418

Hanevik, H., Hestad, K. A., Lien, L., Teglbjaerg, H. S., & Danbolt, L. J. (2013) Expressive art therapy for psychosis: A multiple case study. *The Arts in Psychotherapy, 40*(3), 312- 321. doi:10.1016/j.aip.2013.05.011

Hannemann (2006). Creativity with Dementia Patients. *Gerontology, 52*(1), 59–65. https://doi.org/ doi:10.1159/000089827

Harlan, B. (1993). The Therapeutic Value of Art for Persons with Alzheimer's Disease and Related Disorders. In M. Lahey, R. Kunstler, A. Grossman, F. Daly, S. Waldman, & F. Schwartz (Eds.), *Recreation, Leisure and Chronic Illness*. Routledge. https://www.taylorfrancis.com/chapters/edit/10.4324/9780203058046-13/therapeutic-value-art-persons-alzheimer-disease-related-disorders-jane-harlan

Harner, H. M., & Riley, S. (2013). The impact of incarceration on Women's mental health: Responses from women in a maximum-security prison. *Qualitative Health Research, 23*(1), 26–42. doi:10.1177/1049732312461452 PMID:23034774

Hartley, L., & Hartley, L. (2004). *Somatic psychology: Body, mind and meaning*. Whurr.

Hasanah, I., Mulatsih, S., Haryanti, F., & Haikal, Z. Effect of music therapy on cortisol as a stress biomarker in children undergoing IV-line insertion. *Journal of Taibah University Medical Sciences, 15*(3), 238-243. https://www.sciencedirect.com/science/article/pii/S1658361220300421

Hass-Cohen, N., & Carr, R. (Eds.). (2008). *Art therapy and clinical neuroscience*. Jessica Kingsley.

Hass-Cohen, N., & Findlay, J. C. (2009). Pain, attachment, and meaning making: Report on an art therapy relational neuroscience assessment protocol. *The Arts in Psychotherapy, 36*(4), 175–184. doi:10.1016/j.aip.2009.02.003

Hays & Lyons. (1981). The bridge drawing: A projective technique for assessment in art therapy. *The Arts in Psychotherapy, 8*(3-4), 207–217. APA PsycInfo. https://psycnet.apa.org/record/1982-26187-001

Heidenreich, V. (2005). Music therapy in war-effected areas. *Intervention, 3*(2), 129–134.

Henderson, P., Rosen, D., & Mascaro, N. (2007). Empirical study on the healing nature of mandalas. *Psychology of Aesthetics, Creativity, and the Arts, 1*(3), 148–154. doi:10.1037/1931-3896.1.3.148

Henley, D. (2007). Naming the Enemy: An Art Therapy Intervention for Children with Bipolar and Comorbid Disorders. *Art Therapy: Journal of the American Art Therapy Association, 24*(3), 104–110. doi:10.1080/07421656.2007.10129421

Herman, J. (2023). *Truth and repair: How trauma survivors envision justice*. Basic Books.

Herman, J. L. (1992). *Trauma and Recovery*. Basic Books.

Hillen, M. A., Gutheil, C. M., Strout, T. D., Smets, E. M., & Han, P. K. (2017). Tolerance of uncertainty: Conceptual analysis, integrative model, and implications for healthcare. *Social Science & Medicine, 180*, 62–75. doi:10.1016/j.socscimed.2017.03.024 PMID:28324792

Ho, B. (2012). *The Effect of Art Therapy Chinese Seniors' Quality of Life in a Residential Setting*. Tati. https://www.tati.on.ca/wp-content/uploads/2012/02/Thesis-Proposal-Bonnie-Ho.docx

Holochwost, S. J., Goldstein, T. R., & Wolf, D. P. (2021). Delineating the benefits of arts education for children's socioemotional development. *Frontiers in Psychology, 12*, 624712. doi:10.3389/fpsyg.2021.624712 PMID:34054643

Holston, M. (2004). Paintings of the psyche: An innovative hospital program and museum in Rio has nurtured highly acclaimed artists while revealing the healing power of art. *Americas, 56*(2), 6–13. ProQuest. https://www.proquest.com/docview/1797187731/fulltextPDF/374255DB71A54315PQ/4?accountid=10226

Homer, E. (2015). Piece work: Fabric collage as a neurodevelopmental approach to trauma treatment. *Art Therapy: Journal of the American Art Therapy Association, 32*(1), 20–26. doi:10.1080/07421656.2015.992824

Hongo, A., Katz, A., & Valenti, K. (2015). Art: Trauma to Therapy for Aging Female Prisoners. *Traumatology*, *21*(3), 201–207. https://www.researchgate.net/publication/281537684_Art_Trauma_to_Therapy_for_Aging_Female_Prisoners. doi:10.1037/trm0000042

Hosea, H. (2006). The Brush's Footmarks": Parents and infants paint together in a small community art therapy group. *International Journal of Art Therapy*, *11*(2), 69–78. doi:10.1080/17454830600980317

Howe, D. (1999). Attachment theory. *Social Work Theories and Methods*, 75.

Huang, S. (2020, Nov 3). *Attachment styles.* Simply Psychology. www.simplypsychology.org/attachment-styles.html

Hudson, A. L. (2013). Career mentoring needs of youths in foster care: Voices for change. *Journal of Child and Adolescent Psychiatric Nursing*, *26*(2), 131–137. doi:10.1111/jcap.12032 PMID:23607825

Hughes, K. C., & Shin, L. M. (2011). Functional neuroimaging studies of post-traumatic stress disorder. *Expert Review of Neurotherapeutics*, *11*(2), 275–285. doi:10.1586/ern.10.198 PMID:21306214

Ignacio, A., & Cupchik, G. (2021). Therapeutic benefits of adult doll play. *Imagination, Cognition and Personality*, *41*(1), 5–30.. doi:10.1177/0276236621989227

Ikonomopoulos, J., Cavazos-Vela, J., Vela, P., Sanchez, M., Schmidt, C., & Catchings, C. V. (2017). Evaluating the effects of creative journal arts therapy for survivors of domestic violence. *Journal of Creativity in Mental Health*, *12*(4), 496–512. doi:10.1080/15401383.2017.1328290

Ilali, E. S., Mokhtary, F., Mousavinasab, N., & Tirgari, A. H. (2018). Impact of art-based life review on depression symptoms among older adults. *Art Therapy: Journal of the American Art Therapy Association*, *35*(3), 148–155. doi:10.1080/07421656.2018.1531276

Improv Therapy Group. (2022). *Our mission.* Improv Therapy Group. https://improvtherapygroup.com/empathy-emotional-intelligence/

Jacobsen, H., Bergsund, H. B., Wentzel, T., Smith, L. L., & Moe, V. (2020). Foster children are at risk for developing problems in social-emotional functioning: A follow-up study at 8 years of age. *Children and Youth Services Review*, *108*, 104603. doi:10.1016/j.childyouth.2019.104603

James, D., & Glaze, L. (2006). *Mental health problems of prisons and jail inmates*. U.S. Department of Justice. http://bjs.ojp.usdoj.gov/content/pub/pdf/mhppji.pdf

Jett, L. (2018). Nursing Homes with Dementia Special Care Units Provide Better Quality of Care. *Harvard Medical School*. https://hcp.hms.harvard.edu/news/nursing-homes-dementia-special-care-units-provide-better-quality-care

Johnson, L. M. (2007). Jail wall drawings and jail art programs. *International Journal of Criminal Justice Sciences*, *2*(2), 66–84. https://citeseerx.ist.psu.edu/document?repid=rep1&type=pdf&doi=5368e93862bd61fd4898fa6de09cde0bb100273b

Johnson, L. M. (2007). Jail Wall Drawings and Jail Art Programs: Invaluable Tools for Corrections. *International Journal of Criminal Justice*, *2*(2), 66–84. https://www.sascv.org/ijcjs/jhonsonijcjsjuly2007.pdf

Joyce, N. R., McGuire, T. G., Bartels, S. J., Mitchell, S. L., & Grabowski, D. C. (2018). The Impact of Dementia Special Care Units on Quality of Care: An Instrumental Variables Analysis. *Health Services Research*, *53*(5), 3657–3679. doi:10.1111/1475-6773.12867 PMID:29736944

Junge, M. B. (2010). *The modern history of art therapy in the United States*. Charles C Thomas Publisher.

Kahn-Denis, K. B. (1997). Art Therapy with Geriatric Dementia Clients. *Art Therapy: Journal of the American Art Therapy Association*, *14*(3), 194–199. doi:10.1080/07421656.1987.10759281

Kaimal, G., & Arslanbek, A. (2020). Indigenous and traditional visual artistic practices: Implications for art therapy clinical practice and research. *Frontiers in Psychology*, *11*, 1320. doi:10.3389/fpsyg.2020.01320 PMID:32612560

Kaimal, G., & Ray, K. (2016). Free art-making in an art therapy open studio: Changes in affect and self-efficacy. *Arts & Health*, *9*(2), 154–166. doi:10.1080/17533015.2016.1217248

Kamar, O. (1997). Light and death: Art therapy with a patient with - ProQuest. *American Journal of Art Therapy*, *35*(4). ProQuest. https://www.proquest.com/docview/199488748?pq-origsite=gscholar&fromopenview=true

Kandarakis, E., Bourguignon, J., Giudice, L., Hauser, R., Prins, G., Soto, A., Zoeller, R. T., & Gore, A. (2009). Endocrine-disrupting chemicals: an endocrine society scientific statement. *National Library of Medicine*, *30*(4), 293-342, https://www.ncbi.nlm.nih.gov/pmc/articles/PMC2726844/

Kapitan, L., Litell, M., & Torres, A. (2011). Creative art therapy in a community's participatory research and social transformation. *Art Therapy: Journal of the American Art Therapy Association*, *28*(2), 64–73. doi:10.1080/07421656.2011.578238

Karlsson, M. E., & Zielinski, M. J. (2020). Sexual Victimization and Mental Illness Prevalence Rates Among Incarcerated Women: A Literature Review. *Trauma, Violence & Abuse*, *21*(2), 326–349. doi:10.1177/1524838018767933 PMID:29661117

Katzman, J., & O'Connor, D. (2018). *Life unscripted: Using improv principles to get unstuck, boost confidence and transform your life*. North Atlantic Books.

Kaye, J. A., Swihart, T., Howieson, D., Dame, A., Moore, M. M., Karnos, T., Camicioli, R., Ball, M., Oken, B., & Sexton, G. (1997). Volume loss of the hippocampus and temporal lobe in healthy elderly persons destined to develop dementia. *Neurology*, *48*(5), 1297–1304. doi:10.1212/WNL.48.5.1297 PMID:9153461

Kedem-Tahar, E., & Felix-Kellermann, P. (1996). Psychodrama and drama therapy: A comparison. *The Arts in Psychotherapy, 23*(1), 27–36. doi:10.1016/0197-4556(95)00059-3

Kiely, D. K., Simon, S. E., Jones, R. N., & Morris, J. N. (2000). The Protective Effect of Social Engagement on Mortality in Long-Term Care. *Journal of the American Geriatrics Society, 48*(11), 1367–1372. doi:10.1111/j.1532-5415.2000.tb02624.x PMID:11083310

Kifer, M., Hemmens, C., & Stohr, M. K. (2003). The Goals of corrections: Perspectives from the line. *Criminal Justice Review, 28*(1), 47–69. doi:10.1177/073401680302800104

Killick, K., & Schaverien, J. (1997). *Art, Psychotherapy, and Psychosis*. Routledge.

Kim, H.-K., Kim, K. M., & Nomura, S. (2016). The effect of group art therapy on older Korean adults with neurocognitive disorders. *The Arts in Psychotherapy, 47*, 48–54. doi:10.1016/j.aip.2015.11.002

Kim, S.-Y., Lee, J. S., & Choi, H. (2023). The Effects of art therapy on anxiety and distress for Korean–Ukrainian refugee: Quasi-experimental design study. *Health Care, 11*(4), 466. doi:10.3390/healthcare11040466 PMID:36833000

Kira, I. A., Ahmed, A., Wasim, F., Mahmoud, V., Colrain, J., & Rai, D. (2012). Group therapy for refugees and torture survivors: Treatment model innovations. *International Journal of Group Psychotherapy, 62*(1), 69–88. doi:10.1521/ijgp.2012.62.1.69 PMID:22229369

Kirk, A. B., & Madden, L. L. (2003). Trauma related critical incident debriefing for adolescents. *Child & Adolescent Social Work Journal, 20*(2), 123–134. doi:10.1023/A:1022816731082

Klein. (1987). When the brain betrays the body. *Tel Aviv: Sifriat HaPoalim.*

Kochersberger, G., Hielema, F., & Westlund, R. (1994). Rehabilitation in the nursing home: how much, why, and with what results. *Public Health Reports (Washington, D.C: 1974), 109*(3), 372–376. https://www.ncbi.nlm.nih.gov/pmc/articles/PMC1403501/?page=3

Koch, S. C., Mehl, L., Sobanski, E., Sieber, M., & Fuchs, T. (2015). Fixing the mirrors: A feasibility study of the effects of dance movement therapy on young adults with autism spectrum disorder. *Autism, 19*(3), 338–350. doi:10.1177/1362361314522353 PMID:24566716

Kolanowski, A., & Litaker, M.Kolanowski & Litaker. (2006). Social Interaction, Premorbid Personality, and Agitation in Nursing Home Residents With Dementia. *Archives of Psychiatric Nursing, 20*(1), 12–20. doi:10.1016/j.apnu.2005.08.006 PMID:16442470

Kolb, B., & Whishaw, I. Q. (1998). Brain Plasticity and Behavior. *Annual Review of Psychology, 49*(1), 43–64. doi:10.1146/annurev.psych.49.1.43 PMID:9496621

Kometiani, M. K., & Farmer, K. W. (2020). Exploring resilience through case studies of art therapy with sex trafficking survivors and their advocates. *The Arts in Psychotherapy, 67*, 101582. doi:10.1016/j.aip.2019.101582

Koontz, A. (2019, March). The circuitry of creativity: How our brains innovate thinking. *Cal Tech Letters*.

Kovach, C. R., Noonan, P. E., Schlidt, A. M., & Wells, T. (2005). A Model of Consequences of Need-Driven, Dementia-Compromised Behavior. *Journal of Nursing Scholarship, 37*(2), 134–140. Sigma. https://doi.org/ doi:10.1111/j.1547-5069.2005.00025_1.x

Kraft, K. E., Jaschke, A. C., Ravensbergen, A. G., Feenstra-Weelink, A., van Goor, M., de Kroon, M., Reijneveld, S. A., Bos, A. F., & van Dokkum, N. H. (2021). Maternal anxiety, infant stress, and the role of live-performed music therapy during NICU stay in the Netherlands. *International Journal of Environmental Research and Public Health, 18*(13), 7077. doi:10.3390/ijerph18137077 PMID:34281014

Kramer, O. (2001). Art as Therapy: Collected Papers. In *Google Books*. Jessica Kingsley Publishers.

Kramer, E. (1958). *Art therapy in a children's community: A study of the function of art therapy in the treatment program of Wiltwyck School for Boys*. Charles C Thomas Publisher.

Krantz, A. M. (1999). Growing into Her Body: Dance/Movement therapy for women with eating disorders. *American Journal of Dance Therapy, 21*(2), 81–103. doi:10.1023/A:1022104603189

Krueger, D. W., & Schofield, E. (1986). Dance/movement therapy of eating disordered patients: A model. *The Arts in Psychotherapy, 13*(4), 323–331. doi:10.1016/0197-4556(86)90033-X

Krystyniak, J. (2020). *The Use of Dolls and Figures in Therapy: A Literature Review*. [Thesis, Lesley University]. 321. https://digitalcommons.lesley.edu/expressive_theses/321

Kudrowitz, B. M. (2010). *Haha and aha!: Creativity, idea generation, improvisational humor, and product design* (Unpublished doctoral dissertation). Massachusetts Institute of Technology, Massachusetts.

Lagorio, R. (1989). Art therapy for battered women. *Advances in Art Therapy*, 92-113.

Landreth, G. L. (2002). *Play therapy: The art of the relationship* (2nd ed.). Brunner-Routledge.

Landy, R. J. (2003). Drama therapy with adults. *Play Therapy with Adults*, 15-33.

Larrieu, S., Letenneur, L., Orgogozo, J. M., Fabrigoule, C., Amieva, H., Le Carret, N., Barberger-Gateau, P., & Dartigues, J. F. (2002). Incidence and outcome of mild cognitive impairment in a population-based prospective cohort. *Neurology, 59*(10), 1594–1599. doi:10.1212/01.WNL.0000034176.07159.F8 PMID:12451203

Lavik, E. (2021). Thermo in the Time of COVID-19: Using improvisation to foster discussion and translating the experience to online learning. *Biomedical Engineering Education, 1*(1), 133–138. doi:10.100743683-020-00022-z PMID:35141717

Lee, K. H., Boltz, M., Lee, H., & Algase, D. L. (2017). Does Social Interaction Matter Psychological Well-Being in Persons With Dementia? *American Journal of Alzheimer's Disease and Other Dementias, 32*(4), 207–212. doi:10.1177/1533317517704301 PMID:28417644

Lee, S.-Y. (2013). "Flow" in art therapy: Empowering immigrant children with adjustment difficulties. *Art Therapy: Journal of the American Art Therapy Association, 30*(2), 56–63. doi:10.1080/07421656.2013.786978

Lee, S.-Y. (2015). Flow indicators in art therapy: Artistic engagement of immigrant children with acculturation gaps. *Art Therapy: Journal of the American Art Therapy Association, 32*(3), 120–129. doi:10.1080/07421656.2015.1060836

Lefebvre, A. D. (2008). *Art Therapy Interventions with an Adolescent with Bipolar Disorder.* [Thesis, Ohio]. OhioLINK Electronic Theses and Dissertations Center. https://rave.ohiolink.edu/etdc/view?acc_num=urs1210794791

Lemons, G. (2005). When the horse drinks: Enhancing everyday creativity using elements of improvisation. *Creativity Research Journal, 17*(1), 25–36. doi:10.120715326934crj1701_3

Levenson, J. S., & Willis, G. M. (2019). Implementing trauma-informed care in correctional treatment and supervision. *Journal of Aggression, Maltreatment & Trauma, 28*(4), 481–501. doi:10.1080/10926771.2018.1531959

Leveson, M., & Patterson, D. (Creators). (1998). Whose line is it anyway? [Television series]. Hollywood, CA: Hat Trick Productions.

Levine-Madori. (2013). Utilizing a thematic approach to art therapy with seniors: Enhancing cognitive abilities and social interactions. In P. Howie, S. Prasad, & J. Kristel (Eds.), *Using Art Therapy with Diverse Populations: Crossing Cultures and Abilities* (pp. 317–327). Jessica Kingsley Publishers.

Lewinsohn, P. M., Seeley, J. R., Roberts, R. E., & Allen, N. B. (1997). Center for Epidemiological Studies-Depression Scale (CES-D) as a screening instrument for depression among community-residing older adults. *Psychology and Aging, 12*(2), 277–287. doi:10.1037/0882-7974.12.2.277 PMID:9189988

Lewis, C., & Lovatt, P. J. (2013). Breaking away from set patterns of thinking: Improvisation and divergent thinking. *Thinking Skills and Creativity, 9*, 46–58. doi:10.1016/j.tsc.2013.03.001

Lie, D. C., Song, H., Colamarino, S. A., Ming, G., & Gage, F. H. (2004). Neurogenesis in the Adult Brain: New Strategies for Central Nervous System Diseases. *Annual Review of Pharmacology and Toxicology, 44*(1), 399–421. doi:10.1146/annurev.pharmtox.44.101802.121631 PMID:14744252

Linden, D. E. (2006). How psychotherapy changes the brain – the contribution of functional neuroimaging. *Molecular Psychiatry, 11*(6), 528–538. doi:10.1038j.mp.4001816 PMID:16520823

Lindquist, L. A., Liggett, A., Muhammad, R., Seltzer, A., Kim, K. Y. A., Barish, B., & Ramirez-Zohfeld, V. (2021). Effects of improv training on older adults in a long term care facility. *Gerontology & Geriatric Medicine, 7*. doi:10.1177/23337214211016111 PMID:34104682

Linehan, M. M. (1997). Validation and psychotherapy. In A. C. Bohart & L. S. Greenberg (Eds.), *Empathy reconsidered: New directions in psychotherapy* (pp. 353–392). American Psychological Association. doi:10.1037/10226-016

Linesch, D., Quezada, P., Acevedes, P., Trochez, M., & Zuniga, E. (2012). An art therapy exploration with Latino families. *Art Therapy: Journal of the American Art Therapy Association*, *29*(3), 120–126. doi:10.1080/07421656.2012.701603

Liu, H., Zhang, Z., Choi, S., & Langa, K. M. (2020). Marital Status and Dementia: Evidence from the Health and Retirement Study. *The Journals of Gerontology. Series B, Psychological Sciences and Social Sciences*, *75*(8), 1783–1795. doi:10.1093/geronb/gbz087 PMID:31251349

Loewenstein, D. A., Acevedo, A., Czaja, S. J., & Duara, R. (2004). Cognitive Rehabilitation of Mildly Impaired Alzheimer Disease Patients on Cholinesterase Inhibitors. *The American Journal of Geriatric Psychiatry*, *12*(4), 395–402. doi:10.1097/00019442-200407000-00007 PMID:15249277

Logsdon, R. G., McCurry, S. M., & Teri, L. (2008). Time-Limited Support Groups for Individuals with Early Stage Dementia and Their Care Partners. *Clinical Gerontologist*, *30*(2), 5–19. Taylor & Francis Online. doi:10.1300/J018v30n02_02

Luanaigh, C. Ó., & Lawlor, B. A. (2008). Loneliness and the health of older people. *International Journal of Geriatric Psychiatry*, *23*(12), 1213–1221. doi:10.1002/gps.2054 PMID:18537197

Lusebrink, V. (2004). Art Therapy and the Brain: An Attempt to Understand the Underlying Processes of Art Expression in Therapy. *Art Therapy: Journal of the American Art Therapy Association*, *21*(3), 125–135. doi:10.1080/07421656.2004.10129496

Lyshak-Stelzer, F., Singer, P., Patricia, S. J., & Chemtob, C. M. (2007). Art therapy for adolescents with posttraumatic stress disorder symptoms: A pilot study. *Art Therapy: Journal of the American Art Therapy Association*, *24*(4), 163–169. doi:10.1080/07421656.2007.10129474

Mahncke, H. W., Connor, B. B., Appelman, J., Ahsanuddin, O. N., Hardy, J. L., Wood, R. A., Joyce, N. M., Boniske, T., Atkins, S. M., & Merzenich, M. M. (2006). Memory enhancement in healthy older adults using a brain plasticity-based training program: A randomized, controlled study. *Proceedings of the National Academy of Sciences of the United States of America*, *103*(33), 12523–12528. doi:10.1073/pnas.0605194103 PMID:16888038

Malchiodi, C. A. (2003). Art therapy and the brain. Handbook of Art Therapy, 16-24.

Malchiodi, C. (2003). *Handbook of art therapy*. The Guilford Press.

Malchiodi, C. A. (2012). *Handbook of Art Therapy*. The Guilford Press.

Maslow, A. H. (1943). A theory of human motivation. *Psychological Review*, *50*(4), 370–396. doi:10.1037/h0054346

Mayeux, R., & Stern, Y. (2012). Epidemiology of Alzheimer Disease. *Cold Spring Harbor Perspectives in Medicine*, *2*(8), a006239–a006239. doi:10.1101/cshperspect.a006239 PMID:22908189

McGarry, L. M., & Russo, F. A. (2011). Mirroring in dance/movement therapy: Potential mechanisms behind empathy enhancement. *The Arts in Psychotherapy*, *38*(3), 178–184. doi:10.1016/j.aip.2011.04.005

McGinn, T., Taylor, B., McColgan, M., & Lagdon, S. (2016). Survivor Perspectives on IPV Perpetrator Interventions: A Systematic Narrative Review. *Trauma, Violence & Abuse*, *17*(3), 239–255. doi:10.1177/1524838015584358 PMID:25964277

McLeod, S. A. (2018, May 21). *Maslow's hierarchy of needs.* Simply Psychology. https://www.simplypsychology.org/maslow.html

McNeilly, G. (1983). Directive and non-directive approaches in art therapy. *The Arts in Psychotherapy*, *10*(4), 211–219. https://psycnet.apa.org/record/1984-23708-001. doi:10.1016/0197-4556(83)90021-7

Meekums, B. (2005). Responding to the embodiment of distress in individuals defined as obese: Implications for research. *Counselling & Psychotherapy Research*, *5*(3), 246–255. doi:10.1080/17441690500317119

Meekums, B., Vaverniece, I., Majore-Dusele, I., & Rasnacs, O. (2012). Dance movement therapy for obese women with emotional eating: A controlled pilot study. *The Arts in Psychotherapy*, *39*(2), 126–133. doi:10.1016/j.aip.2012.02.004

Mendis, K., Gardner, F., & Lehmann, J. (2015). The education of children in out-of-home care. *Australian Social Work*, *68*(4), 483–496. doi:10.1080/0312407X.2014.963134

Merriam, A. E., Aronson, M. K., Gaston, P., Wey, S.-L., & Katz, I. (1988). The Psychiatric Symptoms of Alzheimer's Disease. *Journal of the American Geriatrics Society*, *36*(1), 7–22. doi:10.1111/j.1532-5415.1988.tb03427.x PMID:3335733

Merrick, M. T., Ford, D. C., Ports, K. A., Guinn, A. S., Chen, J., Klevens, J., Metzler, M., Jones, C. M., Simon, T. R., Daniel, V. M., Ottley, P., & Mercy, J. A. (2019). Vital signs: Estimated proportion of adult health problems attributable to adverse childhood experiences and implications for prevention — 25 States, 2015–2017. *MMWR. Morbidity and Mortality Weekly Report*, *68*(44), 999–1005. doi:10.15585/mmwr.mm6844e1 PMID:31697656

Mignon, S. (2016). Health issues of incarcerated women in the United States. *Ciencia & Saude Coletiva*, *21*(7), 2051–2060. doi:10.1590/1413-81232015217.05302016 PMID:27383339

Miller. (1984). Art therapy with the elderly and the terminally ill. In *Art as Therapy* (pp. 128–129).

Miller, N. A., & Najavits, L. M. (2012). Creating trauma-informed correctional care: A balance of goals and environment. *European Journal of Psychotraumatology*, *3*(1), 17246. doi:10.3402/ejpt.v3i0.17246 PMID:22893828

Milman, D., & Goldman, G. (1987). *Techniques of Working with Resistance*. Jason Aronson.

Milton, A., Hambleton, A., Roberts, A., Davenport, T., Flego, A., Burns, J., & Hickie, I. (2021). Body-image distress and its associations from an international sample of men and women across the adult life span: Web-based survey study. *JMIR Formative Research*, *5*(11), e25329. Advance online publication. doi:10.2196/25329 PMID:34734831

Mitchell, S. L., Mor, V., Gozalo, P. L., Servadio, J. L., & Teno, J. M. (2016). Tube Feeding in US Nursing Home Residents With Advanced Dementia, 2000-2014. *Journal of the American Medical Association, 316*(7), 769. doi:10.1001/jama.2016.9374 PMID:27533163

Montag, C., Haase, L., Seidel, D., Bayerl, M., Gallinat, J., Herrmann, U., & Dannecker, K. (2014). A pilot RCT of psychodynamic group art therapy for patients in acute psychotic episodes: Feasibility, impact on symptoms and mentalizing capacity. *PLoS One, 9*(11), e112348. doi:10.1371/journal.pone.0112348 PMID:25393414

Monti, D. A., Peterson, C., Kunkel, E. J. S., Hauck, W. W., Pequignot, E., Rhodes, L., & Brainard, G. C. (2006). A randomized, controlled trial of mindfulness-based art therapy (MBAT) for women with cancer. *Psycho-Oncology, 15*(5), 363–373. doi:10.1002/pon.988 PMID:16288447

Moreno, J. L. (1946). Psychodrama and group psychotherapy. *Sociometry, 9*(2/3), 249–253. doi:10.2307/2785011

Morinville, A., Miranda, D., & Gaudreau, P. (2013). Music listening motivation is associated with global happiness in Canadian late adolescents. *Psychology of Aesthetics, Creativity, and the Arts, 7*(4), 384–390. doi:10.1037/a0034495

Morrissey, J. P., Steadman, H. J., Dalton, K. M., Cuellar, A., Stiles, P., & Cuddeback, G. S. (2006). Medicaid enrollment and mental health service use following release of jail detainees with severe mental illness. *Psychiatric Services (Washington, D.C.), 57*(6), 809–815. doi:10.1176/ps.2006.57.6.809 PMID:16754757

Morse, L. A., Xiong, L., Ramirez-Zohfeld, V., Anne, S., Barish, B., & Lindquist, L. A. (2018). Humor doesn't retire: Improvisation as a health-promoting intervention for older adults. *Archives of Gerontology and Geriatrics, 75*, 1–5. doi:10.1016/j.archger.2017.10.013 PMID:29156247

Mor, V., Branco, K., Fleishman, J., Hawes, C., Phillips, C., Morris, J., & Fries, B. (1995). The Structure of Social Engagement among Nursing Home Residents. *The Journals of Gerontology. Series B, Psychological Sciences and Social Sciences, 50B*(1), 1–P8. doi:10.1093/geronb/50B.1.P1 PMID:7757818

Moya-Raggio, E. (1984). —Arpilleras||: Chilean culture of resistance. *Feminist Studies, 10*(2), 277–290. doi:10.2307/3177867

Mujica, B. (1997). Tapestries of hope, threads of love: The arpillera movement in Chile 1974-1994/Ashes of revolt. *Americas, 49*(5), 62–63.

Murman, D. (2015). The impact of age on cognition. *Seminars in Hearing, 36*(03), 111–121. doi:10.1055-0035-1555115 PMID:27516712

Myers, D. G. (2015). Psychology (11th edition in modules). New York: Worth Publishers. .

Nair, S., McGreevy, J. E., Hutchinson-Colas, J., Turock, H., Chervenak, F., & Bachmann, G. (2021). Pregnancy in incarcerated women: Need for national legislation to standardize care. *Journal of Perinatal Medicine, 49*(7), 830–836. doi:10.1515/jpm-2021-0145 PMID:34167182

Najavits, L. (2002). *Seeking safety: A treatment manual for PTSD and substance abuse*. Guilford Press.

Nambiar, N., & Joy, M. (2020). Impact of Art Therapy on Emotional Wellness among Incarcerated Women. *International Journal for Research in Engineering Application & Management*, *6*(3), 1–6.

Nash, J. (2022, October 16). *Expressive arts therapy: 15 Creative Activities and Techniques*. PositivePsychology.com. https://positivepsychology.com/expressive-arts-therapy/

National Institute on Aging. (2017). *What Happens to the Brain in Alzheimer's Disease?* National Institute on Aging. https://www.nia.nih.gov/health/what-happens-brain-alzheimers-disease

National Institute on Aging. (2018). *How Is Alzheimer's Disease Treated?* National Institute on Aging. https://www.nia.nih.gov/health/how-alzheimers-disease-treated

Novotney, A. (2013). Music as medicine. *American Psychological Association, 44*(10), 46. https://www.apa.org/monitor/2013/11/music

Oren, E. M. D. R., & Solomon, R. (2012). EMDR therapy: An overview of its development and mechanisms of action. *European Review of Applied Psychology*, *62*(4), 197–203. doi:10.1016/j.erap.2012.08.005

Packard, S. (1980). The history of art therapy education. *Art Education*, *33*(4), 10–13. doi:10.2307/3192416

Palmiero, M., Di Giacomo, D., & Passafiume, D. (2012). Creativity and dementia: A review. *Cognitive Processing*, *13*(3), 193–209. doi:10.100710339-012-0439-y PMID:22438178

Panza, F., Lozupone, M., Sardone, R., Battista, P., Piccininni, M., Dibello, V., La Montagna, M., Stallone, R., Venezia, P., Liguori, A., Giannelli, G., Bellomo, A., Greco, A., Daniele, A., Seripa, D., Quaranta, N., & Logroscino, G. (2018). Sensorial frailty: Age-related hearing loss and the risk of cognitive impairment and dementia in later life. *Therapeutic Advances in Chronic Disease*, *10*, 204062231881100. doi:10.1177/2040622318811000 PMID:31452865

Paula, J. J., Albuquerque, M. R., Lage, G. M., Bicalho, M. A., Romano-Silva, M. A., & Malloy-Diniz, L. F. (2016). Impairment of fine motor dexterity in mild cognitive impairment and Alzheimer's disease dementia: Association with activities of daily living. *Revista Brasileira de Psiquiatria (Sao Paulo, Brazil)*, *38*(3), 235–238. doi:10.1590/1516-4446-2015-1874 PMID:27508398

Perey, I., & Cook-Cottone, C. (2020). Eating disorders, embodiment, and yoga: A conceptual overview. *Eating Disorders*, *28*(4), 315–329. doi:10.1080/10640266.2020.1771167 PMID:32964817

Peterson, C. (2014). Mindfulness-based art therapy. *Mindfulness and the art therapies. Theory into Practice*, 42–58.

Phillips Sheesley, A., Pfeffer, M., & Barish, B. (2016). Comedic improv therapy for the treatment of social anxiety disorder. *Journal of Creativity in Mental Health, 11*(2), 157–169.

Pifalo, T. (2006). Art therapy with sexually abused children and adolescents: Extended research study. *Art Therapy: Journal of the American Art Therapy Association, 23*(4), 181–185. doi:10.1080/07421656.2006.10129337

Pifalo, T. (2007). Jogging the cogs: Trauma-focused art therapy and cognitive behavior therapy with sexually abused children. *Art Therapy: Journal of the American Art Therapy Association, 24*(4), 170–175. doi:10.1080/07421656.2007.10129471

Poissant, D. (2018). 'Yes, and': Overcoming anxiety with improv. *UCF Forum,* 1-4.

Potter, L. M., Grealy, M. A., & O'Connor, R. C. (2009). Healthy ageing, perceived motor-efficacy, and performance on cognitively demanding action tasks. *British Journal of Psychology, 100*(1), 49–70. doi:10.1348/000712608X304478 PMID:18447971

Pratt, R. R. (2004). Art, dance, and music therapy. *Physical Medicine and Rehabilitation Clinics of North America, 15*(4), 827–841. doi:10.1016/j.pmr.2004.03.004 PMID:15458755

Quest, A. D., Fullerton, A., Geenen, S., & Powers, L. (2012). Voices of youth in foster care and special education regarding their educational experiences and transition to adulthood. *Children and Youth Services Review, 34*(9), 1604–1615. doi:10.1016/j.childyouth.2012.04.018

Radloff, L. S. (1977). The CES-D scale: A self report depression scale for research in the general population. *Applied Psychological Measurement, 1*(3), 385–401. doi:10.1177/014662167700100306

Raglio, A., Bellelli, G., Traficante, D., Gianotti, M., Ubezio, M. C., Villani, D., & Trabucchi, M. (2008). Efficacy of Music Therapy in the Treatment of Behavioral and Psychiatric Symptoms of Dementia. *Alzheimer Disease and Associated Disorders, 22*(2), 158–162. doi:10.1097/WAD.0b013e3181630b6f PMID:18525288

Ragneskog, H., Asplund, K., Kihlgren, M., & Norberg, A. (2001). Individualized music played for agitated patients with dementia: Analysis of video-recorded sessions. *International Journal of Nursing Practice, 7*(3), 146–155. Wiley Online Library. https://doi.org/ doi:10.1046/j.1440-172X.2001.00254.x

Rao, Y. L., Ganaraja, B., Murlimanju, B. V., Joy, T., Krishnamurthy, A., & Agrawal, A. (2022). Hippocampus and its involvement in Alzheimer's disease: a review. *3 Biotech, 12*(2). doi:10.1007/s13205-022-03123-4

Rauch, S. L., van der Kolk, B. A., & Fisler, R. E. (1996). A symptom provocation study of posttraumatic stress disorder using positron emission tomography and script-driven imagery. *Archives of General Psychiatry, 53*(5), 380–387. doi:10.1001/archpsyc.1996.01830050014003 PMID:8624181

Reading, R., & Rubin, L. R. (2011). Advocacy and empowerment: Group therapy for LGBT asylum seekers. *Traumatology, 17*(2), 86–98. doi:10.1177/1534765610395622

Reid-Wisdom, Z., & Perera-Delcourt, R. (2022). Perceived effects of improv on psychological wellbeing: A qualitative study. *Journal of Creativity in Mental Health, 17*(2), 246–263. doi:10.1080/15401383.2020.1856016

Reynolds, F. (2004). Conversations about creativity and chronic illness II: Textile artists coping with long-term health problems reflect on the creative process. *Creativity Research Journal, 16*(1), 79–89. doi:10.120715326934crj1601_8

Rice, K., & Jennings, J. L. (2014). The ROC program. *Journal of Correctional Health Care, 20*(1), 59–69. doi:10.1177/1078345813505067 PMID:24226289

Richedson, N. & Neill, J. (2004). *Therapeutic recreation music intervention to decrease mealtime agitation and increase food intake in older adults with dementia.* Scientific Publishing.

Rickerl, K. (1996). Quilting a new tradition. *Journal of Psychosocial Nursing and Mental Health Services, 34*(4), 40–43. https://search-proquestcom.ezproxy.philau.edu/docview/1024133953. doi:10.3928/0279-3695-19960401-14

Riley, S. (2001). *Group process made visible: Group art therapy.* Brunner-Routledge.

Rodin, J. (1986). Aging and health: effects of the sense of control. *Science, 233*(4770), 1271–1276. doi:10.1126/science.3749877

Rodin, J. (1989). Sense of Control: Potentials for Intervention. *The ANNALS of the American Academy of Political and Social Science, 503*(1), 29–42. https://doi.org/ doi:10.1177/0002716289503001003

Rogers, C. R. (1959). A theory of therapy, personality, and interpersonal relationships as developed in the client-centered framework. In S. Koch (Ed.), *Psychology: A study of a science. Formulations of the person and the social context* (Vol. 3, pp. 184–256). McGraw-Hill.

Roje, J. (1995). LA '94 earthquake in the eyes of children: Art therapy with elementary school children who were victims of disaster. *Art Therapy: Journal of the American Art Therapy Association, 12*(4), 237–243. doi:10.1080/07421656.1995.10759171

Rosal, M. L. (2018). *Cognitive Behavioral Art Therapy from Behaviorism to the Third Wave. Routledge, Taylor &amp.* Francis Group. doi:10.4324/9781315459257

Rosen Saltzman, M., Matic, M., & Marsden, E. (2013). Adlerian Art Therapy with Sexual Abuse and Assault Survivors. *Journal of Individual Psychology, 69*(3).

Rosenberg, M. (1965). *Rosenberg Self-Esteem Scale (RSES)* [Database record]. APA PsycTests., doi:10.1037/t01038-000

Rubin, J. (1982). Art therapy: What it is and what it is not. *American Journal of Art Therapy, 21*(2), 57–58. APA PsycInfo. https://psycnet.apa.org/record/1984-31877-001

Rubin, J. (Ed.). (2001). *Approaches to art therapy: Theory & technique* (2nd ed.). Brunner-Routledge.

Rubin, J. A. (2010). *Introduction to art therapy: Sources & resources* (2nd ed.). Routledge.

Rubin, J. A. (2015). Psychoanalytic Art Therapy. In D. E. Gussak & M. L. Rosal (Eds.), *The Wiley Handbook of Art Therapy*., doi:10.1002/9781118306543.ch3

Ruddy, R., & Milnes, D. (2005). Art therapy for schizophrenia or schizophrenia-like illnesses. *Cochrane Database of Systematic Reviews*, (4), CD003728. Advance online publication. doi:10.1002/14651858.CD003728.pub2 PMID:16235338

Rusted, J., Sheppard, L., & Waller, D. (2016). A Multi-centre Randomized Control Group Trial on the Use of Art Therapy for Older People with Dementia. *Group Analysis, 39*(4). Sage Journals. doi:10.1177/0533316406071447

Sachs, G. A., Shega, J. W., & Cox-Hayley, D. (2004). Barriers to excellent end-of-life care for patients with dementia. *Journal of General Internal Medicine, 19*(10), 1057–1063. doi:10.1111/j.1525-1497.2004.30329.x PMID:15482560

Sadeghi, S. (2018). *Photovoice, a Long of Belonging Among Iranian Immigrants*. [Thesis, Notre Dame de Namur University]. ProQuest Dissertations & Theses Global. (2377675269). https://www.proquest.com/dissertations-theses/photovoice-long-belonging-among-iranian/docview/2377675269/se-2

Salom, A. (2015). Weaving potential space and acculturation: *Art therapy at the museum. Journal of Applied Arts & Health, 6*(1), 47–62. doi:10.1386/jaah.6.1.47_1

Samaritter, R., & Payne, H. (2013). Kinaesthetic intersubjectivity: A dance informed contribution to self-other relatedness and shared experience in non-verbal psychotherapy with an example from autism. *The Arts in Psychotherapy, 40*(1), 143–150. doi:10.1016/j.aip.2012.12.004

Santamaría, M. L. (2019*). Creating Connection: Group Expressive Arts Therapy with Incarcerated Women.* [Capstone Thesis, Graduate School of Arts and Social Sciences]. Expressive Therapies Capstone Theses.

Sarokhani, D., Parvareh, M., Hasanpour Dehkordi, A., Sayehmiri, K., & Moghimbeigi, A. (2018). Prevalence of Depression among Iranian Elderly: Systematic Review and Meta-Analysis. *Iranian Journal of Psychiatry, 13*(1), 55–64. PMID:29892318

Savidaki, M., Demirtoka, S., & Rodríguez-Jiménez, R.-M. (2020). Re-inhabiting one's body: A pilot study on the effects of dance movement therapy on body-image and alexithymia in eating disorders. *Journal of Eating Disorders, 8*(1), 22. Advance online publication. doi:10.118640337-020-00296-2 PMID:32426135

Schouten, K. A., de Niet, G. J., Knipscheer, J. W., Kleber, R. J., & Hutschemaekers, G. J. M. (2015). The Effectiveness of Art Therapy in the Treatment of Traumatized Adults: A Systematic Review on Art Therapy and Trauma. *Trauma, Violence & Abuse, 16*(2), 220–228. doi:10.1177/1524838014555032 PMID:25403446

Schwenke, D., Dshemuchadse, M., Rasehorn, L., Klarhölter, D., & Scherbaum, S. (2021). Improv to improve: The impact of improvisational theater on creativity, acceptance, and psychological well-being. *Journal of Creativity in Mental Health, 16*(1), 31–48. doi:10.1080/15401383.2020.1754987

Schwiezer, C., Knorth, E. J., Van Yperen, T. A., & Spreen, M. A. (2020). Evaluation of "Images of Self," an art therapy program for children diagnosed with autism spectrum disorders (ASD). *Children and Youth Services Review, 116*, 105207. https://doi.org/10.1016/j.childyouth.2020.105207. doi:10.1016/j.childyouth.2020.105207

Scrine, E. (2021). The limits of resilience and the need for resistance: Articulating the role of music therapy with young people within a shifting trauma paradigm. *Frontiers in Psychology, 12*, 26. doi:10.3389/fpsyg.2021.600245 PMID:33584471

Seifert, K., Spottke, A., & Fliessbach, K. (2017). Effects of sculpture based art therapy in dementia patients—A pilot study. *Heliyon, 3*(11), e00460. doi:10.1016/j.heliyon.2017.e00460 PMID:29264417

Seppänen, S., Toivanen, T., Makkonen, T., Jääskeläinen, I. P., Anttonen, M., & Tiippana, K. (2020). Effects of improvisation training on student teachers' behavioral, neuroendocrine, and psychophysiological responses during the Trier Social Stress Test. *Adaptive Human Behavior and Physiology, 6*(3), 356–380. doi:10.100740750-020-00145-1

Shafir, T., Orkibi, H., Baker, F. A., Gussak, D., & Kaimal, G. (2020). Editorial: The state of the art in creative arts therapies. *Frontiers in Psychology, 11*, 68. doi:10.3389/fpsyg.2020.00068 PMID:32116898

Shechtman, Z., & Tsegahun, I. (2004). Phototherapy to enhance self-disclosure and client–therapist alliance in an intake interview with Ethiopian immigrants to Israel. *Psychotherapy Research, 14*(3), 367–377. doi:10.1093/ptr/kph030

Shin, L. M., McNally, R. J., Kosslyn, S. M., Thompson, W. L., Rauch, S. L., Alpert, N. M., Metzger, L. J., Lasko, N. B., Orr, S. P., & Pitman, R. K. (1999). Regional cerebral blood flow during script-driven imagery in childhood sexual abuse-related PTSD: A PET investigation. *The American Journal of Psychiatry, 156*(4), 575–584. doi:10.1176/ajp.156.4.575 PMID:10200737

Shmerling, R. H. (2020). *Autoimmune diseases and stress: is there a link?* Harvard Health Publishing. https://www.health.harvard.edu/blog/autoimmune-disease-and-stress-is-there-a-link-2018071114230

Sholt, M., & Gavron, T. (2006). Therapeutic Qualities of Clay-work in Art Therapy and Psychotherapy: A Review. *Art Therapy: Journal of the American Art Therapy Association, 23*(2), 66–72. doi:10.1080/07421656.2006.10129647

Shore (1997). Promoting Wisdom: The Role of Art Therapy in Geriatric Settings. *Art Therapy, 14*(3), 172–177. https://doi.org/ doi:10.1080/07421656.1987.10759278

Shore, A. (2014). Art therapy, attachment, and the divided brain. *Art Therapy: Journal of the American Art Therapy Association, 31*(2), 91–94. doi:10.1080/07421656.2014.903827

Siliezar, J. (2019, May 1). Improv can boost social and professional skills, students find. *The Harvard Gazette.* https://news.harvard.edu/gazette/story/2019/05/improv-skills-can-translate-to-social-and-professional-skills/

Simon, B. H. (2015). Music as medicine. *The American Journal of Medicine, 128*(2), 208–210. doi:10.1016/j.amjmed.2014.10.023 PMID:25448175

Sitzer, D. I., Twamley, E. W., & Jeste, D. V. (2006). Cognitive training in alzheimer's disease: A meta-analysis of the literature. *Acta Psychiatrica Scandinavica, 114*(2), 75–90. doi:10.1111/j.1600-0447.2006.00789.x PMID:16836595

Skop, M., Darewych, O. H., Root, J., & Mason, J. (2022). Exploring intimate partner violence survivors' experiences with group art therapy. *International Journal of Art Therapy, 27*(4), 159–168. doi:10.1080/17454832.2022.2124298

Slayton, S. C., D'Archer, J., & Kaplan, F. (2010). Outcome Studies on the Efficacy of Art Therapy: A Review of Findings. *Art Therapy: Journal of the American Art Therapy Association, 27*(3), 108–118. doi:10.1080/07421656.2010.10129660

Smolarski, K., Leone, K., & Robbins, S. J. (2015). Reducing negative mood through drawing: Comparing venting, positive expression, and tracing. *Art Therapy: Journal of the American Art Therapy Association, 32*(4), 197–201. doi:10.1080/07421656.2015.1092697

Sommers-Flanagan, J., & Sommers-Flanagan, R. (1995). Intake interviewing with suicidal patients: A systematic approach. *Professional Psychology, Research and Practice, 26*(1), 41–47. doi:10.1037/0735-7028.26.1.41

Souillard-Mandar, W., Davis, R., Rudin, C., Au, R., Libon, D. J., Swenson, R., Price, C. C., Lamar, M., & Penney, D. L. (2015). Learning classification models of cognitive conditions from subtle behaviors in the digital clock drawing test. *Machine Learning, 102*(3), 393–441. doi:10.100710994-015-5529-5 PMID:27057085

Spiegel, D., Malchiodi, C., Backos, A., & Collie, K. (2006). Art therapy for combat-related PTSD: Recommendations for research and practice. *Art Therapy: Journal of the American Art Therapy Association, 23*(4), 157–164. doi:10.1080/07421656.2006.10129335

Spolin, V. (1963). *Improvisation for the theater.* Northwestern University Press.

Springer, S. A. (2010). Improving healthcare for incarcerated women. *Journal of Women's Health, 19*(1), 13–15. doi:10.1089/jwh.2009.1786 PMID:20088653

Stace, S. M. (2014). Therapeutic doll making in art psychotherapy for complex trauma. *Art Therapy: Journal of the American Art Therapy Association, 31*(1), 12–20. doi:10.1080/07421656.2014.873689

Steenbakkers, A., Van Der Steen, S., & Grietens, H. (2018). The needs of foster children and how to satisfy them: A systematic review of the literature. *Clinical Child and Family Psychology Review*, *21*(1), 1–12. doi:10.100710567-017-0246-1 PMID:29075894

Stensrud, R. H., Gilbride, D. D., & Bruinekool, R. M. (2019). The Childhood to prison pipeline: Early childhood trauma as reported by a prison population. *Rehabilitation Counseling Bulletin*, *62*(4), 195–208. doi:10.1177/0034355218774844

Stevenson, M., & Orr, K. (2013). Art therapy: Stimulating non-verbal communication. *Nursing and Residential Care*, *15*(6), 443–445. doi:10.12968/nrec.2013.15.6.443

Stevens, R., & Spears, E. (2009). Incorporating photography as a therapeutic tool in counseling. *Journal of Creativity in Mental Health*, *4*(1), 3–16. doi:10.1080/15401380802708767

Stewart (2004). Art Therapy and Neuroscience Blend: Working with Patients Who Have Dementia. *Art Therapy, 21*(3), 148–155. https://doi.org/ doi:10.1080/07421656.2004.10129499

Stewart, A., Kathawalla, U., Wolfe, A., & Everson-Rose, S. (2018). Women's heart health at mid-life: what is the role of psychosocial stress. *National Library of Medicine, 4*(11). https://www.ncbi.nlm.nih.gov/pmc/articles/PMC6297972/

Stohr, M. K., & Walsh, A. (2020). Corrections: From research, to policy, to practice. *Sage (Atlanta, Ga.)*.

Stoner, A. M., Leon, S. C., & Fuller, A. K. (2015). Predictors of reduction in symptoms of depression for children and adolescents in foster care. *Journal of Child and Family Studies*, *24*(3), 784–797. doi:10.100710826-013-9889-9

Suzuki, R., Lee, J., & Rudovic, O. (2017, March). Nao-dance therapy for children with ASD. *Proceedings of the Companion of the 2017 ACM/IEEE International Conference on Human-Robot Interaction*, 295-296. 10.1145/3029798.3038354

Swain, G. (2019). The Healing Power of Art in Intergenerational Trauma: Race, Sex, Age and Disability. *Canadian Journal of Disability Studies*, *8*(1), 15–31. doi:10.15353/cjds.v8i1.469

Tadros, E., Barbini, M., & Kaur, L. (2021). Collaborative healthcare in incarcerated settings. *International Journal of Offender Therapy and Comparative Criminology*, *0*(0), 0306624X2110589. doi:10.1177/0306624X211058952 PMID:34784803

Teixeira-Machado, L. (2015). Dance therapy in autism: A case report. *Fisioterapia e Pesquisa*, *22*, 205–211.

Teixeira-Machado, L., Azevedo-Santos, I., & DeSantana, J. M. (2017). Dance improves functionality and psychosocial adjustment in cerebral palsy: A randomized controlled clinical trial. *American Journal of Physical Medicine & Rehabilitation*, *96*(6), 424–429. doi:10.1097/PHM.0000000000000646 PMID:27820729

Teplin, L. A., Abram, K. M., & McClelland, G. M. (1996). Prevalence of psychiatric disorders among incarcerated women. I. Pretrial jail detainees. *Archives of General Psychiatry*, *53*(6), 505–512. doi:10.1001/archpsyc.1996.01830060047007 PMID:8639033

Tomaino, C. M. (2015). Music therapy and the brain. *Music Therapy Handbook*, 40-50.

TomaszewskiC.BelotR. A.EssadekA.Onumba-BessonnetH.ClesseC. (2022). Therapeutic impact of dance therapy on adult individuals with psychological trauma: a systematic review. medRxiv. doi:10.1101/2022.10.27.22281614

Trably, F., Gorwood, P., & Di Lodovico, L. (2022). Art therapy in eating disorders. A systematic review of literature. *European Psychiatry*, *65*(S1), S151. Advance online publication. doi:10.1192/j.eurpsy.2022.405

Tramer, B. (2008). *Case Study: Geriatric Group Art Therapy in a Nursing Home.* [Thesis, Ursuline College]. https://etd.ohiolink.edu/apexprod/rws_etd/send_file/send?accession=urs1210555128&disposition=inline

Tripp, T. (2007). A short-term therapy approach to processing trauma: Art therapy and bilateral stimulation. *Art Therapy: Journal of the American Art Therapy Association*, *24*(4), 178–183. doi:10.1080/07421656.2007.10129476

Tulving, E. (2002). Episodic memory: From mind to brain. *Annual Review of Psychology*, *53*(1), 1–25. doi:10.1146/annurev.psych.53.100901.135114 PMID:11752477

Tutty, L. M., Babins-Wagner, R., & Rothery, M. A. (2016). You're not alone: Mental health outcomes in therapy groups for abused women. *Journal of Family Violence*, *31*(4), 489–497. doi:10.100710896-015-9779-6

Tyano, S. (2003). Post-traumatic stress disorder in Israeli children. *International Psychiatry : Bulletin of the Board of International Affairs of the Royal College of Psychiatrists*, *1*(2), 7–8. doi:10.1192/S1749367600006421 PMID:31507661

Tyng, C. M., Amin, H. U., Saad, M. N., & Malik, A. S. (2017). The influences of emotion on learning and memory. *Frontiers in Psychology*, *8*, 1454. doi:10.3389/fpsyg.2017.01454 PMID:28883804

U.S. Department of Health and Human Services. (2019). *The AFCARS Report: Preliminary FY1 2018 Estimates as of August 22, 2019* (No. 26). https://www.acf.hhs.gov/sites/default/files/documents/cb/afcarsreport26.pdf

University of Minnesota Libraries. (n.d.). *The purposes of punishment.* https://open.lib.umn.edu/criminallaw/chapter/1-5-the-purposes-of-punishment/

Uttley, L., Scope, A., Stevenson, M., & Rawdin, A. (2015). The clinical and cost effectiveness of group art therapy for people with non-psychotic mental health disorders: A systematic review and cost-effectiveness analysis. *BMC Psychiatry*, *15*(1), 151. doi:10.118612888-015-0528-4 PMID:26149275 van der Kolk, B. (2000). Posttraumatic stress disorder and the nature of trauma. *Dialogues in Clinical Neuroscience*, *2*(1), 7–22. doi:10.31887/DCNS.2000.2.1/bvdkolk PMID:22034447

Van der Kolk, B. (2014). *The Body Keeps the Score: Brain, mind and body in the healing of trauma*. Viking.

van der Kolk, B. A. (1996). The body keeps the score: Approaches to the psychobiology of post-traumatic stress disorder. In B. A. van der Kolk, A. C. McFarlane, & L. Weisaeth (Eds.), *Traumatic stress: The effects of overwhelming experience on mind, body and society* (pp. 214–241). Guilford Press.

van der Meulen, E., & Omstead, J. (2021). The Limits of Rehabilitation and Recidivism Reduction: Rethinking the Evaluation of Arts Programming in Prisons. *The Prison Journal*, *101*(1), 102–122. doi:10.1177/0032885520978477

Vernooij-Dassen, M., Vasse, E., Zuidema, S., Cohen-Mansfield, J., & Moyle, W. (2010). Psychosocial interventions for dementia patients in long-term care. *International Psychogeriatrics*, *22*(07), 1121–1128. doi:10.1017/S1041610210001365 PMID:20813074

Vespa, J. (2021, October 9). *The U.S. joins other countries with large aging populations*. Census.gov. https://www.census.gov/library/stories/2018/03/graying-america.html

Vick, R. M. (1999). Utilizing prestructured art elements in brief group art therapy with adolescents. *Art Therapy: Journal of the American Art Therapy Association*, *16*(2), 68–77. doi:10.1080/07421656.1999.10129670

Wadeson, H. (2010). *Art Psychotherapy* (2nd ed.). John Wiley & Sons, Inc.

Wald (1986). Fusion of Symbols, Confusion of Boundaries: Percept Contamination in the Art Work of Alzheimer's Disease Patients. *Art Therapy*, *3*(2), 74–80. https://doi.org/ doi:10.1080/07421656.1986.10758827

Walker, L. E. A., Pann, J. M., Shapiro, D. L., & Van Hasselt, V. B. (2016). A Review of best practices for the treatment of persons with mental illness in jail. In: Best Practices for the Mentally Ill in the Criminal Justice System. SpringerBriefs in Psychology (BRIEFSBC). Springer, Cham. doi:10.1007/978-3-319-21656-0_5

Wallace, A. (2021, March 2). *Supporting student success through afterschool program*. NCSL. https://www.ncsl.org/research/education/expanding-learning-opportunities-through-afterschool-programs.aspx

Walton, A. P. (2003). The impact of interpersonal factors on creativity. *International Journal of Entrepreneurial Behaviour & Research*, *9*(4), 146–162. doi:10.1108/13552550310485120

Wang, J.-J., Hsieh, P.-F., & Wang, C.-J. (2013). Long-term Care Nurses' Communication Difficulties with People Living with Dementia in Taiwan. *Asian Nursing Research*, *7*(3), 99–103. doi:10.1016/j.anr.2013.06.001 PMID:25030246

Wang, Q.-Y., & Li, D.-M. (2016). Advances in art therapy for patients with dementia. *Clinical Nursing Research, 3*(3), 105–108. doi:10.1016/j.cnre.2016.06.011

Winfrey, O. & Perry, B. D. (2021) *What Happened to You? Conversations on Trauma, Resilience, and Healing*. Flatiron Books: An Oprah Book.

Winslow, L. E. (2018). *Creating reminiscence through art therapy doll making with older women*. [Thesis, Notre Dame University]. ProQuest Dissertations & Theses Global. (2164378232). https://www.proquest.com/dissertations-theses/creating-reminiscence-through-art-therapy-doll/docview/2164378232/se-2

Winters, A. F. (2008). Emotion, embodiment, and mirror neurons in dance/movement therapy: A connection across disciplines. *American Journal of Dance Therapy, 30*(2), 84–105. doi:10.100710465-008-9054-y

Witte, M. D., Pinho, A., Stams, G. J., Moonen, X., Bos, A. E. R., & van Hooren, S. (2020). Music therapy for stress reduction: A systematic review and meta-analysis. *Health Psychology Review, 16*(1), 134–159. https://www.tandfonline.com/doi/full/10.1080/17437199.2020.1846580

Wolff, K. (2018, March 18). *Materiality*. Society for Cultural Anthropology. https://culanth.org/fieldsights/materiality#:~:text=Materiality

World Health Organization. (2022, September 20). *Dementia*. World Health Organization. https://www.who.int/news-room/fact-sheets/detail/dementia

Wraith, R. (2000). Children and debriefing. *Psychological debriefing: Theory, practice and evidence*, 195.

Young, J. T. N., & Haynie, D. L. (2022). Trusting the untrustworthy: The Social organization of trust among incarcerated women. *Justice Quarterly, 39*(3), 553–584. doi:10.1080/07418825.2020.1807588

Young, M. E., & Bemak, F. (1996). The Role of Emotional Arousal and Expression in Mental Health Counseling. *Journal of Mental Health Counseling, 18*(4), 316–332.

Zarit, S. H., Femia, E. E., Watson, J., Rice-Oeschger, L., & Kakos, B. (2004). Memory Club: A Group Intervention for People With Early-Stage Dementia and Their Care Partners. *The Gerontologist, 44*(2), 262–269. doi:10.1093/geront/44.2.262 PMID:15075423

Zgola. (1987). Doing Things: A Guide to Programming Activities for Persons with Alzheimer's Disease and Related Disorders. In *Google Books*. JHU Press.

# About the Contributors

**Nava R. Silton**, Ph.D. is a Developmental Psychologist with a B.S. from Cornell University and an M.A. and Ph.D. from Fordham University. She is a Full Professor at Marymount Manhattan College, where she teaches classes in Child Development, Cognition, Personality, Creativity, Children's Media and has won numerous Teaching, Research and Advising Awards. She has worked at Nickelodeon, Sesame Workshop and has consulted for Disney, Netflix, Apple, Blue's Clues & You, 9Story Media Group and The Autism Seaver Center. She also serves as a Developmental Psychologist for Gan Aliya and Manhattan Day School. She has appeared over 150 times on Fox 5 News as a Parenting and Developmental Expert, and has appeared on Good Day New York, Good Day Street Talk and NBC. Silton has written over 36 peer-reviewed journal articles, over 20 chapters, book reviews and encyclopedia entries and has edited seven full textbooks, and this is her eighth. Her first two books discuss innovative technologies for individuals with autism and other disabilities, her third delves into creativity, her fourth into family dynamics and romantic relationships, her fifth explores the constructs of happiness, gratitude, kindness, empathy and well-being, her sixth text discusses best parenting and child development practices for the 21st century, her seventh discusses the impact of COVID-19 on children, adolescents and adults and her eighth discusses the benefits of creative arts therapies for children, adolescents and adults. Silton also created The Realabilities Educational Comic Book Series (), which offers 18 comics (12 on disabilities and 6 on mental health disorders) and two instructional manuals for use in classrooms across the world. The disabilities-based series, which received The Reader's Favorite Award and was a Page Turner Awardee has now been translated into Hebrew and Spanish and is currently being translated into Chinese and French, as well. Due to the popularity of The Realabilities Educational Series in the schools, Silton created Addy & Uno, The First Family Musical about Disabilities, Bullying and Kindness. Addy & Uno, which was nominated for an Off-Broadway Alliance Award, ran Off-Broadway for over 18 months at Theatre Row on 42nd Street in Manhattan () and is now being developed by the Jim Henson Company for TV. She also is developing another show with LeVar Burton Entertainment. In addition, Silton created a

Child Development and Parenting Podcast, entitled A Cup of Java with Dr. Nava. She also created Bashert, , a brand-new card game which helps individuals connect and forge meaningful relationships with others. Finally, Nava recently penned four feature screenplays, Pure, The Prof, Jackpot and Toycoon. All four screenplays have already achieved significant recognition (Finalist, Semifinalist and Quarterfinalist designations) in over twenty screenplay contests. Most recently, Silton was identified as one of the Top 50 screenwriters on the ISA Fellowship slate. Silton is married to Dr. Ariel Brandwein and has five children; three boys and two little girls.

* * *

**Zach Biron** is a student at Marymount Manhattan College pursuing a Bachelors in Psychology with an expected graduation of May 2024. He is passionate about Clinical Psychology, furthering his education through an Art Therapy minor, and works under the mentorship of his Advisor, Nava Silton, to pursue further research opportunities.

**Rachel Brandoff**, Ph.D., LCAT, LPAT, is a Registered, Board-Certified Art Therapist (ATR-BC) and credentialed supervisor (ATCS). She is an Associate Professor and Coordinator of the Art Therapy Concentration in the Community and Trauma Counseling program at Thomas Jefferson University. Dr. Brandoff maintains a clinical practice specializing in working with individuals who are coming out of crises and coping with trauma. She provides supervision and consultation to art therapists and professional counselors. Dr. Brandoff has served on the boards of various professional organizations and is a regular presenter at regional and national conferences. Her first book, "Quick and Creative Art Projects for Creative Therapists with (Very) Limited Budgets", was published in 2019.

**Kayleen Cabrera** is an aspiring therapist from Bronx, NY, and graduated from Marymount Manhattan College in 2023 with a B.A. in Psychology and a minor in Art Therapy. She has worked with groups such as those with developmental disabilities, the elderly, and teenagers. Additionally, having worked at Duke University and The Student Leadership Network, providing services and information to families and adolescents in crisis intervention, the offset of underage pregnancies, and college readiness. Witnessing the benefits and healing factors that mental health services provide to numerous demographics has become the driving force behind her passion in Psychology. She has been recognized with various leadership awards, including being inducted into the Psi Chi Honors Society. She was a spokesperson for one of the largest national conferences in North America; the National Student Leadership Diversity Convention, where she discussed the importance of diversity, equity, and inclusion on college campuses in the U.S. As a first generational college graduate, Cabrera is pursuing a masters degree in social work and public health. She is preparing to give back to underserved communities like the one she grew up in. Her focus on advocating for those in need aids her in working with marginalized groups and others alike.

**Giselle B Caraballo Matos** received her B.A. from Marymount Manhattan College in 2022. Her research interests include the intersections between psychology and the legal system, the promotion of access to mental health facilities in low-income communities, and the use of creative arts in therapy settings. Since graduating from MMC, Caraballo Matos worked as an advocacy legal intern at Covenant House, an organization dedicated to providing legal services and education to immigrants in the NYC community, and currently works as a Human Resources Coordinator at her alma mater.

**Marisa T. Cohen** is a relationship researcher, marriage, and family therapist, and teaches college level psychology courses. She is also the author of From First Kiss to Forever: A Scientific Approach to Love, a book that relates relationship science research to everyday experiences and real relationship issues confronted by couples. Dr. Cohen is passionate about discovering and sharing important relationship research from the field, and has given guest lectures at locations including the 92nd Street Y, Strand Bookstore, and the New York Hall of Science. She is also a 2021 TEDx Speaker, has appeared in segments for Newsweek, and is the subject of a piece focusing on her work, which aired on BRIC TV. Her work has been quoted in publications such as Bustle, Good Housekeeping, The Cut, InStyle, The Washington Post, Men's Health, and Women's Health. She has also appeared on many podcasts and radio shows to discuss the psychology of love and ways in which we can improve our relationships.

**Jacqui Johnson**, LPC, ATR-BC, NCC, CCMHC, PMH-C, is the Founder and Clinical Director of Sankofa Healing Studio in Philadelphia. She is a Social-Justice Art Therapist who specializes in trauma-specific treatment within marginalized communities, using a holistic approach. As a trained art therapist and play therapist, Jacqui integrates art, story-telling, hip-hop therapy, parts of self, and body awareness, using EMDR, Brainspotting, and energy-based practices (e.g. Sound & Energy Healing, Reiki) to create holistic healing-centered spaces. Jacqui provides consultation to newly trained EMDR and Brainspotting clinicians seeking certification and is a training facilitator for EMDR in Color. Jacqui teaches in the Community and Trauma Counseling program at Thomas Jefferson University, and lectures widely around the country. Her clinical work and research center around working with people in the

Black community who have been impacted by childhood, racial, and generational traumas, as well as mass incarceration and systemic trauma.

**Heather Kroesche** grew up in Detroit, Michigan and moved to New York City to attend Marymount Manhattan College where she received a B.F.A in Dance, a B.A. in Psychology, and a minor in Art Therapy 2023.

**Jenna Rivera**'s interest in the field of psychology stemmed from assisting in special education dance classes in high school where she worked with children with Autism, ADHD, Down Syndrome, and Cerebral Palsy. She aided in teaching basic motor skills, memory skills, and social/communication skills. Jenna graduated Marymount Manhattan College in 2023 with a Bachelor of Arts, as a double major in Psychology and Business, with a minor in Dance Education. As a first-generation college student, she was invited into the College Honors Program and received the Academic Achievement Award for outstanding scholastic accomplishments. She is an achieved member of three international honors societies: Alpha Chi, Psi Chi, and Sigma Beta Delta. Jenna also became a teaching assistant for Experimental Psychology at MMC where she facilitated classroom management and met with students one-on-one to aid in their research and advancement in the course. Jenna is currently pursuing a Master's degree in Special Education with a concentration in Applied Behavioral Analysis.

**Mónica Sánchez**, MS, ATR-BC, LCAT, is the Director of Mental Health Services at LSA Family Health Service (LSA). As a Latina immigrant woman, she is committed to developing and providing high-quality therapeutic interventions for immigrant women survivors of trauma. She has developed the mental health program at LSA to include a holistic blend of individual, dyad, and group psychotherapy and art therapy, and she works primarily with women of childbearing age who have histories of significant and complex trauma. She presents her work widely at regional and national universities and conferences and works to partner with various community services to broaden the reach of her program.

**Deanna Villetto**, LMSW is a social worker who graduated from Columbia University School of Social Work. She graduated with a Master's Degree in 2019, and received a Bachelor's Degree in 2017 from Marymount Manhattan College.

# Index

# D



# E



# F

## N



## O



## P



## R



## S

# T



# U



# V

www.ingramcontent.com/pod-product-compliance
Lightning Source LLC
LaVergne TN
LVHW081333300926
849161LV00008B/1961